Otolaryngology: Current Concepts and Techniques in Head and Neck Surgery

Otolaryngology: Current Concepts and Techniques in Head and Neck Surgery

Editor: Adrien Butler

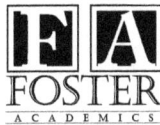

FA FOSTER ACADEMICS

www.fosteracademics.com

www.fosteracademics.com

FA
FOSTER
ACADEMICS

Cataloging-in-Publication Data

Otolaryngology : current concepts and techniques in head and neck surgery / edited by Adrien Butler.
 p. cm.
Includes bibliographical references and index.
ISBN 978-1-63242-772-4
1. Otolaryngology, Operative. 2. Head--Surgery. 3. Neck--Surgery. 4. Otolaryngology. I. Butler, Adrien.
RF51 .O86 2019
617.51--dc23

Foster Academics,
118-35 Queens Blvd., Suite 400,
Forest Hills, NY 11375, USA

ISBN 978-1-63242-772-4 (Hardback)

Contents

Permissions

List of Contributors

Index

Preface

Otolaryngology is a surgical field of medicine which studies the conditions associated with the parts of the head and neck, including the ear, nose and throat. It also deals with the treatment of various tumors and cancers, including the ones affecting the head and neck. One of the most common surgical methods used to treat such cancers is microvascular head and neck reconstruction. The tissue which is usually moved during the surgical process is from the back, arms and legs. In the process, the transfer of the tissue to the head and neck allows the head and neck surgeons in rebuilding the patient's jaw and reconstructing the throat. This book explores all the important aspects of otolaryngology in the present day scenario. It attempts to understand the current concepts and techniques that fall under the discipline of head and neck surgery and how such concepts have practical applications. For all those who are interested in otolaryngology, this book can prove to be an essential guide.

This book has been the outcome of endless efforts put in by authors and researchers on various issues and topics within the field. The book is a comprehensive collection of significant researches that are addressed in a variety of chapters. It will surely enhance the knowledge of the field among readers across the globe.

It gives us an immense pleasure to thank our researchers and authors for their efforts to submit their piece of writing before the deadlines. Finally in the end, I would like to thank my family and colleagues who have been a great source of inspiration and support.

Editor

Comparison of the mechanical properties of different skin sites for auricular and nasal reconstruction

M. F. Griffin[1,2,3*], B. C. Leung[1,3], Y. Premakumar[2], M. Szarko[2] and P. E. Butler[1,3]

Abstract

Background: Autologous and synthetic nasal and auricular frameworks require skin coverage. The surgeon's decides on the appropriate skin coverage for reconstruction based on colour matching, subcutaneous tissue thickness, expertise and experience. One of the major complications of placing subcutaneous implants is the risk of extrusion (migration through the skin) and infection. However, knowledge of lessening the differential between the soft tissue and the framework can have important implications for extrusion. This study compared the mechanical properties of the skin commonly used as skin sites for the coverage in auricular and nasal reconstruction.

Methods: Using ten fresh human cadavers, the tensile Young's Modulus of the skin from the forehead, forearm, temporoparietal, post-auricular and submandibular neck was assessed. The relaxation rate and absolute relaxation level was also assessed after 90 min of relaxation.

Results: The submandibular skin showed the greatest Young's elastic modulus in tension of all regions (1.28 MPa ±0.06) and forearm showed the lowest (1.03 MPa ±0.06). The forehead demonstrated greater relaxation rates among the different skin regions (7.8 MPa^{-07} ± 0.1). The forearm showed the lowest rate of relaxation (4.74 MPa^{-07} ± 0.1). The forearm (0.04 MPa ±0.004) and submandibular neck skin (0.04 MPa ±0.005) showed similar absolute levels of relaxation, which were significantly greater than the other skin regions ($p < 0.05$).

Conclusions: This study provides an understanding into the biomechanical properties of the skin of different sites allowing surgeons to consider this parameter when trying to identify the optimal skin coverage in nasal and auricular reconstruction.

Keywords: Biomechanics skin, Skin flap, Nasal, Auricular, Young elastic modulus

Background

Craniofacial auricular and nasal cartilage defects including those caused by cancer, trauma, burns or congenital deformities are restored by transferring autologous cartilage from elsewhere in the body and shaping the tissue for the specific anatomical defect [1]. However, due to limitations in availability of suitable tissue, resorption of the tissue with time, surgeons have utilised synthetic materials to replace the cartilage defect [1]. Several materials have been investigated to replace the cartilaginous framework including silicone, porous polyethylene (Medpor ®) and polyfluorethylene

(Gore-tex) with different mechanical properties [1]. However, research is still on going to develop materials to replace the cartilaginous frameworks due to the high levels of infection and extrusion with currently available materials [1]. Whether surgeons use autologous or allografts, the cartilaginous framework requires soft tissue coverage. Surgeons choose their skin coverage based on colour match, tissue availability, pedicle quality and personal experience and expertise [2]. Currently, used skin flaps to cover an auricular implants include the temporoparietal and postauricular mastoid due to the good colour match being anatomically close to the ear [3, 4]. For nasal reconstruction the forehead is the gold standard due to the close colour match and subcutaneous thickness. The forearm skin flap can also be used if the forehead flap is unavailable [5, 6].

---

* Correspondence: 12michellegriffin@gmail.com
[1]Division of Surgery & Interventional Science, University College London (UCL), London, UK
[2]Anatomy Department, St Georges University, London, UK
Full list of author information is available at the end of the article

Implant extrusion is a devastating complication of using allografts, where the implant migrates through the subcutaneous skin meaning the patient requires further surgical intervention [7]. The cause of extrusion of implants is unpredictable and not well understood. The mechanism of implant extrusion has been suggested to result from infection, patient co-morbidities and implant characteristics [7, 8].

One technique implemented by craniofacial surgeons when utilising synthetic materials for auricular or nasal reconstruction is stress shielding. This involves wrapping the implant with a layer of autologous tissue to reduce the contact stress subjected to the overlying skin by the implant. Several reports have shown that fascia covered frameworks reduce the stress of the implant on the surrounding skin tissue and aid in the prevention of extrusion [8, 9].

Similarly, it has been shown that if an implant is manufactured with similar mechanical properties to the surrounding tissues, then shear stress can be avoided, preventing micro-movement, risk of infection and extrusion of the implant [10–12]. Therefore, for researchers developing new auricular and nasal implants, it would be important to consider the mechanical properties of the skin coverage that is going to be utilised by the surgeon to cover the implant [10, 11]. However, the mechanical property of the skin of different sites for auricular and nasal reconstruction has not been investigated to date. We have created a reliable and simple protocol to analyse the tensile mechanical properties of human skin tissue [13, 14]. Tensile testing is a standard method of testing mechanical properties of skin tissue [13, 14]. The aim of this study was to analyse the mechanical and histological properties of common skin flaps for coverage in auricular and nasal reconstruction including the forehead, forearm, temporoparietal, post-auricular and submandibular neck.

Methods
Skin sample preparation
A total of ten fresh frozen cadaveric human heads were obtained for skin sampling and full ethnical approval was obtained. The samples included ten males, average age of 84 (range 77 to 94 years), average weight of 102 pounds (range 88 to 130 pounds), Caucasians without with any underlying skin condition or significant comorbidities.

Four regions were selected for skin sampling in each cadaver head: forehead, temporoparietal, post-auricular mastoid and submandibular neck. A total of fourty skin samples were obtained from the ten heads (1 samples per site). Forearms were also taken from the same cadavers. The position and orientation of the skin samples were kept constant, and were designed longitudinally parallel to Langer's lines. Skin samples were 10 mm × 50 mm and accurately measured with digital vernier calipers. The subcutaneous fat is removed from the skin sample, leaving

only the epidermis and dermis. A digital vernier caliper was used to measure the thickness in the different regions prior to mechanical testing.

Skin extraction protocol
The skin samples were marked out on the cadaveric heads using a repeatable method as follows (Additional file 1: Figure S1). The forehead skin was taken 20 mm from the superior nasal bridge indentation and spanned 50 mm across the forehead with a 10 mm height, following the forehead lines. The temporoparietal skin was measured 10 mm above the zygomatic arch and originated 20 mm posterior to the lateral orbital rim, then extended 50 mm posteriorly towards the superior border of the ear with a 10 mm height. The post-auricular mastoid skin was taken from 10 mm posterior to the auricular ear attachment and originated at corner of the ear lobe, then extended towards to the back of head, 50 mm in length and 10 mm in width. The submandibular neck skin was measured 10 mm below and parallel to the submandibular border, extending 50 mm in length and 10 mm in height. The forearm skin was split into anterior, middle and posterior skin. A square paddle was drawn 15 cm posterior from the ulnar styloid and divided into three equal sections (Additional file 1: Figure S1). Anterior forearm was considered the section nearest the wrist joint and posterior was the nearest the elbow joint. Each section was then divided 50 mm in length and 10 mm width per section ($n = 5$ per section of forearm).

Skin samples were immediately stored into 20 ml of Phosphate Buffer solution (PBS) contained in 100 ml bottles after initial cutting and fat stripping, followed by storage in the freezer at −80 °C. The storing process was conducted simultaneously for all the samples, which avoided any shrinkage of the skin. The thawing process prior to the biomechanical testing was carried out by immersing the skin samples in a water bath set at 37.5–38 °C that was checked manually with a digital thermometer, for 15 min. The skin samples were then dried with clean paper towels and were checked for achievement of room temperature, 25–26 °C. Once the skin samples reached room temperature, the samples were then ready for mechanical testing.

Mechanical testing protocol
Biomechanical testing
Skin samples were measured in uniaxial tension using a Mach-1 materials testing machine (Biomomentum, Canada) as described by our institution, Wood et al., 2012 [13]. Each skin sample was orientated and immobilised between two clamps, one fixed to a 10 kg load cell and the other to the immovable base plate. No slippage was observed as the samples were fixed in a commercial jig suing 'finger tight' tightness. The resulting area to be tested is

then stable of 1 cm by 4 cm. The sample was loaded to 3000 g at 1 mm/s. After the 29.42 N load was reached, the tissue was allowed to relax for 1.5 h (a time point sufficient for control skin to reach equilibrium). Calculation of the Young's modulus in tension was then performed as described previously [13] and demonstrated in Additional file 2: Figure S2. The rate of skin relaxation was evaluated by measuring the final 200 s of the experiment (stress (MPa) over time (seconds)) (Additional file 2: Figure S2). The final stress relaxation was calculated by measuring the final skin stress after 90 min (Additional file 2: Figure S2). During experimentation petroleum jelly was applied to prevent desiccation of the skin samples.

Histological analysis

A 1×1 cm^2 samples was taken from the donor before testing. Tissue was formalin-fixed, paraffin-embedded and sectioned at 8 μm. Each section was analysed using H&E, Masson's Trichrome, and Miller's elastin stains were conducted according to standard protocols, then photographed with a Zeiss Axioplan microscope.

Statistical analysis

Inter-treatment comparisons were analysed statistically using one-way analysis of variance (ANOVA) with Tukey HSD post-hoc analysis (JMP, v10; North Carolina, USA). The average and standard deviation (SD) was calculated. Significance was described as $p < 0.05$. Kaleidagraph (v.4.1, Pennsylvania, USA) was used for graphically representing data.

Results

Biomechanical testing

Prior to mechanical analysis, the average thickness of the different skin sites was measured using electronic callipers. Figure 1 shows the forehead (1.4 mm ±0.05 SD) and temporoparietal region (1.39 mm ±0.09 SD) were the thickest of the skin regions. The submandibular neck was the significantly thinnest of all the skin regions (0.87 mm ±0.05 SD). The postauricular mastoid and the forearm region showed similar thickness (PM 1.23 mm ±0.07 SD and FA 1.19 mm ±0.09 SD).

The tensile Young's elastic modulus was varied among the different skin sites (Fig. 2). The submandibular skin showed the greatest Young's elastic modulus of all the regions (1.28 MPa ±0.06 SD, $p < 0.01$). The forearm had a higher Young's modulus than all regions except for the submandibular skin (1.03 MPa ±0.06 SD). The postauricular mastoid had a higher Young's modulus than the forearm (0.86 MPa ±0.05 SD and the temporoparietal skin (0.65 MPa ±0.05 SD). The forehead had the lowest Young's modulus in tension of all the regions (0.33 MPa ±0.04 SD). The Young's elastic modulus of the forearm of the anterior, middle and posterior sections was also evaluated. The

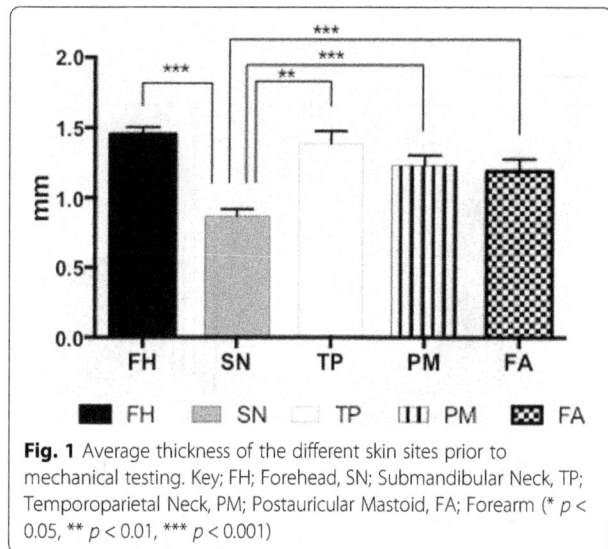

Fig. 1 Average thickness of the different skin sites prior to mechanical testing. Key; FH; Forehead, SN; Submandibular Neck, TP; Temporoparietal Neck, PM; Postauricular Mastoid, FA; Forearm (* $p < 0.05$, ** $p < 0.01$, *** $p < 0.001$)

anterior forearm had a greater Young's elastic modulus than the posterior forearm in tension but showed no significant difference (Additional file 3: Figure S3).

The forehead showed a significantly greater rate of relaxation among the different skin regions (Fig. 3) (7.8 MPa^{-07} ± 0.1 SD, $p < 0.001$). The submandibular neck (5.75 MPa^{-07} ± 0.08 SD), temporoparietal (5.7 MPa^{-07} ± 0.15 SD) and postauricular mastoid (5.7 MPa^{-07} ± 0.07 SD) skin showed similar rates of relaxation. The forearm showed the lowest rate of relaxation among the different skin regions (4.74 MPa^{-07} ± 0.1 SD).

The forearm (0.04 MPa ±0.004 SD) and submandibular neck skin (0.04 MPa ±0.005 SD) showed similar absolute levels of relaxation, which were significantly greater than the other regions of the skin ($p < 0.001$) (Fig. 4). The

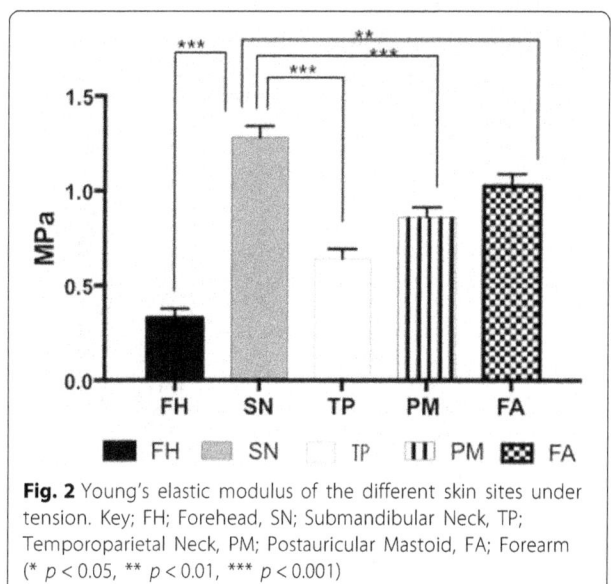

Fig. 2 Young's elastic modulus of the different skin sites under tension. Key; FH; Forehead, SN; Submandibular Neck, TP; Temporoparietal Neck, PM; Postauricular Mastoid, FA; Forearm (* $p < 0.05$, ** $p < 0.01$, *** $p < 0.001$)

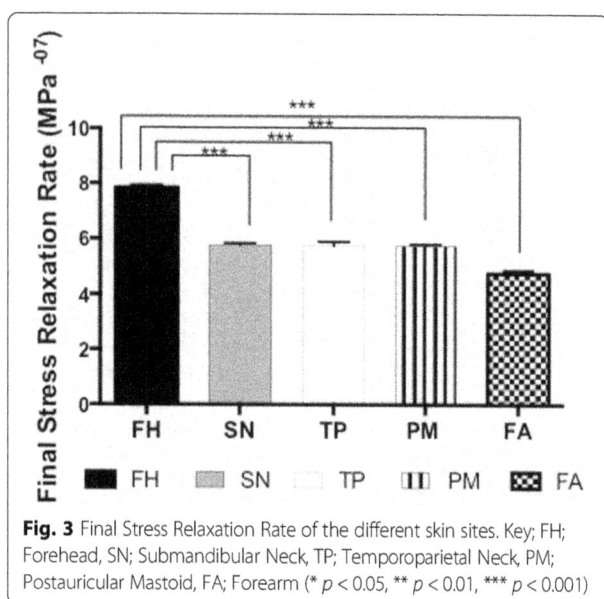

Fig. 3 Final Stress Relaxation Rate of the different skin sites. Key; FH; Forehead, SN; Submandibular Neck, TP; Temporoparietal Neck, PM; Postauricular Mastoid, FA; Forearm (* $p < 0.05$, ** $p < 0.01$, *** $p < 0.001$)

temporoparietal (0.02 MPa ±0.001 SD) and postauricular skin (0.02 MPa ±0.0004 SD), showed similar levels of relaxation. The forehead showed the lowest absolute relaxation level among the different skin regions (0.008 MPa ±0.002 SD).

Histological analysis

The H&E stain was used to subjectively assess the architecture of the skin from the different sites (Additional file 4: Figure S4). All samples showed a similar morphological architecture. The epidermis was a similar size among the skin sites. The papillary dermis and the deeper reticular dermis were also similar. There was also a similar quantity of vasculature in the dermis among the different sites. The submandibular neck showed muscle fibres of platysma, which was not present in the other skin sites.

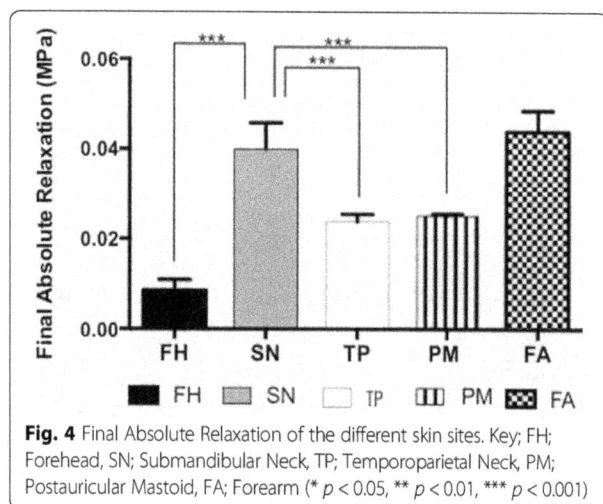

Fig. 4 Final Absolute Relaxation of the different skin sites. Key; FH; Forehead, SN; Submandibular Neck, TP; Temporoparietal Neck, PM; Postauricular Mastoid, FA; Forearm (* $p < 0.05$, ** $p < 0.01$, *** $p < 0.001$)

Massons Trichome was used to subjectively assess the collagen staining in the different skin sites (Additional file 4: Figure S4). Collagen is the predominant constituent in the dermis accounting for 77% of its dry weight [15]. The collagen was stained as green and muscle as red. On subjective assessment the submandibular, post-auricular mastoid and forearm skin showed higher collagen staining than the forehead and temporoparietal regions. The submandibular skin showed think dense collagen bundles in the dermal regions.

Millers Elastin stain was used to subjectively assess the elastin and collagen content in the skin tissue regions (Additional file 4: Figure S4). Elastin fibres were stained black and collagen red. Elastin is responsible for the elasticity and the recoiling of the skin [15]. The elastin in the skin showed a similar pattern to the Massons Trichome where the collagen staining was greater in the submandibular skin, post-auricular mastoid and forearm than the forehead and temporoparietal regions. The elastin staining was also lower in the temporoparietal region than the other skin regions. The forehead showed the greatest level of elastin staining.

Discussion

The aim of this study was to understand the mechanical properties of skin of common sites used for auricular and nasal framework coverage to help surgeons choose skin coverage appropriately to avoid extrusion and infection complications.

The submandibular neck skin demonstrated the highest Young's elastic modulus in tension followed by the forearm skin (Fig. 2). The temporoparietal and post auricular skin showed a similar Young's elastic modulus, which was less than the submandibular and forearm. The forehead skin showed the lowest Young's elastic modulus in tension. Skin is known as an elastic tissue, deforming in response to applied forces [15, 16]. Histology using H&E showed no significant changes in the architecture that may account for these changes.

Collagen fibres are arranged with their long axis parallel to the relax skin tension lines, which are visible on the surface of the skin as the main lines [17]. Collagen fibres within the dermis are responsible for the tensile strength of skin. The submandibular neck, forearm and the temporoparietal skin showed greater staining for collagen using Massons Trichome stain, which may account for the changes in the observed tensile mechanical behaviour.

The relaxation rate was the greatest in the forehead skin (Fig. 3). The submandibular, temporoparietal and post-auricular skin showed similar rates of relaxation. The forearm skin demonstrated the slowest relaxation rate. The absolute relaxation rate was the greatest in the forehead, with similar values among the temporoparietal and neck skin (Fig. 4). The forearm skin demonstrated the lowest absolute relaxation rate (Fig. 4). Elastin is another structural constituent of the skin dermis. Elastin allows for skin's ability to return to its original shape after loading [18]. The forearm showed the greatest elastin content of all the skin regions by Millers Elastin stain, which may account for this region showing the greatest relaxation rate and absolute relaxation level (Additional file 4: Figure S4).

When comparing the biomechanical values for the skin in tension to the literature, there is variation among authors, which is to be expected with biological tissues. The variability may be due to the biological tissue's test conditions and variability between subjects. Ni Annaidh et al. compared the results in the literature to date of excised human skin, reporting the Youngs elastic modulus to range from 2.9 to 150 MPa irrespective of different donor sites [19]. The authors observed that the tensile properties of skin from the human back showed an elastic modulus of 83.3 ± 34.9 MPa [19]. Jacquemond et al. compared the in vitro tension of forehead and arm, observing an elastic modulus of 19.5–87.1 MPa [20]. Other than the reasons already discussed to account for the differences in values in different studies for the biomechanics of skin, it may be due to the properties of the skin changing once removed from the body with different storage and preparation protocols.

They are multiple different nasal and auricular implants available with different mechanical properties [1]. The relevance of our study to the clinical setting is providing knowledge of the mechanical and structural properties of different skin sites to understand which may be more compatible for certain nasal or auricular implants. This study may indicate that submandibular skin would be a suitable choice for reconstruction with a stiff implant as higher stress is likely to be required to cause skin breakdown and consequential implant extrusion. Forearm skin also showed a high Young's modulus and could also be suitable for stiff implants. Forehead skin showed the lowest Young's elastic modulus, demonstrating stiff implants may cause strain on this skin coverage. Forehead skin also showed the greatest rates of relaxation among the regions, which may mean the forehead skin may be able to relax when stressed over implants to a greater degree than other skin sites. Forehead skin also showed the lowest absolute final stress, which could indicate the implants would be under less stress from the skin with this choice of coverage. We have provided a foundation into the understanding of skin site's mechanical properties; however further knowledge of implant mechanics and the interaction with the overlying skin would be required to influence future clinical care. Thus in the future, the mechanical tensile range of the skin sites could be considered along with colour match, hair presence, available skin volume required to better prevent extrusion of nasal and auricular replacements. Our future work will be to further understand how to pair implants with the mechanical properties of the overlying skin coverage.

Due to limitations in sample numbers, future work will be to take into consideration of different cofounding factors that may affect the mechanical properties of the skin including age, comorbidities and different skin types. The preparation of the skin regions included the removal of subcutaneous fat to prevent discrepancies within the data set. Future work will endeavour to account for this layer of skin, as this would be present in skin flaps in the clinical setting and taken into consideration for flap pliability and robustness of the random dermal plexus blood supply. All skin samples underwent two freeze-thaw cycles, which may have affected the mechanical properties. However, compared to other skin preservation methods, such as formaldehyde or embalming, freezing induces the least structural and mechanical changes to the skin [21]. Furthermore, skin has shown to be anisotropic, with Langer demonstrating that in the 1861, skin has natural lines of tension [19]. In this study, to avoid sample bias skin was oriented parallel to Langer lines. In future studies, it will be important to increase the sample size to allow for testing in different directions.

Conclusions

In conclusion, we have demonstrated that human skin from different skin sites for auricular and nasal framework skin coverage behaves differently under tension loads. From this mechanical study, submandibular and forearm skin would be able to cover stiff implants well and forehead skin would cover soft implants well. Surgeons should consider the mechanical behaviour of the skin site in addition to donor site morbidity, colour and surgeon preference when choosing appropriate skin coverage in auricular and nasal reconstruction.

Additional files

Additional file 1: Figure S1. Schematic diagram to illustrate how the skin samples were excised during the study. [A] Forehead excision. [B] Submandibular Neck, Temporoparietal Neck, and Postauricular Mastoid exicision. [C] Forearm excision.

Additional file 2: Figure S2. Loading data of a representative skin samples. [A] Analysis of initial load resistance data allowed the evaluation of the Young's elastic modulus. [B] Measuring the rate of stress relaxation over the last 200 s allowed the determination of the final rate of relaxation, and measuring the stress level at the end of the 90 min relaxation period allowed the calculation of the final absolute relaxation (last point on B).

Additional file 3: Figure S3. Tensile Young's elastic modulus of the different forearm sites including the anterior, middle and posterior sites.

Additional file 4: Figure S4. Histological analysis of the different skin sites by H&E, Massons Trichome and Millers Elastin staining. [A] H&E [B]. Massons Trichome [C]. Millers and Elastin. Key; FH; Forehead, SN; Submandibular Neck, TP; Temporoparietal Neck, PM; Postauricular Mastoid, FA; Forearm. Scale bar = 50 μm.

Acknowledgements
Not applicable.

Funding
We would like to thank the funding from Medical Research Council and Action Medical Research, which provided MG a clinical fellowship to conduct this work, GN 2339.

Authors' contributions
MG collected and analysed data as well as wrote the manuscript. DL collected and analysed data. YP collected and analysed data. PE and MS advised on manuscript preparation.

Authors' information
MG is an academic clinical fellow in plastic surgery undertaking her PhD in ear and nose reconstruction at University College London (UCL). BL completed a MSc under PE in ear and nose reconstruction at UCL. YP is a medical student at St. Georges University. MS is an anatomy senior lecturer at St Georges Anatomy who specialises in biomechanics of cartilage. PE is a Professor of Plastic Surgery at UCL and PhD supervisor of MG.

Competing interests
The authors declare they have no competing interests.

Author details
[1]Division of Surgery & Interventional Science, University College London (UCL), London, UK. [2]Anatomy Department, St Georges University, London, UK. [3]Plastic & Reconstructive Surgery Department, Royal Free Hospital, London, UK.

References
1. Berghaus A. Implants for reconstructive surgery of the nose and ears. GMS Current Topics in Otorhinolaryngology. Head Neck Surg. 2007;6:Doc06.
2. Taghinia AH, Pribaz JJ. Complex nasal reconstruction. Plast Reconstr Surg. 2008;121:15e–27.
3. Simsek T, Eroglu L. Auricle reconstruction with a radial forearm flap prelaminated with porous polyethylene (Medpor®) implant. Microsurgery. 2012;32:627–30.
4. Zhao Y, Wang Y, Zhuang H, Jiang H, Jiang W, Hu X, Hu S, Wang S, Pan B. Clinical evaluation of three total ear reconstruction methods. J Plast Reconstr Aesthet Surg. 2009;62:1550–4.
5. Lee MR, Unger JG, Rohrich RJ. Management of the nasal dorsum in rhinoplasty: a systematic review of the literature regarding technique,outcomes, and complications. Plast Reconstr Surg. 2011;128:538e–50.
6. Guerrerosantos J, Trabanino C, Guerrerosantos F. Multifragmented cartilage wrapped with fascia in augmentation rhinoplasty. Plast Reconstr Surg. 2006;117:804–12. discussion 813–6.
7. Dong L, Hongyu X. Gao ZAugmentation rhinoplasty with expanded polytetrafluoroethylene and prevention of complications. Arch Facial Plast Surg. 2010;12:246–51.
8. Niechajev I. Facial reconstruction using porous high-density polyethylene (medpor): long-term results. Aesthetic Plast Surg. 2012;36:917–27.
9. Monroy A, Kojima K, Ghanem MA, Paz AC, Kamil S, Vacanti CA, Eavey RD. Tissue engineered cartilage "bioshell" protective layer for subcutaneous implants. Int J Pediatr Otorhinolaryngol. 2007;71:547–52.
10. Griffin MF, Premakumar Y, Seifalian AM, Szarko M, Butler PE. Biomechanical characterisation of the human nasal cartilages; implications for tissue engineering. J Mater Sci Mater Med. 2016;27:11.
11. Griffin MF, Premakumar Y, Seifalian AM, Szarko M, Butler PE. Biomechanical Characterisation of the Human Auricular Cartilages; Implications for Tissue Engineering. Ann Biomed Eng. 2016;44(12):3460–7.
12. Silver FH, Kato YP, Ohno M, Wasserman AJ. Analysis of mammalian connective tissue: relationship between hierarchical structures and mechanical properties. J Long Term Eff Med Implants. 1992;2:165–98.
13. Wood JM, Soldin M, Shaw TJ, Szarko M. The biomechanical and histological sequelae of common skin banking methods. J Biomech. 2014;47:1215–9.
14. Griffin MF, Premakumar Y, Seifalian AM, Szarko M, Butler PE. Biomechanical characterization of human soft tissues using indentation and tensile testing. Jove. 2016. In press.
15. Wilkes GL, Brown IA, Wildnauer RH. The biomechanical properties of skin. CRC Crit Rev Bioeng. 1973;1:453–95.
16. Uitto J. Biochemistry of the elasticfibers in normal connective tissues and its alterations in diseases. J Invest Dermatol. 1979;72:1–10.
17. Hussain SH, Limthongkul B, Humphreys TR. The biomechanical properties of the skin. Dermatol Surg. 2013;39:193–203.
18. Silver FH, Freeman JW, DeVore D. Viscoelasticproperties of human skin and processed dermis. Skin Res Technol. 2001;7:18–23.
19. Ní Annaidh A, Bruyère K, Destrade M, Gilchrist MD, Otténio M. Characterization of the anisotropic mechanical properties of excised human skin. J Mech Behav Biomed Mater. 2012;5:139–48.
20. Jacquemoud C, Bruyere-Garnier K, Coret M. Methodology to determine failure characteristics of planar soft tissues using a dynamic tensile test. J Biomech. 2007;40:468–75.
21. Ranamukhaarachchi SA, Lehnert S, Ranamukhaarachchi SL, Sprenger L, Schneider T, Mansoor L, Rai K, Häfeli UO, Stoeber B. A micromechanical comparison of human and porcine skin before and after preservation by freezing for medical device development. Sci Rep. 2016;6:32074.

2

The prevalence of human papillomavirus in pediatric tonsils

Monika Wojtera[1], Josee Paradis[1,2], Murad Husein[1,2], Anthony C. Nichols[1,2], John W. Barrett[1,2], Marina I. Salvadori[1,3] and Julie E. Strychowsky[1,2]*

Abstract

Background: HPV-related head and neck cancer rates have been increasing in recent years, with the tonsils being the most commonly affected site. However, the current rate of HPV infection in the pediatric population remains poorly defined. The objective of this study was to systematically review and evaluate the prevalence and distribution of HPV in the tonsils of pediatric patients undergoing routine tonsillectomy.

Methods and Results: The literature was searched using PubMed, EMBASE, Scopus, CINAHL, Cochrane Library, and ProQuest Dissertations & Theses Global databases (inception to December 2017) by two independent review authors. Inclusion criteria included articles which evaluated the prevalence of HPV in a pediatric cohort without known warts or recurrent respiratory papillomatosis, those which used tonsil biopsy specimens for analysis, and those with six or more subjects and clear outcomes reported. Eleven studies met the inclusion criteria. Using the Oxford Clinical Evidence-based Medicine (OCEBM) guidelines, two reviewers appraised the level of evidence of each study, extracted data, and resolved discrepancies by consensus. The systematic review identified 11 articles ($n = 2520$). Seven studies detected HPV in the subject population, with prevalence values ranging from 0 to 21%. The level of evidence for all included studies was OCEBM Level 3.

Conclusions: HPV may be present in pediatric tonsillectomy specimens; however, the largest included study demonstrated a prevalence of 0%. Future testing should be performed using methods with high sensitivities and specificities, such as reverse transcript real-time PCR or digital droplet PCR.

Keywords: Pediatric, Human papillomavirus, HPV, Tonsils

Background

Human papillomavirus (HPV) is a DNA virus capable of infecting skin or stratified epithelial cells. There are over 100 different types of HPV, of which at least 13 are cancer-causing types deemed 'high-risk'; the most common of these being HPV 16 and 18. The remaining 'low-risk' types cause non-cancerous lesions and diseases, with HPV 6 and 11 infections occurring most frequently. While sexual transmission is the primary method of HPV infection,

vertical transmission, auto-inoculation, and other forms of horizontal transmission have also been considered.

While most HPV infections remain subclinical and are eventually eliminated by the immune system, some cases may persist [1]. In children, this persistence commonly presents as recurrent respiratory papillomatosis (RRP), associated with HPV 6 or 11, or anogenital warts, associated with multiple HPV subtypes. In adults, presentations range from benign skin and anogenital warts due to low-risk subtypes to more serious cervical, anal, and head and neck cancers secondary to high-risk subtypes. The vast majority HPV-related head and neck cancer arises in the oropharynx, with the tonsils being the most commonly affected site [2–4]. Despite the decreasing frequency of tobacco- and alcohol-related oropharyngeal

---

* Correspondence: julie.strychowsky@lhsc.on.ca
[1]Schulich School of Medicine and Dentistry, Western University, 1151 Richmond St, London N6A 5C1, ON, Canada
[2]Department of Otolaryngology-Head and Neck Surgery, Victoria Hospital B3-400, 800 Commissioners Rd E, London N6A 5W9, ON, Canada
Full list of author information is available at the end of the article

squamous cell cancer (OPSCC), the prevalence of HPV-positive cases has been progressively increasing and is now over 70%, due to rising rates of oral infection with HPV [5–9]. Of note, HPV 16 accounts for the majority of cases (> 90%) [10]. Since 6.9% of the adult population has been found to have detectable HPV at any given point in time [5], it is important to delineate both when tonsillar HPV infection is first acquired and how long it remains latent by evaluating its prevalence in the pediatric population. However, the rate of HPV infection in the tonsillar tissue of the pediatric population remains poorly defined. In this manuscript, we endeavor to carry out a systematic review of the prevalence of HPV in pediatric patients undergoing routine tonsillectomy.

Methods

This review was conducted in accordance with the Preferred Reporting Items for Systematic Reviews and Meta-Analyses (PRISMA) 2009 guidelines [11].

Literature search strategy

A comprehensive literature search was performed using PubMed, EMBASE, Scopus, CINAHL, Cochrane Library, and ProQuest Dissertations & Theses Global databases on December 10, 2017. Similar search strategies were applied to search each database. The electronic database search combined disease-specific terms (human papillomavirus, HPV) with anatomic-specific terms (tonsil, throat, pharynx, adenoid, palatine, tubal, lingual) and pediatric-specific terms (pediatric, paediatric, children, kid, youth, teen, preteen, minor, juvenile, virgin, prepubescent, prepubescent, boy, girl, toddler, baby, babies, infant, neonate, newborn). Initially, to ensure the consideration of all relevant published articles in the initial search, the search was not limited in terms of publication date, study design, or language of publication. Relevant articles and abstracts were selected and reviewed, and their reference lists were further searched for additional publications. Next, all studies with abstracts or full articles written in the English language were considered for inclusion.

Study selection criteria

Articles were assessed for eligibility and included if they reported a prevalence of HPV in pediatric tonsils (age < 18 years old), regardless of study design or publication date. Articles were excluded if they did not report results separately for the pediatric population, if they analyzed specimens from anatomic sites other than the palatine tonsils, or if non-biopsy methods of tonsillar testing were used. Where studies analyzed tonsil specimens from adults as well as children, only the pediatric data was used in our analysis. If discerning between the two was not possible, the study was excluded.

To detect tonsillar HPV, studies that utilized tonsillectomy specimens as a sampling method were used. The detection of HPV using swabs of the oral mucosa, tonsillar mucosa, and nasopharynx is inconsistent with the results attained by biopsy, and therefore these sampling methods were excluded. It is theorized that HPV tends to localize to the epithelium of tonsillar crypts, which would account for the unreliability of tonsillar swabs as a method of detection [12]. In cases where oropharyngeal scrapings were used as opposed to tonsillar scraping or biopsy, that study or portion of the study was excluded [13].

Articles in a foreign language were included as long as an abstract was available in the English language and if the abstract described the method of specimen acquisition and reported the prevalence of HPV [13, 14].

Data analysis

The methodological quality of identified studies was appraised using the Oxford Center for Evidence-Based Medicine (OCEBM) 2011 Levels of Evidence [15] and the Newcastle-Ottawa Scale modified for cross-sectional studies [16]. Relevant data was extracted from included studies following tables developed a priori by two independent review authors (M.W. and J.S.). Disagreement was resolved by consensus. Data collected included the country of study, number of patients, age range, mean age, reported prevalence of HPV, testing method, types of HPV tested, and types of HPV detected. Qualitative and quantitative synthesis of results was performed when applicable. A pooled proportion of the prevalence of HPV in pediatric tonsils was considered.

Results

Six hundred twenty-six studies were identified during the initial literature search (Fig. 1). Four hundred seventy-nine studies remained for consideration after duplicate publications were removed. The titles and abstracts of these studies were screened for the inclusion and exclusion criteria, and 433 studies were eliminated because of excluded records. The remaining 46 full-text articles were reviewed in their entirety. Eleven studies with a total of 2520 patients met the inclusion criteria and were included in the analysis. Among these, nine were full-text articles in English while two were abstracts in English with the full-text articles in another language.

Study and patient characteristics are reported in Table 1. The number of patients enrolled in each study ranged from 8 to 1670. HPV was detected in seven studies, and the prevalence of HPV ranged from 0 to 21%. The geographic distribution is illustrated in Fig. 2. The HPV subtypes that were detected varied: subtype 6 (two studies) [14, 17], 11 (three studies) [14, 17, 18], 16 (four studies) [17, 19–21], and 31 (one study) [17]. There was

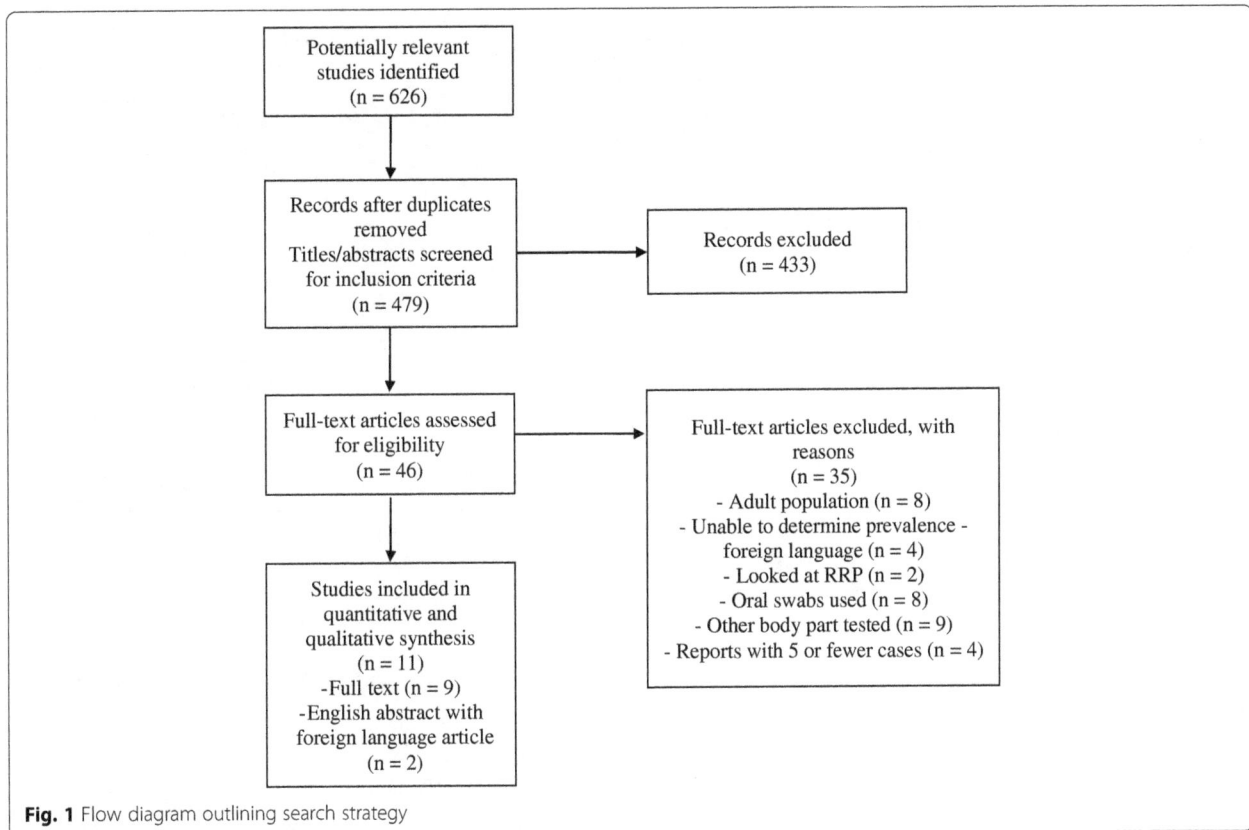

Fig. 1 Flow diagram outlining search strategy

variability in testing methods and HPV subtypes tested, with the majority of studies using conventional PCR with broad-spectrum probes (8/11 studies, 72%), with four studies following up this initial screen with type-specific probes. Three studies used real-time PCR (qPCR), and none used reverse-transcriptase qPCR (RT-qPCR). Reporting and subgroup analysis of the ages and genders of HPV-positive samples was considered, but was not possible as most included studies did not provide these details.

The OCEBM level of evidence for all 11 included studies was Level 3. Quality assessment according to the Newcastle-Ottawa Scale modified for cross-sectional studies is reported in Table 2.

Although a pooled statistical analysis was considered for the collected data, the variability in sample size, geographic distribution, HPV testing methods, and types of HPV tested would limit generalizability of possible pooled analyses. Due to this heterogeneity, a pooled analysis of the data was not performed.

Discussion

To our knowledge, this is the first comprehensive analysis of the prevalence of HPV in pediatric tonsillar tissue. Based on this systematic review of the literature, the prevalence ranges from 0 to 21%.

Study limitations

The wide variability in the prevalence of HPV between studies warrants discussion. While each of the studies used biopsy specimens for testing, the majority used conventional PCR and broad-spectrum GP5+/6+ or MY09/11 primers. Conventional PCR has been noted to exhibit poor specificity and consequently a high false positive rate when testing for HPV, which may explain some of the high prevalence findings reported [22]. qPCR is more accurate, with an improved ability to discriminate between positive and negative samples based the cycle threshold [23]. However, the gold standard is RT-qPCR, which amplifies signals based on the presence of viral transcripts and demonstrates the expression of early viral proteins, as the significance of the presence of HPV DNA in the absence of viral expression is unclear [23]. A newer technique is digital droplet PCR (ddPCR), which may prove to be a more sensitive technique for HPV viral load quantification [24]. The unreliability of conventional PCR and lack of controls in some studies may explain the differences observed. Only three studies [20, 25, 26] used qPCR for analysis, and none employed RT-qPCR or ddPCR.

It is also of value to note that although the overall prevalence of HPV ranged from 0 to 21%, the largest study [27], encompassing 1670 patients, was unable to

Table 1 Summary of included studies

First Study Author & Year of Publication[a]	Country	# of Patients	Age Range (Years) [mean]	Prevalence of HPV[a]	Testing Method	Types of HPV Tested	Types of HPV Found
Cockerill, CC (2016) [25] [full text] [b]	USA	129	1–12 [NR]	0%	Biopsy + swabs + Roche Cobas Amplicor test qPCR & E6/E7 Gene-Probe Aptima HPV test	16, 18, 31, 33, 35, 39, 45, 51, 52, 56, 58, 59, 66, 68	None
Palmer, E (2014) [27] [full text]	United Kingdom	1670	0–18 [NR]	0%	Biopsy + GP5+/6+ primer PCR enzyme immunoassay + PCR E6 gene targeting for HPV16	20 types (unspecified), 14 high-risk and 6 low-risk	None
Xue, XC (2014) [26] [full text]	China	42	3–12 [6.8]	0%	Biopsy + MY09/11 primer qPCR	6, 11, 16, 18, 26, 31, 33–35, 39, 40, 42–45, 51–59, 61, 66–73, 81–84	None
Sun, YF (2012) [abstract] [article in Chinese] [14] [full text]	China	177	NR[NR]	1%	Biopsy + PCR (unspecified)	NR	6, 11
Duray, A (2011) [19] [full text]	Belgium	42	0–15 [NR]	21%	Biopsy + GP5+/GP6+ primer PCR + E6/E7 type-specific qPCR for multiple HPV subtypes	6, 11, 16, 18, 31, 33, 35, 39, 45, 51, 52, 53, 56, 58, 59, 66, 68	16, NR
Baloglu, H (2010) [17] [full text]	Turkey	165	5–21 [11.9]	7%	Biopsy + MY/GP PCR + E6/E7 type-specific PCR	6, 11, 16, 18, 31, 33, 35, 39, 42, 43, 44, 45, 51, 52, 56, 58, 59, 66, 68	6, 11, 16, 31
Soldatskiĭ, IuA (2009) [abstract] [article in Russian] [13]	Russia	8	2–14 [6.8]	13%	PCR	6, 11, 16, 18, 31, 33	NR
Mammas, IN (2006) [20] [full text]	Greece	64	2–14 [7.1]	9%	Biopsy + GP5+/6+ primer PCR + type-specific PCR for multiple HPV subtypes	11, 16, 18, 33	16, NR
Sisk, J (2006) [18] [full text]	USA	50	3–12 [NR]	4%	Biopsy + MY09/11 primer PCR	NR	11
Ribeiro, KM (2006) [37] [full text]	Brazil	100	2–13 [NR]	0%	Biopsy + MY09/11 primer PCR	NR	None
Chen, R (2005) [21] [full text]	Finland	73	1–16 [8.3]	8%	Biopsy + GP5+/6+ & MY09/11 primer PCR + type-specific testing	NR	16

HPV human papillomavirus, *NR* not reported in the study or for the tonsillectomy portion
[a] Articles published in English unless otherwise specified
[b] This study only assessed high-risk HPV subtypes. This was also the only study to report that some patients had been vaccinated against HPV; 6 (4.7%) of patients had received the vaccine

detect the virus. In total, four studies found a 0% prevalence of HPV, comprising 1941 of this review's 2520 patients. Studies with positive results were all completed on a smaller scale; the largest patient sample from a study with a positive result consisted of 177 patients, with a prevalence of only 1% [14], suggesting potential sampling or selection bias. It is also important to consider that in all cases, tonsillar hypertrophy and chronic tonsillitis were the indications for tonsillectomy. Although these conditions are not known to be related to HPV infection, it is possible that they may be confounders.

Geographical considerations

An alternate possibility for the variation in prevalence of pediatric tonsillar HPV infection is that this infection has a geographical distribution, as illustrated in Fig. 2, with the highest prevalence in Belgium. HPV-related cervical lesions have been found to have a geographical distribution [28, 29], supporting the notion of such a pattern in tonsillar HPV. However, it does not appear as though worldwide oropharyngeal cancer incidence rates have a parallel distribution (Fig. 3) [30]. Country-specific prevalence rates could not be determined based on currently-available data. Of note, the highest rates for both pediatric HPV prevalence and oropharyngeal cancer incidence among the countries identified was Belgium; however, there is no obvious pattern beyond this. This lack of correlation could be simply because there is no relationship between pediatric tonsillar HPV infection and later adult oropharyngeal cancer; perhaps pediatric patients are more easily able to eliminate the infection, or prior HPV infection protects against future infection. Alternately, a correlation between childhood infection and adult cancer may exist, but be difficult to discern at this time due to the currently limited literature.

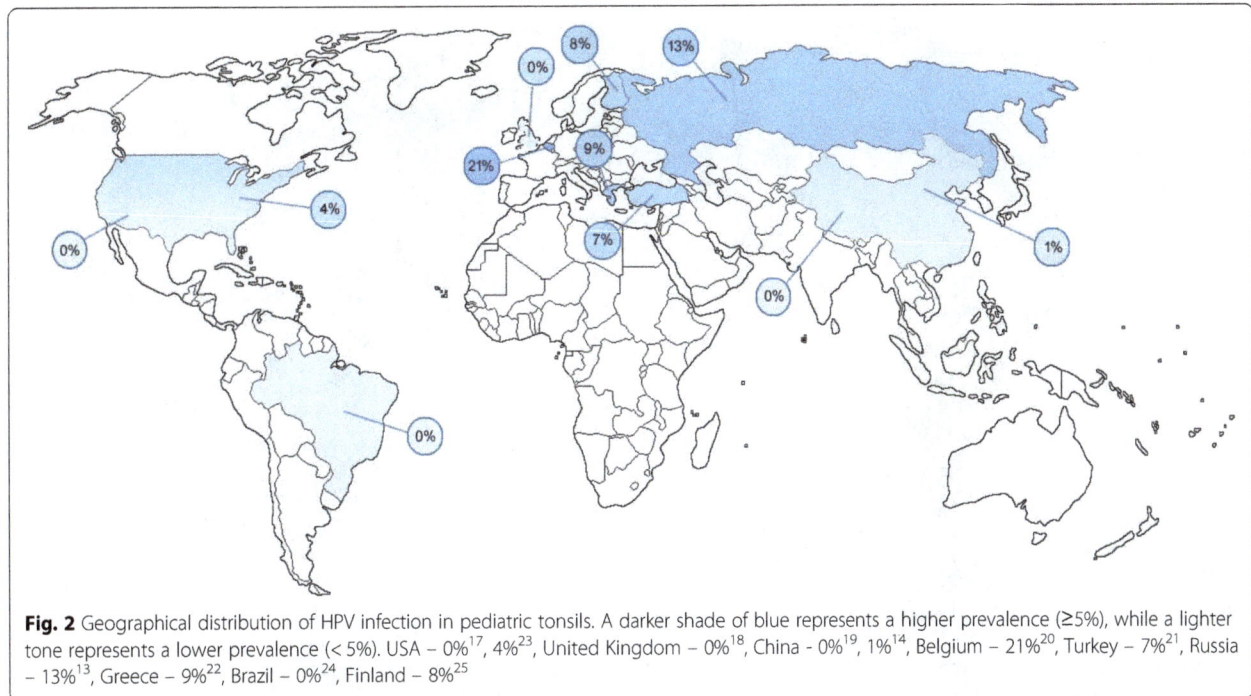

Fig. 2 Geographical distribution of HPV infection in pediatric tonsils. A darker shade of blue represents a higher prevalence (≥5%), while a lighter tone represents a lower prevalence (< 5%). USA – 0%[17], 4%[23], United Kingdom – 0%[18], China - 0%[19], 1%[14], Belgium – 21%[20], Turkey – 7%[21], Russia – 13%[13], Greece – 9%[22], Brazil – 0%[24], Finland – 8%[25]

Subtypes of Tonsillar HPV

Of the HPV subtypes identified among the patients included in this study ($n = 28$), HPV 6, 11, 16, and 31 were observed, with HPV 16 being the most prevalent (78.6%). High-risk HPV 16 is the subtype most frequently associated with OPSCC, with an average age of diagnosis of 61 years old [7]. This suggests that the subclinical HPV infection detected in childhood may be a pre-malignant lesion with a long-term course, representing a risk factor for the development of tonsillar cancer in adulthood. No studies reported long-term follow-up to determine the incidence of possible malignant transformation.

Whether this pediatric infection eventually progresses to symptomatic disease or cancer, remains dormant for the lifespan of the patient, or is eventually eliminated by the host's immune system, is currently unknown. An interesting parallel is the pathogenesis of HPV infection in the cervix, wherein persistent and often asymptomatic HPV infection can lead to intraepithelial neoplasia and the eventual accumulation of mutations, resulting in cancerous invasion and metastasis [31]. A similar cycle

Table 2 Quality assessment using a version of the Newcastle-Ottawa modified for cross-sectional studies

Author (Year)	Selection (Maximum 4 Stars)	Comparability (Maximum 2 Stars)	Exposure (Maximum 3 Stars)	Total (Maximum 9 Stars)
Cockerill, CC (2016) [25]	**	*	*	****
Palmer, E (2014) [27]	***	*	**	******
Xue, X-C (2014) [26]	**	*	**	*****
Sun, YF (2012) [abstract] [article in Chinese] [14]	**	**	*	*****
Duray, A (2011) [19]	**	*	*	****
Baloglu, H (2010) [17]	**	*	*	****
Soldatskiĭ, IuA (2009) [abstract] [article in Russian] [13]	*	*	*	**
Mammas, IN (2006) [20]	**	**	**	******
Sisk, J (2006)[18]	**	**	**	******
Ribeiro, KM (2006)[37]	**	*	*	****
Chen, R (2005)[21]	*	*	*	***

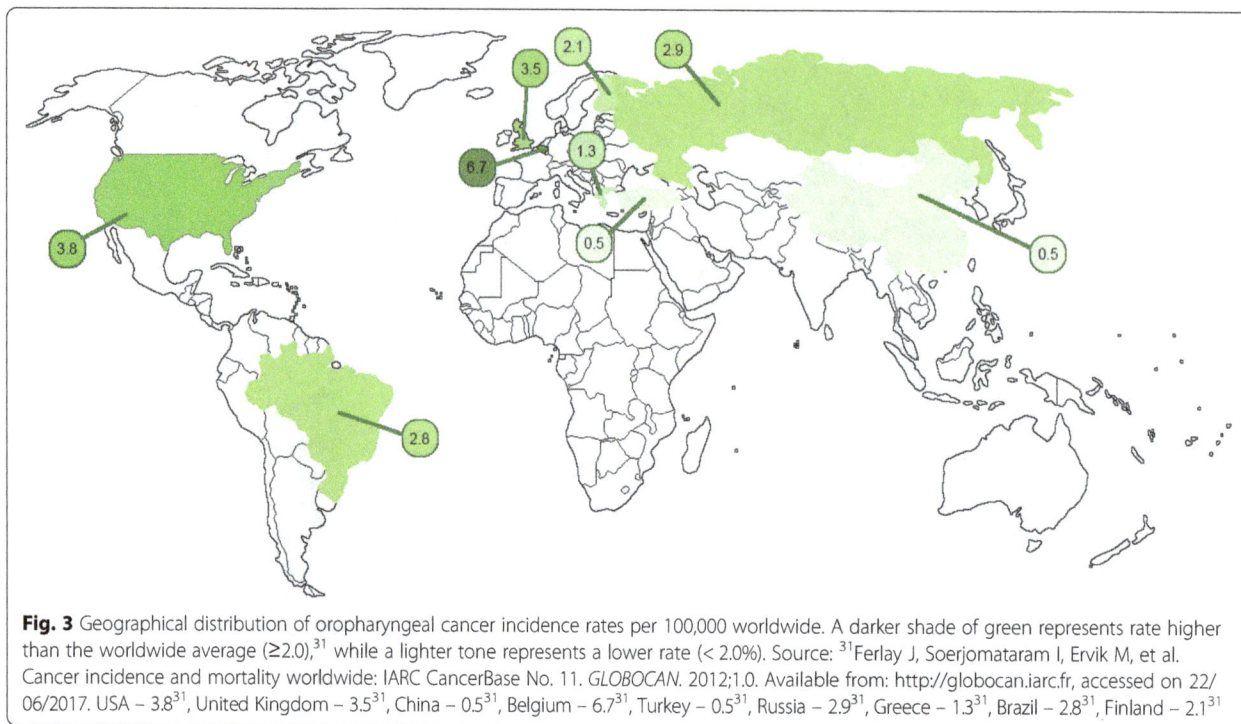

Fig. 3 Geographical distribution of oropharyngeal cancer incidence rates per 100,000 worldwide. A darker shade of green represents rate higher than the worldwide average (≥2.0),[31] while a lighter tone represents a lower rate (< 2.0%). Source: [31]Ferlay J, Soerjomataram I, Ervik M, et al. Cancer incidence and mortality worldwide: IARC CancerBase No. 11. *GLOBOCAN*. 2012;1.0. Available from: http://globocan.iarc.fr, accessed on 22/06/2017. USA – 3.8[31], United Kingdom – 3.5[31], China – 0.5[31], Belgium – 6.7[31], Turkey – 0.5[31], Russia – 2.9[31], Greece – 1.3[31], Brazil – 2.8[31], Finland – 2.1[31]

may occur with tonsillar HPV infection, emphasizing the importance of early detection of HPV.

HPV transmission and implications

The presence of HPV in the tonsils of pediatric patients suggests that consideration must be given for a mode of transmission other than sexual transmission. While sexual transmission through early sexual activity or sexual abuse remains a possibility [32–34], the detection of HPV in infants and in high rates among youth in some studies suggests that sexual exposure is unlikely to account for all cases. As such, vertical and horizontal transmission must also be considered.

HPV vaccination

Both bivalent and quadrivalent vaccines against HPV are currently available on the world market, and a 9-valent vaccine has also been introduced in some areas. The bivalent vaccine is effective at preventing the high-risk HPV 16 and 18 subtypes, and the quadrivalent vaccine adds protection against HPV 6 and 11. As of 2014, 58 countries had introduced one or both versions of the HPV vaccine into their national immunization programs for girls, and countries such as Canada, the USA, Australia, and Austria also currently advocate its use in boys [22, 35].

Despite the availability of a publicly-funded vaccine against HPV infection in Canada, immunization rates for HPV remain far below those of other vaccine-preventable diseases [36]. This study calls into questions the preconception that HPV is solely a sexually-

transmitted disease, and may be used to further vaccination campaigns in locations where stigma against vaccination for a sexually transmitted infection is still a barrier for larger-scale immunization campaigns.

Conclusion

HPV 6, 11, 16, and 31 may be present in some pediatric tonsils, and their prevalence ranges from 0 to 21%. The largest study demonstrated a prevalence of 0%. A geographical distribution could account for these discrepancies, but does not appear to correlate with adult oropharyngeal cancer incidence rates. Whether these infections are a pre-malignant state, a transient infection, or a latent infection that will ultimately lead to malignant disease is yet to be determined. Further adequately powered studies utilizing qPCR, the gold-standard RT-qPCR, or the newer and more sensitive ddPCR for detection of HPV are warranted to determine the true prevalence of HPV in the pediatric population.

Abbreviations
ddPCR: Digital droplet PCR; HPV: Human papillomavirus; OCEBM: Oxford clinical evidence-based medicine; OPSCC: Oropharyngeal squamous cell cancer; PRISMA: Preferred reporting items for systematic reviews and meta-analyses; qPCR: Real-time PCR; RRP: Recurrent respiratory papillomatosis; RT-qPCR: Reverse-transcriptase qPCR

Acknowledgements
Not applicable.

Funding
Not applicable.

Authors' contributions

MW: Designed the data collection instruments, performed the literature search and data extraction, appraised the levels of evidence, carried out the initial analyses and interpretation of data, and drafted the initial manuscript. P, H, N, B and S: Assisted with study design and critically reviewed and revised the manuscript. JES: Conceptualized the study, performed the literature search and data extraction, appraised the levels of evidence, and critically reviewed and revised the manuscript. All authors approved the final manuscript as submitted and agree to be accountable for all aspects of the work.

Competing interests

The authors declare that they have no competing interests.

Author details

[1]Schulich School of Medicine and Dentistry, Western University, 1151 Richmond St, London N6A 5C1, ON, Canada. [2]Department of Otolaryngology-Head and Neck Surgery, Victoria Hospital B3-400, 800 Commissioners Rd E, London N6A 5W9, ON, Canada. [3]Department of Paediatrics, Children's Hospital at London Health Sciences Centre, 800 Commissioners Rd E, London, ON N6A 5W9, Canada.

References

1. Koutsky L. Epidemiology of genital human papillomavirus infection. Am J Med. 1997;102(5):3–8.
2. Gillison ML, Shah KV. Human papillomavirus-associated head and neck squamous cell carcinoma: mounting evidence for an etiologic role for human papillomavirus in a subset of head and neck cancers. Curr Opin Oncol. 2001;13(3):183–8.
3. Koskinen WJ, Chen RW, Leivo I, et al. Prevalence and physical status of human papillomavirus in squamous cell carcinomas of the head and neck. Int J Cancer. 2003;107(3):401–6.
4. Klussmann JP, Weissenborn SJ, Wieland U, et al. Prevalence, distribution, and viral load of human papillomavirus 16 DNA in tonsillar carcinomas. Cancer. 2001;92(11):2875–84.
5. Gillison ML, Broutian T, Pickard RK, et al. Prevalence of oral HPV infection in the United States, 2009-2010. JAMA. 2012;307(7):693–703.
6. Hocking JS, Stein A, Conway EL, et al. Head and neck cancer in Australia between 1982 and 2005 show increasing incidence of potentially HPV-associated oropharyngeal cancers. Br J Cancer. 2011;104(5):886–91.
7. Chaturvedi AK, Engels EA, Anderson WF, Gillison ML. Incidence trends for human papillomavirus-related and -unrelated oral squamous cell carcinomas in the United States. J Clin Oncol. 2008;26(4):612–9.
8. Mehanna H, Beech T, Nicholson T, et al. Prevalence of human papillomavirus in oropharyngeal and nonoropharyngeal head and neck cancer—systematic review and meta-analysis of trends by time and region. Head Neck. 2013;35(5):747–55.
9. Syrjänen S. HPV infections and tonsillar carcinoma. J Clin Pathol. 2004; 57(5):449–55.
10. Herrero R, Castellsagué X, Pawlita M, et al. Human papillomavirus and oral cancer: the International Agency for Research on Cancer multicenter study. J Natl Cancer Inst. 2003;95(23):1772–83.
11. Liberati A, Altman DG, Tetzlaff J, et al. The PRISMA statement for reporting systematic reviews and meta-analyses of studies that evaluate healthcare interventions: explanation and elaboration. BMJ. 2009;339:b2700.
12. Begum S, Cao D, Gillison M, Zahurak M, Westra WH. Tissue distribution of human papillomavirus 16 DNA integration in patients with tonsillar carcinoma. Clin Cancer Res. 2005;11(16):5694–9.
13. IuA S, Onufrieva EK, Pogosova IE, IuV S, Diudia AV. Infection of the upper respiratory tract with human papilloma virus in children without clinical signs of respiratory papillomatosis [in Russian]. Vestn Otorinolaringol. 2009; (1):16–9.
14. Sun YF, Wu YD, Wu L, et al. Detection of human papillomavirus in the upper respiratory tract in children without recurrent respiratory papillomatosis [in Chinese]. Zhonghua Er Bi Yan Hou Tou Jing Wai Ke Za Zhi. 2012;47(12):974–7.
15. OCEBM Levels of Evidence Working Group. The Oxford levels of evidence 2. Oxford Centre Evid Based Med. http://www.cebm.net/blog/2016/05/01/ocebm-levels-of-evidence/. Accessed 21 July 2016.
16. BioMed Central. Newcastle-Ottawa Scale adapted for cross-sectional studies website. http://journals.plos.org/plosone/article/file?type=supplementary&id=info:doi/10.1371/journal.pone.0147601.s001. Accessed 21 July 2016.
17. Baloglu H, Kucukodaci Z, Gungor A, et al. Human papilloma virus prevalence in hyperplastic tonsils and adenoids in children and young adults. Turkiye Klinikleri J Med Sci. 2010;30(2):528–32.
18. Sisk J, Schweinfurth JM, Wang XT, Chong K. Presence of human Papillomavirus DNA in tonsillectomy specimens. Laryngoscope. 2006;116(8):1372–4.
19. Duray A, Descamps G, Bettonville M, et al. High prevalence of high-risk human papillomavirus in palatine tonsils from healthy children and adults. Otolaryngol Head Neck Surg. 2011;145(2):230–5.
20. Mammas IN, Sourvinos G, Michael C, Spandidos DA. Human papilloma virus in hyperplastic tonsillar and adenoid tissues in children. Pediatr Infect Dis J. 2006;25(12):1158–62.
21. Chen R, Sehr P, Waterboer T, et al. Presence of DNA of human papillomavirus 16 but no other types in tumor-free tonsillar tissue. J Clin Microbiol. 2005;43(3):1408–10.
22. Venuti A, Paolini F. HPV detection methods in head and neck cancer. Head Neck Pathol. 2012;6(suppl 1):S63–74.
23. Jordan RC, Lingen MW, Perez-Ordonez B, et al. Validation of methods for oropharyngeal cancer HPV status determination in US cooperative group trials. Am J Surg Pathol. 2012;36(7):945–54.
24. Lillsunde Larsson G, Helenius G. Digital droplet PCR (ddPCR) for the detection and quantification of HPV 16, 18, 33 and 45 – a short report. Cell Oncol. 2017;40(5):521–7.
25. Cockerill CC, Orvidas LJ, Moore EJ, et al. Detection of high-risk human papillomavirus infection in tonsillar specimens using 2 commercially available assays. Diagn Microbiol Infect Dis. 2016;86(4):365–8.
26. Xue XC, Chen XP, Yao WH, Zhang Y, Sun GB, Tan XJ. Prevalence of human papillomavirus and Epstein–Barr virus DNA in Chinese children with tonsillar and/or adenoidal hypertrophy. J Med Virol. 2014;86(6):963–7.
27. Palmer E, Newcombe RG, Green AC, et al. Human papillomavirus infection is rare in nonmalignant tonsil tissue in the UK: implications for tonsil cancer precursor lesions. Int J Cancer. 2014;135(10):2437–43.
28. The World Health Organization. Human papillomavirus vaccines: WHO position paper, October 2014. Wkly Epidemiol Rec. 2014;89(43):465–92.
29. De Vuyst H, Clifford G, Li N, Franceschi S. HPV infection in Europe. Eur J Cancer. 2009;45(15):2632–9.
30. Ferlay J, Soerjomataram I, Ervik M, et al. Cancer incidence and mortality worldwide: IARC CancerBase no. 11. GLOBOCAN. 2012;1.0. http://globocan.iarc.fr. Accessed 22 June 2017.
31. Snijders PJ, Steenbergen RD, Heideman DA, Meijer CJ. HPV-mediated cervical carcinogenesis: concepts and clinical implications. J Pathol. 2006; 208(2):152–64.
32. Wingood GM, Seth P, DiClemente RJ, Robinson LS. Association of sexual abuse with incident high-risk human papillomavirus infection among young African-American women. Sex Transm Dis. 2009;36(12):784–6.
33. Stevens-Simon C, Nelligan D, Breese P, Jenny C, Douglas JM Jr. The prevalence of genital human papillomavirus infections in abused and nonabused preadolescent girls. Pediatrics. 2000;106(4):645–9.
34. Gutman LT, St Claire K, Herman-Giddens ME, Johnston WW, Phelps WC. Evaluation of sexually abused and nonabused young girls for intravaginal human papillomavirus infection. Am J Dis Child. 1992;146(6):694–9.
35. Stanley M. HPV vaccination in boys and men. Hum Vaccin Immunother. 2014;10(7):2109–11.
36. Public Health Agency of Canada. Vaccine coverage amongst adult Canadians: results from the 2012 adult National Immunization Coverage (aNIC) survey. http://www.phac-aspc.gc.ca/im/nics-enva/vcac-cvac-eng.php. Accessed 18 June 2016.
37. Ribeiro KM, Alvez JM, Pignatari SS, Weckx LL. Detection of human papilloma virus in the tonsils of children undergoing tonsillectomy. Braz J Infect Dis. 2006;10(3):165–8.

3

Direct cost comparison of minimally invasive punch technique versus traditional approaches for percutaneous bone anchored hearing devices

Yaeesh Sardiwalla[1], Nicholas Jufas[2,3] and David P. Morris[1,2,4*]

Abstract

Background: Minimally Invasive Ponto Surgery (MIPS) was recently described as a new technique to facilitate the placement of percutaneous bone anchored hearing devices.

The procedure has resulted in a simplification of the surgical steps and a dramatic reduction in surgical time while maintaining excellent patient outcomes. Given these developments, our group sought to move the procedure from the main operating suite where they have traditionally been performed. This study aims to test the null hypothesis that MIPS and open approaches have the same direct costs for the implantation of percutaneous bone anchored hearing devices in a Canadian public hospital setting.

Methods: A retrospective direct cost comparison of MIPS and open approaches for the implantation of bone conduction implants was conducted. Indirect and future costs were not included in the fiscal analysis.

A simple cost comparison of the two approaches was made considering time, staff and equipment needs. All 12 operations were performed on adult patients from 2013 to 2016 by the same surgeon at a single hospital site.

Results: MIPS has a total mean reduction in cost of CAD$456.83 per operation from the hospital perspective when compared to open approaches. The average duration of the MIPS operation was 7 min, which is on average 61 min shorter compared with open approaches.

Conclusion: The MIPS technique was more cost effective than traditional open approaches. This primarily reflects a direct consequence of a reduction in surgical time, with further contributions from reduced staffing and equipment costs. This simple, quick intervention proved to be feasible when performed outside the main operating room. A blister pack of required equipment could prove convenient and further reduce costs.

Keywords: Costs and cost analysis, Otologic surgical procedures, Bone conduction, Minimally invasive surgical procedures

Background

Percutaneous bone-anchored hearing devices (BAHD) or bone conduction hearing implants (BCHI) rely on a secure osseointegrated implant first described in the 1970s by Prof. Brånemark [1]. The first BAHD was placed in 1977 by Anders Tjellstrom [1]. The product has found application in the rehabilitation of single sided deafness (SSD) and a range of hearing losses where there is an intolerance of or an inability to wear conventional amplification [2]. BAHD transmit sound directly through the temporal bone to the inner ear. The three main components are the osseointegrated screw or fixture, the skin penetrating abutment and the removable sound processor that connects externally to the abutment [3]. The implantation of the device has been shown to be safe in both adults and children with many publications demonstrating beneficial effects on hearing [2, 4].

* Correspondence: drdavidpmorris@gmail.com
[1]Faculty of Medicine, Dalhousie University, Halifax, NS, Canada
[2]Division of Otolaryngology – Head and Neck Surgery, Dalhousie University, Halifax, NS, Canada
Full list of author information is available at the end of the article

A number of open techniques have been described where the drilling stages of the surgery are performed under direct vision. Traditional approaches have varied in the style of initial incision but most of them involved significant soft tissue undermining and excision in order to obtain the thin, hairless and immobile implant site that was deemed optimal for long term stability [5]. Such techniques were time-consuming and were often associated with significant bleeding. Many were previously performed under general anaesthesia at our institution for precisely these reasons.

In more recent years there has been a move to less soft tissue reduction and simplified linear incisions that in turn demanded the use of longer abutments [6]. As the surgical technique has become less invasive and surgical times have reduced, the procedures have been exclusively performed under local anaesthetic in our operating room.

In 2011, Hultcrantz et al. described the Minimally Invasive Ponto Surgery (MIPS) procedure using a 5 mm dermal punch to remove the limited tract of soft tissue needed to accommodate the Ponto (Oticon, Copenhagen, Denmark) abutment [7]. The drilling procedure was then completed in seconds, through a cannula placed to protect the skin and soft tissues while holding cooling fluid. MIPS heralds a departure from the traditional "open approach" to percutaneous fixture placement. Soft tissue preservation and longer abutments placed in a few simple surgical steps mark a natural evolution in technique where technical simplification appears possible without compromise to patient care. Early evidence suggests that techniques preserving soft tissue result in favorable outcomes [5].

In our series, we saw the significant reduction in surgical time and procedural invasiveness as a logistical opportunity to move such cases out of the main operating room. Our motivation to do so was driven by our desire to reduce the impact of this surgical intervention on our patients while maintaining a high standard of care and safety. As medical professionals we are constantly striving to deliver high quality, patient-centered care, balancing optimal outcomes from our interventions with the efficient use of finite resources [8].

Although direct, indirect and future costs should be considered to fully evaluate the monetary value of a health care intervention, this study focuses on direct costs. Direct costs include those of the surgeon, anesthesiologist, nursing staff, hospital resources and equipment costs. The objective of this study was to conduct a direct cost analysis comparing MIPS performed outside the OR to the traditional more open techniques in an OR setting at the Queen Elizabeth II Health Sciences Centre in Halifax, Nova Scotia. This is the first cost analysis of this type to be reported.

Methods
Patient information

A cost difference analysis of open approaches and MIPS procedures was performed using a retrospective analysis of direct costs. A total of 12 adult patients operated on by a single surgeon as day case procedures were evaluated. Indirect and future costs were excluded. There were 6 patients who received an abutment implant prior to July 2015 using the open approach in the OR setting. This sample was compared 6 MIPS procedures performed outside of the OR under local anesthetic. A minor procedures room (brachytherapy suite) that conformed to Infection Prevention and Control standards, particularly that of adequate air exchange, was used for the operation during this transition. A convenience sampling approach was used for patients in each group.

Cost analysis

A cost difference approach was used to evaluate the total costs of each procedure. The relevant resources to be evaluated were identified by mapping the patient's health journey. Costs that were similar between open approaches and MIPS procedures were negated in the analysis. The negated costs included pre-operative workup and consultation, hospital admission, as well as post-operative follow up (see Discussion for clarification). As a result, only costs associated with the operative procedure itself were included in this direct cost analysis.

The costs and resources evaluated in this study were broken down in four major groups:

1. Surgeon's fee
2. Nurses' fees
3. Anesthesiologist's fee
4. Operative set-up/equipment

Costs associated with the two procedures were obtained from the Queen Elizabeth II Health Sciences Centre Business Department and relevant nursing staff following the guidance of previously published studies from our institution [9]. The average hourly salary for the health care providers involved in the operations was calculated. Billing codes through Medical Services Insurance (MSI) were used to determine the annual salary of surgeons, and divided by the average number of hours worked each week to yield an average hourly salary [9]. The cost of sterilization and preparation of equipment trays for each procedure were itemized and priced by the business department. The costs of the anaesthetic items were not able to be included in the calculations due to limitations at our institution.

All costs were reported in Canadian Dollars (CAD).

Procedure mean time

For open approaches, OR records were sourced and the operating time was determined by subtracting the end time (patient leaving OR) from the start time (first incision). The MIPS time was calculated prospectively from the moment of skin punch, to the moment the healing cap had been placed.

Results

The mean time for the MIPS procedure was 5 min and 55 s (0.10 h) and 1 h and 7 min (1.13 h) for the open approaches. The cost of staffing was $44.72 per hour for nursing, $140.00 per hour for the surgeons and $125.00 per hour for the anesthesiologist at our facility. Two additional nurses and a single anesthesiologist were required for the open approaches in the OR versus MIPS. Total mean intraoperative costs for the open approach were $451.05 and $18.22 for MIPS. The MIPS technique therefore produced a cost saving of $432.83 compared to the open approaches in terms of provider cost. Intraoperative costs are summarized in Table 1.

The total cost for sterilization of the equipment tray used in the MIPS procedure was found to be $24.00 less than the standard open approaches. Costs of disposables and anesthesia resources were not available for our facility and therefore not included.

The MIPS technique produced a $456.83 total cost saving when compared to open approaches for insertion of percutaneous bone anchored hearing devices. The cost saving can be broken down into the equipment and provider costs.

Discussion

As clinicians we are primarily driven by safety and quality of care measures when faced with the choice of a new intervention for our patients. Once satisfied that these have been demonstrated, logistical issues of cost become our next responsible consideration. MIPS offers the opportunity of cost saving with no suggested negative impact to patient care [5, 7].

We confirmed a total cost saving of $456.83 for MIPS compared the open approaches. The comparative cost saving calculated is independent of surgical venue meaning that the cost saving will be evident at institutions where moving MIPS outside the main OR is not possible. Our attempts to quantify costs associated with the preparation and sterilization of the MIPS equipment tray was somewhat challenging. We were only able to show a small cost saving of $24.00 for equipment costs as bulk sterilization in our centre that has both large turnover and capacity is likely to under-estimate the potential savings that exist in a smaller facility or office setting.

It is intuitive and entirely feasible that equipment costs can be reduced even further in the future. Once out of the operating room setting, we reviewed the items required for this short procedure. The arrangement shown below (Fig. 1) is a significant departure from the previous requirement to open a full surgical tray. When soft tissue reduction was required, bleeding was the rule not the exception and cautery was essential. If the small dissector could be made disposable it could be included with a skin punch as additions to the currently offered blister-packed set. In short, the drill would be the only piece of equipment requiring sterilization. These proposals have clear implications both for costs associated with initial outlay to purchase items and equipment and for the subsequent costs of sterilizing and maintaining such equipment.

Small incidental costs that are no greater than those associated with the traditional approach include limited hair-shave, infiltration of local anaesthetic (at which stage skin thickness can be estimated) and sterile preparation and drape. A syringe with an attached plastic cannula and a bottle of cold saline are required for irrigation. Ribbon gauze with ointment can be left to the surgeon's discretion or a sponge disc could be a further addition to the blister pack.

In moving MIPS out the main suite of operating rooms, continued patient safety was our top priority. In close consultation with the infection control teams at our institution, the MIPS procedures were performed in a treatment room that still met particular specifications. Importance was placed on adequacy of air exchange. All supplies were removed from the room, appropriate

Table 1 The costs and number of healthcare providers (HCP) required for MIPS versus open techniques

Procedure type	HCP	Number of HCP	Hourly wage ($/h)	Hours	Total cost ($)
MIPS	Nurse	1	44.72	0.10	4.41
	Surgeon	1	140.00	0.10	13.81
				Total Provider Cost	18.22
Open/Incision	Nurse	3	44.72	1.13	151.60
	Surgeon	1	140.00	1.13	158.20
	Anaesthesiologist	1	125.00	1.13	141.25
				Total Provider Cost	451.05

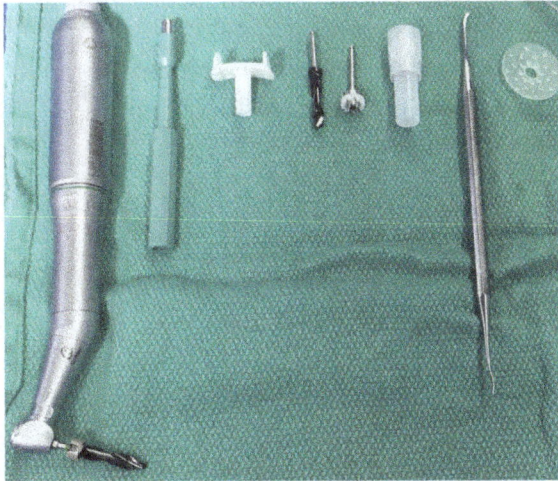

Fig. 1 Proposed reduction in surgical tray. From *left*: Drill with bit, skin punch, cannula, countersink drill bit, handpiece connector, combined abutment and fixture, raspatorium/ dissector, healing cap

data of MIPS outcomes from other groups will soon be made available [11, 12]. Institutionalized memory of earlier more bloody techniques used for implant placement may need to be faced and discussed during such a transition (Fig. 2).

This study employed a simple cost difference analysis only taking into account measurable direct costs. The simplicity of this approach made the cost calculations easy to compute. The only direct cost that was not captured was that of anaesthetic resources during the operation due to facility constraints except for the anesthesiologist's fee. These would be expected to be greater in the open approach not least as many such cases are performed using general anaesthetic requiring intubation, monitoring and recovery. The cost saving of $456.83 could therefore grossly underestimate the total direct cost saving.

An inherent shortcoming of a direct cost analysis is that it fails to capture future and indirect costs. Indirect costs could be categorized as those borne by the patient or those assumed by the health service. Reduced aftercare is likely to represent a further potential cost saving. In our experiences so far, MIPS has offered a faster recovery time as there is little to heal and this is consistent with results that involved less soft tissue undermining [5].

Indirect cost savings to the healthcare system include the benefit of regaining over two hours of prime operating time including procedure and turnaround that frees up facilities and staff to allow for other more urgent operations to be completed. In addition to this, the logistical consideration of performing MIPS procedures as day cases is that a hospital bed is not required. Procedures will not be cancelled due to a lack of overnight hospital bed availability. Hospital resources can be channeled more efficiently for surgical procedures that necessitate an overnight bed. Follow-up studies examining patient satisfaction, recovery time, quality of life, medical outcomes and functionality have not yet been published but are much anticipated and currently ongoing [11, 12].

Personal Protective Equipment (PPE) was worn, there was an external sink for surgical scrub, the door was not opened during the procedure and a terminal clean was performed between cases.

There are theoretical concerns regarding any procedure where dura, brain tissue or cerebrospinal fluid (CSF) might be encountered and equally so where surgical procedures might generate a blood and bone dust aerosol. There is precedent for procedures such as burr hole drilling for intracranial pressure monitoring being performed at the bed side with proven safety [10]. We propose that surgical venue is not the most important factor in determining operative risk, provided that correct protocols are followed, and sterility concerns are satisfied. There have been no long-term complications such as fixture failures in our cohort and all devices are still being worn by patients. Our group will be publishing a case-series evaluation of this cohort and long-term

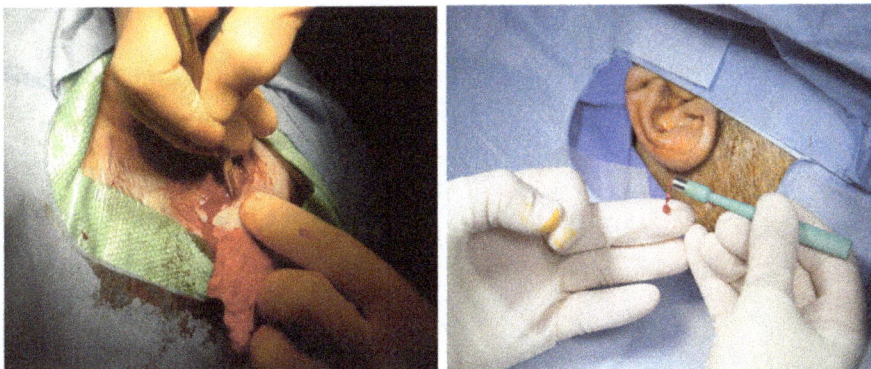

Fig. 2 Bleeding and dissection are strikingly reduced with the MIPS approach (*right*) compared to the more intrusive open approach (*left*)

A limitation of this study relates to imperfect case matching between MIPS and open approach surgeries. Patient demographics and patient comorbidities likely affect surgical duration, and this was not strictly controlled for in our study, but randomization was likely with our convenience sampling approach. Larger patient numbers, matching for measurable characteristics or systematic randomization in a prospective study could mitigate the potential for bias in future analysis. Despite this, there is a clear and intuitive trend of the opportunity for cost saving.

As medical professionals, we have a responsibility to ensure that the services we provide are safe, high quality and economically efficient. When alternative procedures to the current standards have been demonstrated to show those qualities, they should be considered as changes to normal practice. This study has demonstrated the obvious economic benefit of taking the simplified MIPS technique out of the main operating suite. We have confirmed that MIPS has a reduced mean time of operation and staff costs. Equipment cost savings have not been fully captured in this study and are likely to have been under-estimated.

Conclusion

This is the first published study documenting the direct cost benefits of the MIPS procedure compared to open approaches. Lower equipment costs and reduced healthcare professional fees make this true regardless of where the procedure is performed. The study has also demonstrated the suitability of performing MIPS outside the traditional operating room setting, as it is quicker and less invasive. In moving MIPS out of our main OR suite we were able to better utilize facilities and staff to allow for other more pressing operations to be completed. This study has calculated a considerable direct cost saving of at least $456.83 per operation. This figure likely grossly underestimates the true total cost saving to the health care system and the individual patient when all direct, indirect and future costs are considered.

Abbreviations
BAHD: Bone anchored hearing devices; BCHI: Bone conduction hearing implants; CAD: Canadian Dollars; CSF: Cerebrospinal fluid; HCP: Healthcare providers; MIPS: Minimally Invasive Ponto Surgery; MSI: Medical Services Insurance; OR: Operating room; PPE: Personal Protective Equipment

Acknowledgements
The authors gratefully acknowledge the assistance of the following individuals who were instrumental in helping us to navigate the transition of the MIPS procedure from the main OR suite:
Elizabeth Gilfoy RN (Operating Room nurse Victoria General Hospital, Halifax)
Daphne Murray RN ICP CIC (Cobequid Community Health Centre)
Alyson Lamb RN MN MHA (Health Services Manager, Victoria General Hospital, Halifax).

Funding
None.

Authors' contributions
YS was responsible for the preparation of the manuscript, conducting the cost analysis, literature review, liaising with hospital departments and analyzing the data. NJ was involved in the preparation and editing of the manuscript, and was the Fellow for all of the MIPS cases. DPM was the lead surgeon responsible for all MIPS cases and contributed and edited the manuscript. All authors read and approved the final manuscript.

Authors' information
YS is a second year medical student at Dalhousie University. NJ was an otology fellow at Dalhousie University and currently a consulting ENT surgeon in Sydney, Australia. DPM is a staff physician at the Queen Elizabeth II Health Science Center and assistant professor at Dalhousie University.

Competing interests
DPM has participated in scientific meetings and workshops arranged by Oticon Medical where travel and accommodation costs were provided. YS and NJ have none to declare.

Author details
[1]Faculty of Medicine, Dalhousie University, Halifax, NS, Canada. [2]Division of Otolaryngology – Head and Neck Surgery, Dalhousie University, Halifax, NS, Canada. [3]Discipline of Surgery, Sydney Medical School, University of Sydney, Sydney, Australia. [4]QEII Health Science Center - VG Site Otolaryngology, 5820 University Ave - Rm 3037, Halifax, NS B3H 2Y9, Canada.

References
1. Lustig LR, et al. Hearing rehabilitation using the BAHA bone-anchored hearing aid: results in 40 patients. Otol Neurotol. 2001;22:328–34.
2. Bento RF, Kiesewetter A, Ikari LS, Brito R. Bone-anchored hearing aid (BAHA): Indications, functional results, and comparison with reconstructive surgery of the ear. Int Arch Otorhinolaryngol. 2012;16:400–5.
3. Westerkull P, The Ponto bone- anchored hearing system. Adv Otorhinolaryngol. 2011;71:32–40.
4. Secreteriat MA. Bone anchored hearing aid: an evidence based analysis. Ont Health Technol Assess Ser. 2002;2:1–47.
5. Johansson M, Holmberg M, Hultcrantz PM. Bone anchored hearing implant surgery with tissue preservation – a systematic literature review. Oticon Med Rev. 2015;M52107INT.
6. Woolford T, Morris D, Saeed S, Rothera M. The implant-site split-skin graft technique for the bone-achored hearing aid. Clin Otolaryngol. 1999;24:177–80.
7. Hultcrantz M. Outcome of the bone-anchored hearing aid procedure without skin thinning: a prospective clinical trial. Otol Neurotol. 2011;32:1134–9.
8. Halvorson G. Understanding the trade-offs of the Canadian health system. Healthc Financ Manage. 2007;61:82–4.
9. Forner D, Phillips T. Submental island flap reconstruction reduces cost in oral cancer reconstruction compared to radial forearm free flap reconstruction: a case series and cost analysis. J Otolaryngol Head Neck Surg. 2016;45:1–8.
10. Bochicchio M, Latronico N, Zappa S, Beindorf A, Candiani A. Bedside burr hole for intracranial pressure monitoring performed by intensive care physicians. A 5-year experience. Intensive Care Med. 1996;22:1070–4.
11. Johansson M, Holmberg M. Design and clinical evaluation of MIPS – a new perspective on tissue preservation. Oticon Med. 2014;1–12. doi:10.13140/RG. 2.1.3624.7762.
12. Calon TGA, et al. Minimally Invasive Ponto Surgery compared to the linear incision technique without soft tissue reduction for bone conduction hearing implants: study protocol for a randomized controlled trial. Trials. 2016;17:540.

4

Endoscopically-assisted transmastoid approach to the geniculate ganglion and labyrinthine facial nerve

Nicholas Jufas[1,2,3]* (iD) and Manohar Bance[1]

Abstract

Background: Endoscopic transcanal approaches to the facial nerve allow excellent exposure of the tympanic facial nerve. This approach becomes limited when access is required to the more proximal geniculate ganglion and labyrinthine portion of the facial nerve. The aim of this report was to determine the feasibility of a transmastoid endoscopically assisted approach to the geniculate ganglion and labyrinthine facial nerve. This is an endoscopic cadaveric dissection and video review at a university anatomical laboratory.

Methods: A total of 12 endoscopic cadaveric dissections were performed. A cortical mastoidectomy and perilabyrinthine air cell removal was performed using an operating microscope. Beyond this, dissection was performed with an endoscope.

Results: In all dissections, an endoscopically assisted transmastoid approach allowed complete access to the geniculate ganglion, and at least 1.5 mm of the distal labyrinthine facial nerve. Further transcrusal drilling through the anterior crus of the superior semicircular canal allowed access to the entire labyrinthine facial nerve.

Conclusions: The entire geniculate ganglion and labyrinthine facial nerve is difficult to access with microscopic techniques. Adding endoscopic visualization allows for complete visualization of the geniculate ganglion. Clinical reports will further strengthen these preliminary cadaveric results.

Keywords: Surgical Procedure, Endoscopic, Geniculate Ganglion, Decompression, Surgical, Facial Nerve, Semicircular Canals

Background

The geniculate ganglion and labyrinthine segment of the facial nerve are of importance as they are challenging to access surgically and can be affected by disease. The most common pathologies affecting this region of the facial nerve include inflammation, traumatic injury, cholesteatoma and neoplasms.

This area can be accessed by both the middle fossa and transmastoid approach, each with their own limitations. The transmastoid approach obviates the need for a craniotomy, but is difficult in a poorly pneumatised

temporal bone and has been shown able to access the entire labyrinthine segment of the facial nerve in only 60% of patients, mainly through the superior semicircular canal [1].

Although the middle fossa approach offers an alternative, the scarce anatomical landmarks on the floor of the middle cranial fossa can lead to disorientation. Additionally, the inherent craniotomy and temporal lobe retraction to permit an adequate view risks sensorineural and conductive hearing loss, intracranial bleeding, cerebrospinal fluid (CSF) leak and seizures. In addition, in the acute trauma situation, the middle fossa approach may be contra-indicated, if there is concomitant brain injury.

Endoscopic transcanal approaches to the facial nerve provides the most direct approach with minimal bone removal needed allow excellent exposure of the tympanic facial nerve, tympanic portion of the geniculate ganglion

* Correspondence: drnicholasjufas@gmail.com
[1]Division of Otolaryngology – Head and Neck Surgery, Dalhousie University, 3rd Floor Dickson Building, VG Site, QE II Health Sciences Centre, 5820 University Ave, Halifax, NS B3H 2Y9, Canada
[2]Kolling Deafness Research Centre, University of Sydney and Macquarie University, Sydney, Australia
Full list of author information is available at the end of the article

and greater superficial petrosal nerve. However the transcanal approach is limited anteriorly by the anterior canal wall and limitation would be expected in visualizing the labyrinthine portion of the geniculate ganglion and the labyrinthine facial nerve. The additional anterior exposure afforded by an extended epitympanotomy may be useful to access these structures. Although an endoscopic transcanal suprageniculate corridor has been recently described, the extent of labyrinthine facial nerve exposure was not quantified [2, 3].

The primary aim of this report was to determine the feasibility of a transmastoid endoscopically assisted approach to the geniculate ganglion and labyrinthine facial nerve. In particular, we wished to evaluate how much of the labyrinthine segment could be visualized without violating the superior semicircular canal. The secondary aim was to analyse the relationship of the geniculate ganglion to the cochleariform process.

Methods

Approval was obtained under institutional anatomical licencing for cadaveric research for medical and scientific purposes. Six human fresh-frozen cadaveric heads were obtained from an in-house human body donation program. The cadavers had no history of ear surgery, ear disease or trauma.

Using microscopic visualization, a wide post-auricular incision was performed and soft tissues elevated. An extensive cortical mastoidectomy was performed, outlining the otic capsule and exposing the epitympanic portion of the malleus and incus.

Zero, 30 and 45 degree, 3 mm diameter, 14 cm endoscopes, with a SPIES H3-Z three-chip full High Definition (HD) camera, Image1 Connect Processing Module and full HD monitor (Karl Storz Gmbh & Co. KG, Tuttlingen, Germany) were used for visualization. The incudostapedial joint was divided, malleus nipped at the neck and tensor tympani divided. The incus and head of the malleus were removed.

Bony removal of the superior aspect of the facial nerve canal above the cochleariform process was then performed using a 2 mm curved diamond burr (Medtronic Inc., Fridley, MN, USA). The epineurium of the facial nerve was exposed proximally along its course to include the entire first genu. Drilling then proceeded proximally along the labyrinthine segment of the facial nerve. Initially the superior semicircular canal was blue-lined but not entered to the maximum extent possible (Fig. 1).

Further drilling occurred after breaching the anterior crus of the superior semicircular canal in order to attempt to expose the entire labyrinthine portion of the facial nerve via a transcrusal approach. This necessitated, in all cases, a transcrusal approach through the anterior crus of the superior semicircular canal. Exposure along

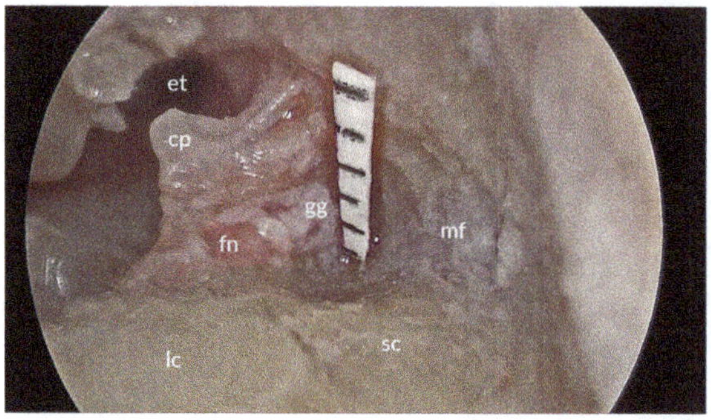

Fig. 1 Endoscopic view of specimen (*right ear*), with view of tympanic and labyrinthine facial nerve and geniculate ganglion. Measurement is taken of exposed labyrinthine facial nerve after blue-lining of and prior to entry into the superior semicircular canal. et, Eustachian tube; cp, cochleariform process; fn, facial nerve; gg, geniculate ganglion; lc, lateral semicircular canal; sc, superior semicircular canal; mf, middle cranial fossa dura

the entire segment was confirmed by noting the dilation of the facial canal as the meatal segment is entered (Fig. 2).

The following aspects of the dissection were noted and measurements taken using a surgical ruler (DeRoyal Industries Inc., Powell, TN, USA) that had been cut into appropriate strips to the nearest 0.25 mm. Two measurements were taken for each, and the results averaged:

- The length of the precochleariform segment, defined as refers to the portion of the tympanic facial nerve lying superiorly and anteriorly to the posterior bony limit of the cochleariform process [3].
- The amount of the geniculate ganglion and length of labyrinthine segment of the facial nerve that could be exposed without breaching the semicircular canals.
- The subsequent length of labyrinthine segment of facial nerve that could be exposed once the superior semicircular canal was breached.

Results

In all 12 ears dissected, the use of angled endoscopes assisted in increasing the proportion of the geniculate ganglion and labyrinthine segment of the facial nerve that could be seen without breaching the superior semicircular canal.

In all specimens, the geniculate ganglion was able to be fully exposed on its superior aspect, without breaching the superior semicircular canal. The dura of the floor of the middle cranial fossa approached the geniculate ganglion, but in most cases, a thin bony covering was able to be maintained over the dura. Dissection further forward to expose the greater superficial petrosal nerve would have required complete removal of bone and elevation of dura and this was not performed in this study.

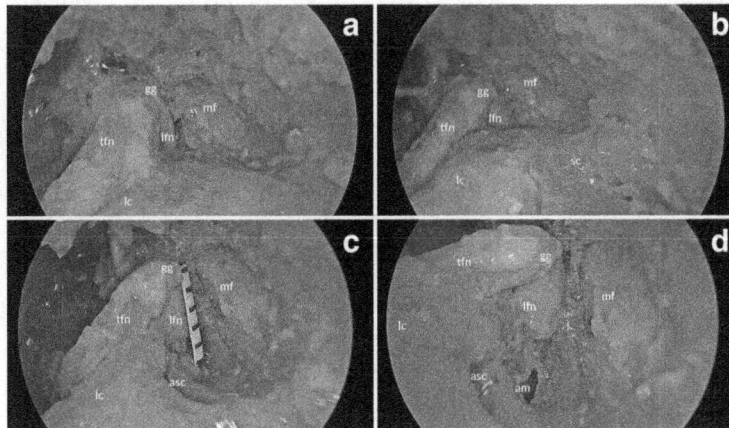

Fig. 2 Sequential endoscopic views (**a-d**) of specimen (*right ear*), showing progress after displaying air cells, a bony spicule and a protympanic spine in the protympanum. tfn, tympanic facial nerve; gg, geniculate ganglion; lfn, labyrinthine facial nerve; lc, lateral semicircular canal; asc, ampulla of superior semicircular canal; mf, middle cranial fossa dura; am, internal auditory meatus

In all specimens, the precochleariform segment was measured from the anterior bony limit of the cochleariform process, anteriorly as far forward as possible along the tympanic portion of the facial nerve on its superolateral aspect. The mean precochleariform segment length was 4.52 mm (range 3.75-5.25 mm; standard deviation (SD) 0.47 mm).

Under endoscopic visualisation, and with bluelining the superior semicircular canal to the maximum extent possible, the mean length of the distal labyrinthine segment of facial nerve visible without breaching the superior semicircular canal was 2.39 mm (range 1.88-2.75 mm; SD 0.30 mm).

After exposing the entire labyrinthine segment of the facial nerve to the fundus of the meatal segment via a transcrusal approach and breaching the anterior crus of the superior semicircular canal, the mean length of the entire labyrtinthine segment of facial nerve visible was 4.30 mm (range 3.63-4.75 mm; SD 0.37 mm).

Discussion

This study has demonstrated that an endoscopically assisted transmastoid approach to the geniculate ganglion and labyrinthine facial nerve is feasible in a cadaver model and defined the limits of accessing the labyrinthine facial nerve with and without transcrusal breach. Exposure of the entire labyrinthine segment requires a transcrusal approach through the superior semicircular canal, whereas just over half of the labyrinthine facial nerve can be exposed without transgression of the labyrinth. This approach may be helpful in treating pathology of this region of the facial nerve, while reducing the risk of complications from more invasive surgery.

Traditional approaches to the geniculate ganglion have either used a transmastoid, middle cranial fossa or a combination of these approaches [4]. Although the middle fossa approach has unique risks and challenges that were discussed earlier, it gives the best chance of hearing preservation as it is the only approach that doesn't disturb the ossicular chain.

Endoscopes are being increasingly used in otology, with significantly more visualization of every subregion of the middle ear when compared with the microscope [5]. Although endoscopic transcanal approaches afford good exposure of the lateral aspect of the geniculate ganglion and greater superficial petrosal nerve [2], they do not adequately access the more medial aspect of the geniculate ganglion and labyrinthine segment of facial nerve without significant breach of the inner ear, where hearing loss would be expected. In cases where there is significant pre-operative hearing loss, a transcanal transpromontorial approach would certainly afford more direct access.

The labyrinthine facial nerve and geniculate ganglion are often involved in facial nerve pathology, in particular idiopathic inflammatory diseases such as Bell's palsy [6] and trauma [7], and could be addressed in surgical decompression. The reasoning for this is likely due to the anatomical dimensions of the labyrinthine segment, being the narrowest section of the bony facial nerve canal [8].

It has been demonstrated in this study that it is possible to expose the entire superior aspect of the geniculate ganglion and an average of 2.39 mm of the distal labyrinthine facial nerve, which is over 50% of the entire segmental length, without breaching the labyrinth. We found it necessary to remove the incus and head of malleus, as would be the case in all transcanal and transmastoid approaches. This would need reconstruction with an OCR or a bone anchored hearing aid to bypass the conductive hearing loss.

Although it has been demonstrated to be possible to provide access to the geniculate ganglion without ossicular disruption in a minority of cases, particularly in a very well pneumatised mastoid [4], the experience of this study suggested it would be prudent to pre-emptively disarticulate the ossicles to ensure protection against drill trauma while attempting to expose the labyrinthine facial nerve.

Avoiding the need for a craniotomy inherent in the middle fossa approach is important as this also avoids a number of significant risks and potential complications. Additionally, preservation of the labyrinth by not utilising translabyrinthine or transcochlear approaches implies that there is not necessarily a certain auditory and vestibular loss on the operated side post operatively. Although this approach has been previously demonstrated microscopically [4], our experience using both methods of visualisation in this study was that that the endoscope was invaluable in ensuring that the superior semicircular canal was not inadvertently entered and that the visualised portion of the distal labyrinthine facial nerve was maximised.

This study demonstrated that it is possible to visualise the entire labyrinthine segment of the facial nerve via a transmastoid approach, without a full translabyrinthine drillout. Removing the anterior crus of the superior semicircular canal allowed access to the whole labyrinthine segment. A mean length of 4.30 mm was found across all specimens, which certainly encompasses the well reported length of the segment at 4 mm [8, 9]. Additional confirmation that the meatal segment of the facial nerve had been reached by noting a widening of the bony canal. As previously noted, this necessitated entering and drilling through the superior semicircular canal. A more extensive variation of this has been previously used for access to the petroclival region and petrous apex, where the posterior and superior semicircular canals are carefully plugged at their ampullated ends and common crus, and subsequently drilled through. Obliteration of the canals begins away from the ampullated end and proceeds with a leading edge maintaining a seal with a combination of either bone dust, bone wax and/ or fibrin sealant. Preservation of serviceable hearing was possible in at least 58% of patients across published studies [10–12]. It is encouraging that even if complete exposure of the labyrinthine segment is required via a transcrusal approach, it may be possible to preserve sensorineural hearing.

The canal wall is typically taken down in transmastoid approaches to the geniculate ganglion, to aid microscopic visualisation. Benefits of preserving the canal wall, as we have been able to do in our study include a greater ease of placing and securing an ossicular reconstructive prosthesis primarily, greater success in fitting hearing aids in the canal and obviating the need for a meatoplasty.

These advantages are minor however and ultimately the decision on whether to take the canal wall down in a transmastoid approach would come down to surgeon experience and preference. If a labyrinthine breach will likely occur either way, then it is arguable whether the more minimal transcrusal approach through the anterior crus of the superior semicircular canal describe herein would provide much advantage. Clinical reports comparing this technique to existing approaches will be needed to clarify this. Nevertheless this paper has been able to define and measure the limits of exposure possible in this novel endoscopically assisted approach.

A final aspect that we wanted to address in this study was the anatomical relationship between the geniculate ganglion and the cochleariform process. There occasionally appears to be a misconception that the geniculate ganglion is superior or immediately anterosuperior to the cochleariform process [13]. This study has shown that while the tympanic segment of the facial nerve is superior, the geniculate ganglion lies on average 4.52 mm, and to a maximum of 5.25 mm more anterior. Although our study had a small sample size of 6 cadavers, this correlates with previous anatomical studies using alternate approaches that have shown a similar result [9, 14].

Conclusion

The entire geniculate ganglion and labyrinthine facial nerve can be visualised utilising a transmastoid approach with endoscopic assistance. In order to expose the entire labyrinthine facial nerve, a transcrusal approach through the superior semicircular canal is necessary. Exposure of slightly more than the distal half of the labyrinthine segment is possible without transgressing the labyrinth. Clinical reports utilising this technique will verify the preliminary findings and hypotheses of this cadaveric study.

Abbreviations
CSF: Cerebrospinal fluid; HD: High definition; SD: Standard deviation

Acknowledgements
The authors would like to acknowledge Karl Storz Gmbh & Co. (Tüttlingen, Germany) for loan of endoscopic equipment for the duration of the study.

Funding
None

Disclosures
Endoscopic equipment described in the study, loaned for the duration of the study by Karl Storz Gmbh.

Authors' contributions
NJ: Study concept and design, cadaveric dissection, data acquisition, data analysis and interpretation, manuscript preparation and revision. MB: Study concept and design, cadaveric dissection, data acquisition, data analysis and

interpretation, manuscript preparation and revision. All authors have read and approve of this manuscript for publication.

Competing interests

The authors declare that they have no competing interests.

Author details

¹Division of Otolaryngology – Head and Neck Surgery, Dalhousie University, 3rd Floor Dickson Building, VG Site, QE II Health Sciences Centre, 5820 University Ave, Halifax, NS B3H 2Y9, Canada. ²Kolling Deafness Research Centre, University of Sydney and Macquarie University, Sydney, Australia. ³Sydney Endoscopic Ear Surgery (SEES) Research Group, Sydney, Australia.

References

1. Bento RF, de Brito RV, Sanchez TG. A rapid and safe middle fossa approach to the geniculate ganglion and labyrinthine segment of the facial nerve. Ear Nose Throat J. 2002;81(5):320–6.
2. Marchioni D, Alicandri-Ciufelli M, Rubini A, Presutti L. Endoscopic transcanal corridors to the lateral skull base: initial experiences. Laryngoscope. 2015; 125(Suppl 5):S1–13.
3. Marchioni D, Alicandri-Ciufelli M, Piccinini A, Genovese E, Monzani D, Tarabichi M, et al. Surgical anatomy of transcanal endoscopic approach to the tympanic facial nerve. Laryngoscope. 2011;121(7):1565–73.
4. Yi H, Liu P, Yang S. Geniculate ganglion decompression of facial nerve by transmastoid-epitympanum approach. Acta Otolaryngol (Stockh). 2013; 133(6):656–61.
5. Bennett ML, Zhang D, Labadie RF, Noble JH. Comparison of middle ear visualization with endoscopy and microscopy. Otol Neurotol. 2016;37(4):1–366.
6. Fisch U, Esslen E. Total intratemporal exposure of the facial nerve: pathologic findings in Bell's palsy. Arch Otolaryngol Head Neck Surg. 1972;95(4):335–41.
7. Felix H, Eby TL, Fisch U. New aspects of facial nerve pathology in temporal bone fractures. Acta Otolaryngol (Stockh). 1991;111(2):332–6.
8. Gupta S, Mends F, Hagiwara M, Fatterpekar G, Roehm PC. Imaging the facial nerve: a contemporary review. Radiol Res Pract. 2013;2013(3):248039–14.
9. Lee HK, Lee EH, Lee WS, Kim WS. Microsurgical anatomy of the perigeniculate ganglion area as seen from a translabyrinthine approach. Ann Otol Rhinol Laryngol. 2000;109(3):255–7.
10. Brandt MG, Poirier J, Hughes B, Lownie SP, Parnes LS. The transcrusal approach: a 10-year experience at one Canadian center. Neurosurgery. 2010;66(5):1017–22.
11. Horgan MA, Delashaw JB, Schwartz MS, Kellogg JX, Spektor S, McMenomey SO. Transcrusal approach to the petroclival region with hearing preservation. J Neurosurg. 2001;94(4):660–6.
12. Kaylie DM, Horgan MA, Delashaw JB, McMenomey SO. Hearing preservation with the transcrusal approach to the petroclival region. Otol Neurotol. 2004;25(4):594–8.
13. Goycoolea MV. Atlas of otologic surgery and magic otology. London: JP Medical Ltd; 2012. p. 802.
14. Goin DW. Proximal intratemporal facial nerve in bell's palsy surgery. A study correlating anatomical and surgical findings. Laryngoscope. 1982;92(3):263–72. John Wiley & Sons, Inc

5

Intraoperative Brief Electrical Stimulation of the Spinal Accessory Nerve (BEST SPIN) for prevention of shoulder dysfunction after oncologic neck dissection: a double-blinded, randomized controlled trial

Brittany Barber[1], Hadi Seikaly[1], K. Ming Chan[2†], Rhys Beaudry[3], Shannon Rychlik[1], Jaret Olson[4], Matthew Curran[4], Peter Dziegielewski[5], Vincent Biron[1], Jeffrey Harris[1], Margaret McNeely[6†] and Daniel O'Connell[1*]

Abstract

Background: Shoulder dysfunction is common after neck dissection for head and neck cancer (HNC). Brief electrical stimulation (BES) is a novel technique that has been shown to enhance neuronal regeneration after nerve injury by modulating the brain-derived neurotrophic growth factor (BDNF) pathways. The objective of this study was to evaluate the effect of BES on postoperative shoulder function following oncologic neck dissection.

Methods: Adult participants with a new diagnosis of HNC undergoing Level IIb +/− V neck dissection were recruited. Those in the treatment group received intraoperative BES applied to the spinal accessory nerve (SAN) after completion of neck dissection for 60 min of continuous 20 Hz stimulation at 3-5 V of 0.1 msec balanced biphasic pulses, while those in the control group received no stimulation (NS). The primary outcome measured was the Constant-Murley Shoulder (CMS) Score, comparing changes from baseline to 12 months post-neck dissection. Secondary outcomes included the change in the Neck Dissection Impairment Index (ΔNDII) score and the change in compound muscle action potential amplitude (ΔCMAP) over the same period.

Results: Fifty-four patients were randomized to the treatment or control group with a 1:1 allocation scheme. No differences in demographics, tumor characteristics, or neck dissection types were found between groups. Significantly lower ΔCMS scores were observed in the BES group at 12 months, indicating better preservation of shoulder function ($p = 0.007$). Only four in the BES group compared to 17 patients in the NS groups saw decreases greater than the minimally important clinical difference (MICD) of the CMS ($p = 0.023$). However, NDII scores ($p = 0.089$) and CMAP amplitudes ($p = 0.067$) between the groups did not reach statistical significance at 12 months. BES participants with Level IIb + V neck dissections had significantly better ΔCMS and ΔCMAP scores at 12 months ($p = 0.048$ and $p = 0.025$, respectively).

Conclusions: Application of BES to the SAN may help reduce impaired shoulder function in patients undergoing oncologic neck dissection, and may be considered a viable adjunct to functional rehabilitation therapies.

(Continued on next page)

* Correspondence: danoconnellmd@gmail.com; dan.oconnell@ualberta.ca
†Equal contributors
[1]Division of Otolaryngology-Head & Neck Surgery, University of Alberta, Edmonton, Canada
Full list of author information is available at the end of the article

(Continued from previous page)

Trial registration: Clinicaltrials.gov (NCT02268344, October 17, 2014).

Keywords: Neck dissection, Electrical stimulation, Head neck cancer, Nerve regeneration, Axonal regeneration, Spinal accessory nerve

Background

Head and neck cancer (HNC) commonly presents in the third and fourth decade of life. Treatment choices in this cancer patient population should consider the potential for many remaining working years [1, 2]. Survivorship, quality of life (QOL), and the goal of returning to life before cancer, have become a major focus in the care of the modern HNC patient.

Advanced HNC may be treated with primary surgical resection including Level IIB with or without Level V neck dissection [3]. Retraction and manipulation of the spinal accessory nerve (SAN) is necessary to access Levels IIb and V [4]. Furthermore, the superior 5 cm of the SAN is often completely devascularized in a Level IIb dissection in order to skeletonize all lymphatic tissues off the nerve [5]. Devascularization and retraction of the SAN can result in axonal injury, which can give rise to shoulder pain and dysfunction postoperatively, even in nerve-sparing procedures [6]. Shoulder pain and dysfunction from SAN injury has pronounced and well-documented negative effects on quality of life [7]. Furthermore, as the majority of HNC patients are still of working age, the potential ramifications of shoulder dysfunction may also result in longstanding socioeconomic consequences [8].

Over the past two decades, it has been demonstrated in both animal models and clinical trials that application of intraoperative brief electrical stimulation (BES) to transected motor and sensory nerves promotes axonal outgrowth and, thereby, enhances reinnervation [9]. In studies of motor nerve regeneration, 60 min of BES applied to the nerve at 20 Hz was shown to be as effective as continuous stimulation for 2 weeks, suggesting that BES should be a clinically viable technique [9].

The aim of this study was to assess the efficacy of BES in reducing postoperative shoulder dysfunction in HNC patients undergoing oncologic Level IIb +/− Level V neck dissection. This is the first randomized controlled trial to examine the effects of an intraoperative intervention of SAN and shoulder function.

Methods

Study design

The BEST SPIN trial was a randomized, double-blind placebo-controlled trial at the University of Alberta, a single tertiary care cancer center in Edmonton, Canada. Patients were recruited after referral for primary surgical treatment for head and neck cancer. Institutional ethical approval was obtained from the Human Research Ethics Board (HREB) (Pro00046671) at the University of Alberta. The trial was registered on Clinicaltrials.gov (NCT02268344, October 17, 2014).

Participants

Participants were identified for eligibility from the Northern Alberta Head and Neck Tumor Board (NAHNTB). NAHNTB is a multidisciplinary group at the University of Alberta that reviews diagnosis and treatment recommendations for all patients treated for HNC within the catchment area of central and northern Alberta, as well as Northern British Columbia and Saskatchewan. Eligible patients were those aged >18 years with a new diagnosis of HNC undergoing oncologic neck dissection including Level IIb. Patients were excluded if they had intraoperative resection of the sternocleidomastoid or trapezius muscle or SAN, previous head and neck surgery or radiation therapy to the neck, pre-existing shoulder dysfunction, an implanted electrical device (eg. pacemaker), or pre-existing neurological or neuromuscular disease. Patients were also ineligible if they required a pectoralis major, latissimus, or scapular flap for reconstruction. Recruitment was undertaken in the University of Alberta Head and Neck Clinic during preoperative surgical education sessions. Informed written consent was obtained from each participant prior to enrolment in the study.

Randomisation and blinding

Eligible participants were block-randomised (1:1) in groups of six to receive: 1) BES, or 2) No Stimulation (NS), on the day of surgery after initiation of general anesthesia. If bilateral oncologic neck dissection including Level IIb was planned, the neck with the most extensive nodal burden was selected for randomisation. This was determined on the basis of preoperative imaging and physical exam findings prior to randomisation. Allocation concealment was by selection from shuffled sealed opaque envelopes. Patients were enrolled by the primary author (BB) according to eligibility criteria, randomisation was performed by the clinical nurse specialist (SR), and intraoperative interventions were performed by BB who was not involved in any of the outcome assessments. SR had no further involvement in the trial. Study participants and response assessors were masked to treatment allocation, and no external cutaneous markings were evident to indicate allocated treatment.

Procedures

Specific parameters of the BES procedure are detailed in Box 1. All patients received therapeutic Level IIb neck dissection. If palpable lymphadenopathy was noted intra-operatively, a frozen pathologic section was submitted for examination. If the lymph node was found to be positive for malignancy, Level V neck dissection was performed. Medtronic NIM® 3.0 ™ 18 mm electrodes, placed intramuscularly on the motor point of the trapezius muscle, were used to monitor electromyographic changes in the muscle before and after neck dissection to determine if a significant injury resulted from the neck dissection. A significant injury was defined as a > 10% decrease in maximum CMAP amplitude (mV) from baseline readings performed upon first identification of the SAN intraoperatively.

Participants randomized to the NS group received no stimulation, and standard skin closure techniques were applied. For participants in the BES group, once neck dissection was complete (Fig. 1a), a 2.0 mm NIM® 3.0 automated periodic stimulation (APS) electrode cuff (Medtronic ENT, Canada) was encircled around the SAN at the proximal aspect of SAN dissection (Fig. 1b). The APS electrode was then connected to a Grass SD9 Stimulator (Grass Technologies, Quincy, MA), and the SAN was stimulated continuously at 20 Hz utilizing 0.1 msec pulses at intensities of 3–5 V for 60 min (Fig. 1c). Voltage was titrated to palpable tetanic trapezius contraction to ensure adequate stimulation. The NIM 3.0 monitoring system allowed for continued ancillary assurance of adequate stimulation. After 60 min of continuous stimulation, the APS electrode was removed and disposed of, and standard skin closure techniques were applied. During this time, other portions of the surgery were conducted. In order to ensure adequate stimulation during this time, the NIM 3.0 monitoring system was monitored, and an alert was provided if stimulation was ceased for any reason.

Prior to surgery, participants underwent baseline evaluation by a blinded physiotherapist using the Constant-Murley Score (CMS), a validated, 100-point clinical assessment scale utilizing both objective and subjective measures of shoulder function, including pain, activities of daily living (ADLs), range of motion, and strength [10, 11]. The minimally important clinical difference (MICD) for the CMS has been previously established as 10.4 points, with a standard deviation of 11 points [12–15]. This was chosen as the primary outcome due to the number of neck dissection studies previously utilizing this assessment tool, and the fact that, as the

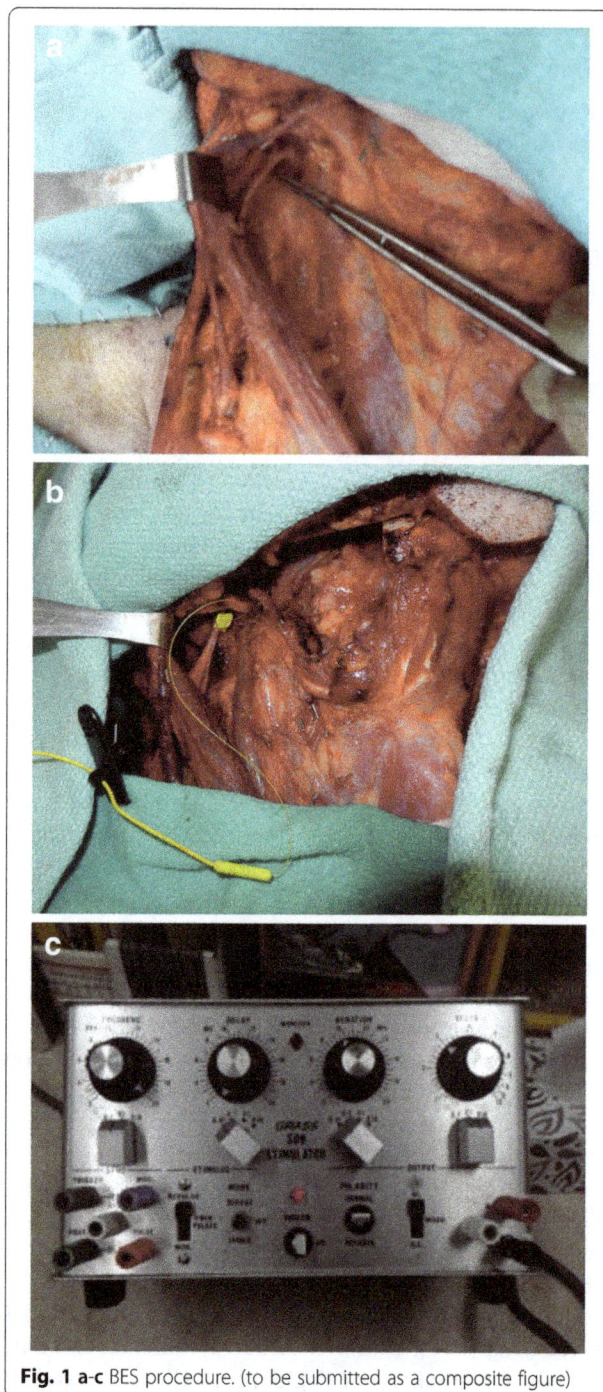

Fig. 1 a-c BES procedure. (to be submitted as a composite figure)

BES technique is thought to affect neuromuscular function, a functional assessment tool would be needed to evaluate this.

The participants were also evaluated with the Neck Dissection Impairment Index (NDII), a validated, 10-item, self-report questionnaire assessing neck dissection-related quality of life including evaluations of recreational, social, and self-care activities [15]. The MICD for the NDII has been previously established as 18.1

from local actuarial data [16]. Lastly, an objective evaluation of baseline SAN function was conducted using an electrophysiological measurement of maximum CMAP by an experienced, blinded neurophysiologist. Follow-up assessments of all outcomes were completed at 6 and 12 months. Twelve months was chosen as the primary endpoint follow-up measure, due to the length of the SAN, the time required for axonal regeneration along the length of this nerve, and the propensity for weakness following adjuvant treatments that may persist up to 1 year.

Outcomes

The primary endpoint was the change in participant CMS score (ΔCMS) from baseline to 12 months after surgical treatment of the randomised shoulder. The number of participants in each group whose score decreased by greater than the MICD of the CMS was also evaluated.

Secondary endpoints included the change in participant NDII score (ΔNDII) and the change in maximum CMAP from baseline to 12 months after surgical treatment for the randomised shoulder. Adverse events (AEs) were monitored by an external Data Safety Monitoring Board (DSMB), who examined independent reports from the theatre nurse and anesthetist present on the day of the surgery. AEs were defined as any arrhythmias occurring after onset of applied BES to the SAN.

Statistical analysis

The study was designed as a superiority study. A sample size of 21 participants in each group was sufficient to detect a difference between the BES and NS groups of 10.4 points, which represents the MICD of the primary outcome, the CMS (power of 80%; significance 5%). To compensate for a potential attrition rate of 30%, the sample size was increased to 27 per group.

Baseline demographic characteristics, tumor features, and neck dissections (Level II vs Levell IIb + V) for the two groups were compared using a Mann-Whitney U-test for continuous data and Chi-square tests for categorical data. The primary and secondary outcomes were compared between the BES and NS groups using a Mann-Whitney U-test analysis. Intention-to-treat and per-protocol analyses were undertaken. The primary outcome was also dichotomized into a ΔCMS above or below the MICD (10.4 points) at the primary endpoint of 12 months. The DSMB reviewed safety data every 6 months. Statistical analysis was performed using SPSS (Version 21.0).

The number needed to treat (NNT) was also calculated. This was performed using the number of patients whose score decreased by more than the MICD to indicate shoulder dysfunction in the NS group as the control

event rate (CER) and the number of patients whose score decreased by more than the MICD in the BES group as the experimental event rate (EER).

Role of the funding source

Funding for the study was provided by the University Hospital Foundation (UHF) Medical Research Grant Competition, a regional peer-reviewed process at the University of Alberta. The funder of the study had no role in study design, data collection, data analysis, data interpretation, or writing of the report. The corresponding author had full access to all the data in the study and had final responsibility for the decision to submit for publication.

Results

Between October 6, 2014 and June 6, 2015, 68 participants were assessed for inclusion in the trial. Ten patients were not eligible due to the presence of exclusion criteria, and four patients refused participation in the trial. The remaining 54 participants were deemed eligible for the study. The median age of all participants was 60.1 years. A CONSORT diagram detailing enrolment is depicted in Fig. 2.

Mean follow-up was 257.7 days (95% CI 222.8 to 292.6, range = 0.0 to 363.0 days, σ = 131.0 days) for all patients, 254.7 (95% CI 207.2 to 302.2, range = 0.0 to 361.0 days, σ = 138.6) for the BES group and 260.5 days (95% CI 208.2 to 312.8, range 0.0 to 361.0 days, σ = 126.1) for the NS group. The most common primary tumor sites were oral cavity (33.3%) and oropharynx (24.1%). Forty-two patients (77.8%) had radiotherapy (37.0% in the BES group, 40.7% in the NS group). Fifteen patients (27.8%) had chemotherapy (18.5% in the BES group, 9.3% in the NS group) (Table 1). None of the patients required pectoralis major, latissimus flaps for wound breakdown.

All 54 patients demonstrated a maximum CMAP decrease >10% to indicate SAN injury and eligibility for intervention. Nine and seven participants were unavailable for final analysis in the BES and NS groups, respectively, at 12 months (Fig. 2). Six-month test values were carried forward to maintain the integrity of the intention-to-treat analysis. The per-protocol analysis was undertaken using only 12-month test values. The remaining 18 and 20 participants were analyzed in the BES and NS groups, respectively. A post-hoc power calculation revealed that, with the final sample size, study power was calculated to be 99.7%.

Demographic factors, including both patient and tumor characteristics, were assessed for the entire cohort and each group separately. In 90.9% of cases, randomised patients underwent major ablative and reconstructive surgery including free tissue transfer. No differences in age, gender, TNM staging, tumor site, or

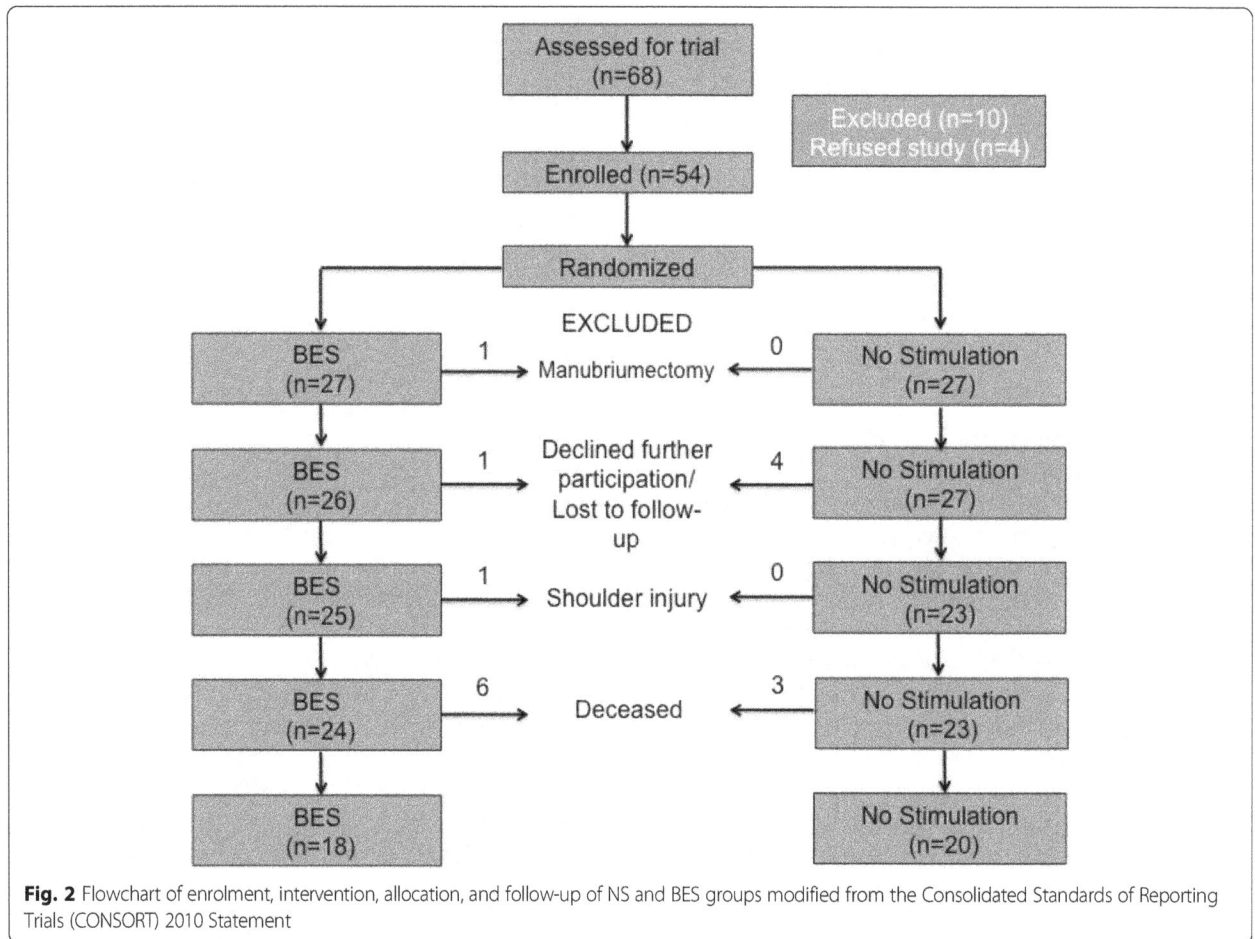

Fig. 2 Flowchart of enrolment, intervention, allocation, and follow-up of NS and BES groups modified from the Consolidated Standards of Reporting Trials (CONSORT) 2010 Statement

Charlson Comorbidity Index (CCI) were observed (Table 1). Prognostic factors known to affect shoulder function were also evaluated between groups, and no significant difference was detected between them (Table 2). There were no significant differences between groups regarding the number of Level IIb + V neck dissections ($p = 0.607$), or the extent of surgery indicated by the number of nodes extirpated ($p = 0.781$) (Table 3).

In the intention-to-treat analysis, mean ΔCMS results 12 months post-neck dissection were −6.82 (95% CI −9.47 to −4.17, σ = 7.02, SE = 1.70) and −25.13 (95% CI −32.73 to −17.53, σ = 20.15. SE = 5.04) points for the BES and NS groups, respectively (Fig. 3). Mann-Whitney U-test demonstrated a significantly higher CMS score in the BES group at 12 months indicating significantly better preservation of shoulder function compared to the NS group ($p = 0.007$) (Fig. 3). Six (BES) and 17 (NS) patients demonstrated a decline in CMS score greater than the MICD. This difference indicates clinically relevant shoulder dysfunction in significantly fewer patients in the BES group ($p = 0.023$) (Fig. 4). The NNT for using BES for preservation of shoulder function after oncologic neck dissection was therefore calculated as 1 patient for

every 2.6 patients treated with BES. In the per-protocol analysis, mean ΔCMS scores were found to be −7.25 (95% CI −9.90 to −4.60, σ = 7.03) and −24.71 (95% CI −32.14 to −17.28, σ = 19.71) for the BES and NS groups, respectively, 12 months post-neck dissection ($p = 0.012$) indicating significantly improved preservation of clinical shoulder function in the BES group ($p = 0.012$).

The mean ΔNDII scores were found to be −10.91 (95% CI −16.72 to −5.10, σ = 15.40) and −24.81 (95% CI −33.50 to −16.12, σ = 23.05) points for the BES and NS groups 12 months post-neck dissection, respectively ($p = 0.089$) (Fig. 5). Four BES and seven NS patients decreased by more than the MICD of the NDII at 12 months in the BES and NS groups, respectively, indicating reduced neck dissection-related quality of life in more patients in the NS group ($p = 0.114$) (Fig. 6). When examined in the per-protocol analysis, mean ΔNDII scores were found to be −11.29 (95% CI −16.96 to −5.62, σ = 15.00) and −31.25 (95% CI −41.76 to −20.74, σ = 27.85) for the BES and NS groups 12 months post-neck dissection ($p = 0.038$) indicating better shoulder-related quality of life in the BES group.

Table 1 Demographic factors in NS and BES groups

Variable	Entire cohort	NS	BES	P-value
Number	54	27	27	–
Age	57.8	57.9	57.8	0.557
Gender				
Males	44 (81.5%)	21 (38.9%)	23 (42.6%)	0.555
Females	11 (20.4%)	6 (11.1%)	5 (9.3%)	
TNM stage				
Early	9 (16.7%)	5 (9.3%)	4 (7.4%)	0.352
Advanced	46 (85.2%)	22 (40.7%)	24 (44.4%)	
Tumor site				
Oral cavity	18 (33.3%)	10 (18.5%)	8 (14.8%)	0.231
Oropharynx	13 (24.1%)	7 (13.0%)	6 (11.1%)	0.532
Larynx	12 (22.2%)	7 (13.0%)	5 (9.3%)	0.323
Other	12 (22.2%)	7 (13.0%)	5 (9.3%)	0.323
Charlson Comorbidity Index	1.57	1.43	1.63	0.754
Smoking (Pack-years)	17.3	16.4	19.7	0.522
BMI (kg)	3.73	4.68	2.98	0.713
Radiotherapy	42 (77.8%)	22 (40.7%)	20 (37.0%)	0.372
Chemotherapy	15 (27.8%)	5 (9.3%)	10 (18.5%)	0.112

NS no stimulation, *BES* brief electrical stimulation, *BMI* body mass index

The mean ΔCMAPs were found to be −2.25 mA (95% CI −4.02 to −0.48, $\sigma = 4.70$) and −3.83 mA (95% CI −5.28 to −2.38, $\sigma = 3.84$) for the BES and NS groups 12 months post-neck dissection, with three and six of the six-month time-points carried forward in the BES and NS groups, respectively ($p = 0.386$) (Fig. 7). When examined in the per-protocol analysis, the mean ΔNCAs were found to be −1.13 mA (95% CI −2.78 to 0.52, $\sigma = 4.38$) and −4.52 mA (95% CI −5.79 to −3.25, $\sigma = 3.36$) for the BES and NS groups 12 months post-neck dissection ($p = 0.067$) indicating better neurophysiologic preservation of function with BES.

A subgroup analysis of ΔCMS, ΔNDII, and ΔCMAP results was undertaken in patients with Level IIb + V neck dissection (Table 3). The mean ΔCMS and ΔCMAP results were significantly higher in the BES group at 12 months ($p = 0.048$ and $p = 0.025$, respectively). No significant difference was observed in ΔNDII between groups at 12 months ($p = 0.097$).

No adverse events were observed as a result of the BES intervention. Two participants died in hospital following surgery from airway obstruction and myocardial infarction. One participant sustained a shoulder injury after an out-of-hospital fall, and one patient required a manubriumectomy for a laryngeal cancer related stomal recurrence. Six patients declined further participation or were lost to follow-up after multiple attempts to contact by the office of the surgeon and research coordinator. Nine patients were deceased at the time of final analysis.

Discussion

The primary objective of this study was to evaluate the effect of intraoperative BES on SAN recovery following traction, compression, and devascularization injury during oncologic neck dissection. Our study demonstrated that BES was effective in reducing clinically significant shoulder dysfunction and optimizing neck dissection in patients undergoing oncologic neck dissection, specifically in those undergoing Level IIb + V neck dissection. The participants who received BES demonstrated significantly higher CMS scores post-neck dissection compared to controls. At 2.6 participants, the NNT suggests that BES is a highly efficacious treatment. Although the differences in the secondary outcomes measured did not reach statistical significance in the intent-to-treat analysis, the ΔNDII was significantly better in the BES group in the per-protocol analysis, which examined only the 12-month results for the remaining patients. As well, the ΔNDII and ΔCMAP values were congruently, if not statistically, improved in the BES group in the intent-to-treat analysis. The lack of statistical significance in the intent-to-treat analysis may be due in part to the relatively small sample size of the study, and/or to the fact that multiple 6-month values were carried forward to maintain the integrity of the intent-to-treat analysis. The study was powered based on the primary outcome measure. The significant results identified in the subgroup analysis of Level IIb + V neck dissection patients must be considered in the context of a limited sample size.

A significant body of evidence has been put forth regarding the success of BES in promoting regeneration following peripheral nerve injuries. To our knowledge, this is the first study to apply intraoperative BES to the SAN for the purposes of preventing shoulder dysfunction, specifically after oncologic neck dissection, and the first study to demonstrate a successful clinical outcome.

The application of BES to a peripheral nerve following injury was initially performed by Nix and Hopf [17] in the soleus nerve of a rabbit after a crush injury. They subsequently reported accelerated recovery of twitch force, tetanic tension, and muscle action potential in the soleus muscle. Thereafter, application of BES to the sciatic nerve proximal to a crush injury demonstrated significantly improved recovery of the toe-spread reflex [18]. Further studies demonstrated that, following application of BES to the rat femoral nerve after transection injury and primary repair, significantly increased numbers of motoneurons regenerated into the nerve branches of the rat femoral nerve when compared to a non-stimulated sham control group. This acceleration of function recovery was found to be due to accelerated sprouting of axons across the nerve repair site and not due to an accelerated rate of regeneration [19]. Subsequent studies have suggested that brain-derived neurotrophic factor (BDNF), a key molecule in activating cyclic adenomonophosphate (cAMP), and protein kinase A (PKA) which leads to downstream protein transcription necessary for neurite outgrowth, may be mediating the effect of BES in accelerating motoneuron regeneration [20]. A randomized control trial in human participants with carpal tunnel syndrome (CTS) was initiated at the University of Alberta. BES was applied for 60 min to the median nerve following carpal tunnel release and compared to a sham control group regarding both motor and sensory conduction studies. Six months after BES was applied, both the terminal motor latency and sensory nerve conduction values improved significantly faster in BES participants than in controls [21]. Thus, the findings of this study are congruent both intrinsically and extrinsically when compared to existing literature.

The NNT for BES to prevent shoulder dysfunction in 1 patient was calculated to be 2.6. For a prophylactic intervention, a widely accepted NNT is less than

40, as indicated by other well-established therapeutic interventions in medicine [22]. The shoulder morbidity incurred after Level IIB + V neck dissections, even in SAN-sparing procedures, has been well-established [23–25]. As such, controversy regarding de-escalating neck dissection techniques has ensued [26, 27]. Conversely, with the discovery of improved survival in Human Papillomavirus (HPV)-related OPC, a shift toward monotherapy in early-stage disease has been discussed, necessitating a thorough surgical approach to neck dissection in patients treated with primary surgery. Thus, the utility of BES in preventing shoulder dysfunction with a thorough dissection technique may be applicable to a larger patient population. As well, concerns often arise regarding interventions that unnecessarily prolong surgical procedures, however, the convenience of applying BES while performing other steps of major ablative and reconstructive surgeries including free tissue transfer, such as in 90.2% of analyzed cases in this study, does not alter the length of overall surgery and makes it clinically viable in the care of HNC patients.

A limitation of our study was the relatively small sample size given the potential heterogeneity in both patient characteristics and surgical procedures among patients. Examining the number of lymph nodes resected in the NS and BES groups as well as strict exclusion criteria did allow us to examine the utility of BES in the most homogenous group possible. As well, the congruency of the results across all measurements supports the

Table 3 ΔCMS, ΔNDII, and ΔNCS results for Level IIb + V neck dissection patients only

Variable	NS	BES	P-value
ΔCMS	−38.8	−6.0	0.048
ΔNDII	−35.0	−11.7	0.097
ΔNCS	−6.31	1.34	0.025

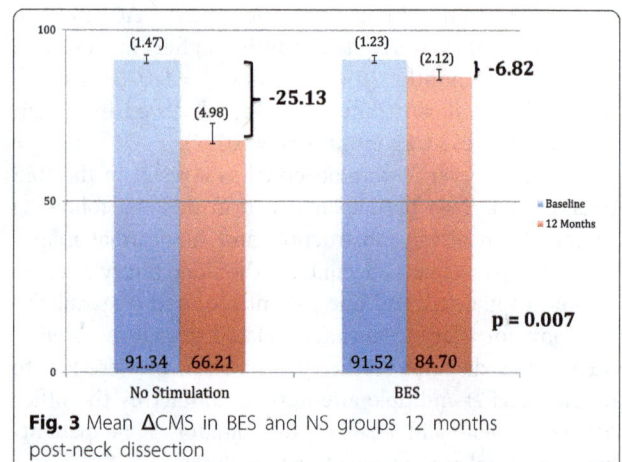

Fig. 3 Mean ΔCMS in BES and NS groups 12 months post-neck dissection

Table 2 Type of neck dissection and extent of surgery in NS and BES groups

Variable	Entire cohort	NS	BES	P-value
N	54	27	27	–
Level IIb only	27 (50.0%)	14 (25.9%)	13 (24.1%)	0.607
Level IIb + Level V	27 (50.0%)	14 (25.9%)	13 (24.1%)	
Nodal yield	32.5	31.3	38.1	0.781

NS no stimulation, *BES* brief electrical stimulation

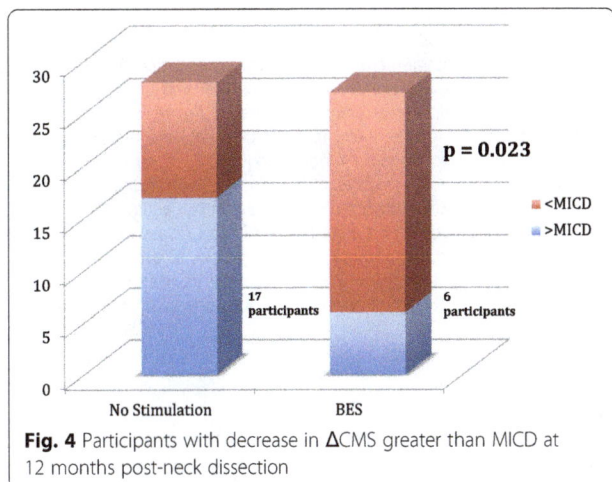

Fig. 4 Participants with decrease in ΔCMS greater than MICD at 12 months post-neck dissection

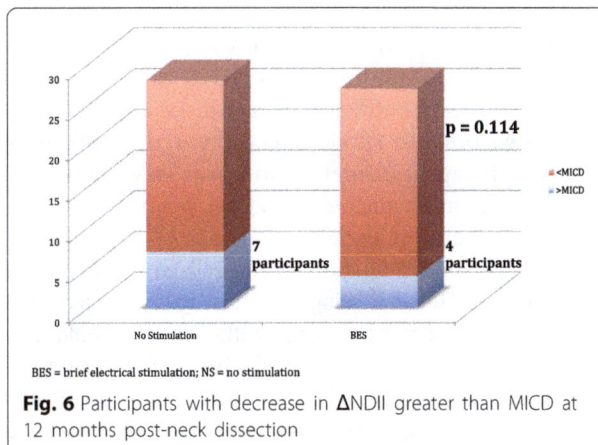

BES = brief electrical stimulation; NS = no stimulation

Fig. 6 Participants with decrease in ΔNDII greater than MICD at 12 months post-neck dissection

significant findings in the study, despite the small sample size. However, determination of the specific effects of BES on subgroup differences, such as those undergoing chemotherapy and/or those sustaining a substantial weight loss, may require a larger sample size. Further studies are needed to target sub-groups undergoing selective or modified radical neck dissection to determine point estimates and measures of variability for the purposes of a larger Phase III study. In addition, the study was powered to detect a minimal important clinically difference (MICD) in the Constant-Murley score of 10.4 points ($\sigma = 11$) based on previous research following post-surgical rotator cuff injuries [12–15, 28, 29]. As the MICD for the Constant-Murley score following neck dissection procedures is currently not known, calculating a neck dissection-specific MICD for the Constant-Murley score is a goal of future studies. A potential confounder in the study is related to pain sustained from operative healing. However, this is unlikely to confound the outcomes, as we anticipate similar levels of pain in both groups. In addition, the intention-to-treat analysis

included six-month values for all outcomes, which are likely to be adversely affected by adjuvant therapies administered within 6 months of the neck dissection. This postulation is supported by the lack of significant outcome findings at 6 months, and subsequent improved clinical shoulder function at 12 months. Lastly, this study was conducted at a single institution. A larger, multi-institutional study will need to be initiated to determine if the effect remains significant.

The clinical impact of this study is multi-dimensional. Previous human trials have demonstrated accelerated axonal regeneration histologically, as well as clinically, in motor and sensory nerves treated with BES after transection or compression injuries. The results shown in this study confirm that BES does have the ability to enhance axonal recovery in a motor nerve (SAN) post-neck dissection. As this study has demonstrated success in improving outcomes after an axonal injury with a devascularization component, BES may enhance regeneration in a more diverse population of peripheral nerve injuries than originally considered. Furthermore and most importantly, as this technique has been shown to be successful in reducing shoulder dysfunction, it

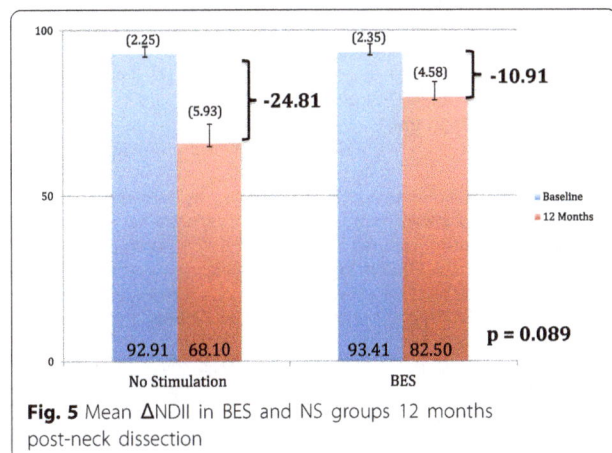

Fig. 5 Mean ΔNDII in BES and NS groups 12 months post-neck dissection

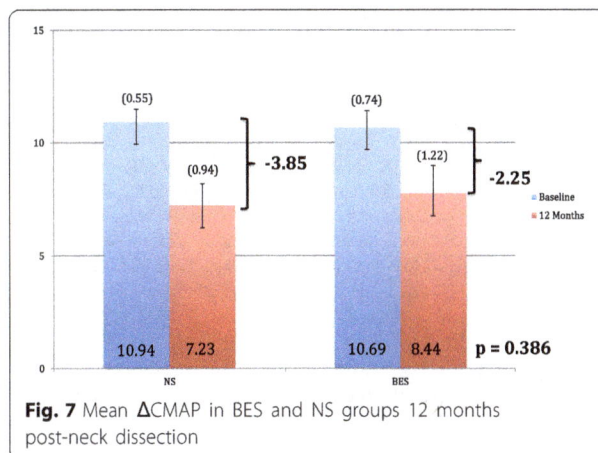

Fig. 7 Mean ΔCMAP in BES and NS groups 12 months post-neck dissection

may provide a useful adjunct to established functional rehabilitation approaches. As lack of treatment compliance with physiotherapy in HNC patients often negatively affects outcomes, a treatment like BES that is initiated prior to surgical recovery and delivered as a single therapeutic intervention may have considerable benefits in an oncologic patient population facing impending adjuvant therapies.

Prior to any consideration of generalized adaptation of intraoperative BES following neck dissection surgery, the reproducibility of these findings within other populations of HNC will need to be confirmed. However, as the equipment necessary to provide BES to the SAN is readily available and inexpensive in comparison to prolonged physiotherapy rehabilitation and/or missed work due to shoulder dysfunction, this can be easily facilitated. Moving forward, multi-institutional studies, cost-effectiveness, and analgesic effects [30] will need to be examined to establish the utility of this technique in preventing shoulder dysfunction in patients undergoing oncologic neck dissections.

Conclusions

Intraoperative BES may reduce shoulder dysfunction in patients undergoing oncologic neck dissection, and can be considered an adjunct to established functional rehabilitation therapies.

Abbreviations
ADL: Activities of daily living; AE: Adverse events; APS: Automated periodic stimulation; BDNF: Brain-derived neurotrophic factor; BES: Brief electrical stimulation; cAMP: Cyclic adenomonophosphate; CCI: Charlson Comorbidity Index; CER: Control event rate; CMAP: Compound muscle action potential; CMS: Constant-Murley Score; CTS: Carpal tunnel syndrome; DSMB: Data safety monitoring board; EER: Experimental event rate; HNC: Head and neck cancer; HPV: Human papillomavirus; HREB: Human research ethics board; MICD: Minimally important clinical difference; NAHNTB: Northern Alberta Head and Neck Tumor Board; NDII: Neck Dissection Impairment Index; NNT: Number needed to treat; NS: No stimulation; PKA: Protein kinase A; QOL: Quality of life; SAN: Spinal accessory nerve; ΔCMAP: Change in compound muscle action potential from baseline to twelve months; ΔCMS: Change in Constant-Murley Score from baseline to twelve months; ΔNDII: Change in Neck Dissection Impairment Index from baseline to twelve months

Acknowledgments
This study was completed as a requirement for the Masters of Surgical Science and Practice (MSc SSP) program at the University of Oxford. The authors would like to acknowledge Dr. Lauren Morgan and Dr. Peter McCulloch for their guidance and tutelage. The authors would also like to acknowledge D.A. O'Connell Professional Corporation and the Alberta Head and Neck Centre for Oncology and Reconstruction (AHNCOR) for their contributions.

Funding
This study was funded by the *University Hospital Foundation Medical Research Grant Competition* at the University of Alberta Hospital.

Authors' contributions
All authors read and approved the final manuscript. KMC assisted with study design, outcomes measurement, and manuscript revision. DAO assisted with study design, ethical approval, funding acquisition and intraoperative procedures, manuscript construction, and manuscript revision. MM assisted with study design, outcomes measurement, and manuscript revision. BB was responsible for funding acquisition, study design, data collection, intraoperative procedures, manuscript construction, and manuscript revision. HS assisted with study design, intraoperative procedures and troubleshooting, data collection, and manuscript revision. JH assisted with intraoperative procedures and manuscript revision. JO assisted with study design and funding acquisition. MC and RB assisted with outcomes measurement and participant scheduling. SR assisted with recruitment and randomization.

Competing interests
DAO is a paid consultant for Medtronic Canada. The other authors declare that they have no competing interests.

Author details
[1]Division of Otolaryngology-Head & Neck Surgery, University of Alberta, Edmonton, Canada. [2]Department of Physical Rehabilitation Medicine, University of Alberta, Edmonton, Canada. [3]Department of Physical Therapy, University of Texas, Arlington, Texas, USA. [4]Division of Plastic Surgery, University of Alberta, Edmonton, Canada. [5]Department of Otolaryngology, University of Florida, Gainesville, FL, USA. [6]Faculty of Rehabilitation Medicine, University of Alberta, Edmonton, Canada.

References
1. Ferreira MB, De Souza JA, Cohen EE. Role of molecular markers in the management of head and neck cancers. Curr Opin Oncol. 2011;23(3):259–64. https://doi.org/10.1097/CCO.0b013e328344f53a.
2. Biron VL, Mohamed A, Hendzel MJ, Alan Underhill D, Seikaly H. Epigenetic differences between human papillomavirus-positive and -negative oropharyngeal squamous cell carcinomas. J Otolaryngol Head Neck Surg. 2012;41(Suppl 1):S65–70.
3. Pfister DG, Ang KK, Brizel DM, Burtness BA, Busse PM, Caudell JJ, et al. Head and neck cancers, version 2.2013. Featured updates to the NCCN guidelines. J Natl Compr Cancer Netw. 2013;11(8):917–23.
4. Umeda M, Shigeta T, Takahashi H, Oguni A, Kataoka T, Minamikawa T, et al. Shoulder mobility after spinal accessory nerve-sparing modified radical neck dissection in oral cancer patients. Oral Surg Oral Med Oral Pathol Oral Radiol Endod. 2010;109(6):820–4. https://doi.org/10.1016/j.tripleo.2009.11.027.
5. Celik B, Coskun H, Kumas FF, Irdesel J, Zarifoglu M, Erisen L, et al. Accessory nerve function after level 2b-preserving selective neck dissection. Head Neck. 2009;31(11):1496–501. https://doi.org/10.1002/hed.21112.
6. van Wilgen CP, Dijkstra PU, van der Laan BF, Plukker JT, Roodenburg JL. Shoulder complaints after nerve sparing neck dissections. Int J Oral Maxillofac Surg. 2004;33(3):253–7. https://doi.org/10.1016/j.ijom.2003.0507.
7. Chepeha DB, Taylor RJ, Chepeha JC, Teknos TN, Bradford CR, Sharma PK, et al. Functional assessment using Constant's Shoulder Scale after modified radical and selective neck dissection. Head Neck. 2002;24(5):432–6. https://doi.org/10.1002/hed.10067.
8. NSW. CI. Cancer in NSW: incidence, mortality and prevalence report 2005. 2005.
9. Gordon T, Brushart TM, Amirjani N, Chan KM. The potential of electrical stimulation to promote functional recovery after peripheral nerve injury–comparisons between rats and humans. Acta Neurochir Suppl. 2007;100:3–11.
10. Razmjou H, Bean A, Macdermid JC, van Osnabrugge V, Travers N, Holtby R. Convergent validity of the constant-murley outcome measure in patients with rotator cuff disease. Physiother Can. 2008;60(1):72–9. https://doi.org/10.3138/physio/60/1/72.
11. Rocourt MH, Radlinger L, Kalberer F, Sanavi S, Schmid NS, Leunig M, et al. Evaluation of intratester and intertester reliability of the Constant-Murley shoulder assessment. J Shoulder Elbow Surg. 2008;17(2):364–9. https://doi.org/10.1016/j.jse.2007.06.024.

12. Christiansen D, Frost P, Falla D, Haahr J, Frich L, Svendsen S. Responsiveness and minimal clinical important change: a comparison between 2 shoulder outcome measures. J Orthop Sports Phys Ther. 2015;45(8):620–5.

13. Kukkonen J, Kauko T, Vahlberg T, Joukainen A, Aarimaa V. Investigating minimal clinically important difference for Constant score in patients undergoing rotator cuff surgery. J Shoulder Elb Surg. 2013;22:1650–5.

14. Henseler J, Kolk A, van der Zwaal P, Nagels J, Vliet Vlieland T, Nelissen R. The minimal detectable change of the Constant score in impingement, full-thickness tears, and massive rotator cuff tears. J Shoulder Elb Surg. 2015;24(3):376–81.

15. Torrens C, Guirro P, Santana F. The minimal clinical important difference for function and strength in patients undergoing reverse shoulder arthroplasty. J Shoulder Elb Surg. 2016;25(2):262–8.

16. Dziegielewski P, McNeely M, O'Connell D, Ashworth N, Allen H, Singh P, Kubrak C, Harris J, Seikaly H. Shoulder function after Level IIb neck dissection: a double-blind, randomizedcontrolled surgical trial. In: American Head & Neck Society (AHNS) Annual Meeting, July 21-25, 2012. Toronto, Canada.

17. Nix W, Hopf H. Electrical stimulation of regenerating nerve and its effect on motor recovery. Brain Res. 1983;272(1):21–5.

18. Pockett S, Gavin RM. Acceleration of peripheral nerve regeneration after crush injury in rat. Neurosci Lett. 1985;59(2):221–4.

19. Al-Majed AA, Neumann CM, Brushart TM, Gordon T. Brief electrical stimulation promotes the speed and accuracy of motor axonal regeneration. J Neurosci. 2000;20(7):2602–8.

20. Al-Majed AA, Brushart TM, Gordon T. Electrical stimulation accelerates and increases expression of BDNF and trkB mRNA in regenerating rat femoral motoneurons. Eur J Neurosci. 2000;12(12):4381–90.

21. Gordon T, Amirjani N, Edwards D, Chan KM. Brief post-surgical electrical stimulation accelerates axon regeneration and muscle reinnervation without affecting the functional measures in carpal tunnel syndrom patients. Exp Neurol. 2010;223(1):192–202.

22. International Study of Infarct Survival (ISIS) Collaboration Group. Randomised trial of intravenous streptokinase, oral aspirin, both, or neither among 17,187 cases of suspected acute myocardial infarction: ISIS-2. Lancet. 1988;13(2):349–60.

23. Caversaccio M, Negri S, Nolte L, Zbaren P. Neck dissection shoulder syndrome: quantification and three-dimensional evaluation with an optoelectronic tracking system. Ann Otolaryngol Rhinol Laryngol. 2003;112:939–46.

24. Inoue H, K-i N, Saito M, et al. Wuality of life after neck dissection. Arch Otolaryngol Head Neck Surg. 2006;132:662–6.

25. McGarvey A, Hoffman G, Osmotherly P, Chiarelli P. Maximizing shoulder function after accessory nerve injury and neck dissection surgery: a multicenter randomized controlled trial. Head Neck 2014;13:1-10.

26. Feng Z, Qin L, Huang X, Li J, Su M, Han Z. Nodal yield: is it a prognostic factor for head and neck squamous cell carcinoma? J Oral Maxillofac Surg. 2015;73(9):1851–9.

27. Agrama M, Reiter D, Topham A, Keane W. Node counts in neck dissection: are they useful in outcomes research? Otolaryngol Head Neck Surg. 2001;124(4):433–5. 24.

28. Grassi FA, Tajana MS. The normalization of data in the Constant-Murley score for the shoulder. A study conducted on 563 healthy subjects. Chirurgia degli Organi di Movimento. 2003;88(1):65–73.

29. Levy O, Haddo O, Massoud S, Mullett H, Atoun E. A patient-derived Constant-Murley score is comparable to a clinician-derived score. Clin Orthop Relat Res. 2014;472(1):294–303. https://doi.org/10.1007/s11999-013-3249-3.

30. Wilson RD, Gunzler DD, Bennett ME, Chae J. Peripheral nerve stimulation compared with usual care for pain relief of hemiplegic shoulder pain: a randomized controlled trial. Am J Phys Med Rehabil. 2014;93(1):17–28. https://doi.org/10.1097/PHM.0000000000000011.

6

Otolaryngology exposure in a longitudinal integrated clerkship setting

Grace Margaret Scott[1*], Corliss Ann Elizabeth Best[2] and Damian Christopher Micomonaco[2]

Abstract

Background: Although 20–40% of primary care complaints are Otolaryngology-Head and Neck Surgery (OtoHNS) related, little emphasis is placed on OtoHNS instruction at the undergraduate medical education level. An OtoHNS clerkship rotation is not required at most Canadian medical schools. Furthermore, at institutions offering an OtoHNS rotation, less than 20% of students are able to complete a placement. Given that a large percentage of medical students in Canada will pursue primary care as a career, there remains a gap in providing OtoHNS clinical training. During the longitudinal integrated clerkship at the Northern Ontario School of Medicine (NOSM), students are assigned to one of 14 sites, and not all have access to an otolaryngologist. This study looks to quantify the level of exposure students are receiving in OtoHNS at NOSM and to assess their comfort level with diagnosing and treating common otolaryngologic conditions.

Methods: A structured 13-item survey was administered to second, third and fourth year medical students at NOSM.

Results: A majority (67.9%) of medical students surveyed had not observed an otolaryngologist. Furthermore, most students (90.6%) reported receiving very little OtoHNS classroom based and clinical instruction during medical school.

Conclusions: A discrepancy exists between the quantity and breadth of OtoHNS training received in undergraduate medical education and the volume of OtoHNS encounters in primary care practice. Although geographic dissemination of students in the distributed learning model may be a challenge, strategies such as standardized objectives and supplemental electronic resources may serve to solidify clinical knowledge.

Keywords: Undergraduate medical education, Curriculum development, Longitudinal integrated clerkship, Primary care, Otolaryngology

Background

Problems related to the ear, nose and throat are frequently encountered across a variety of medical disciplines. In primary care, these conditions represent up to 25% of the practice workload [1]. Notwithstanding the quantity of otolaryngologic concerns, it is generally underrepresented in undergraduate medical education (UME) [2–5]. Furthermore, a recent review found that the majority of final year medical students and junior doctors in the United Kingdom are not confident in managing patients with common Otolaryngology-Head and Neck Surgery (OtoHNS) problems [6].

In Canada, the OtoHNS curriculum is not standardized across medical schools [5, 7]. There is currently great variability in the organization of teaching blocks and clerkship opportunities [5], such that the majority of Canadian medical students are never exposed to a clinical rotation in OtoHNS as part of their training [7]. Adequate exposure may present an increased challenge in a longitudinal integrated clerkship (LIC) model where not all 14 sites have access to an otolaryngologist. The Northern Ontario School of Medicine (NOSM) in Canada is the first medical school in which all students undertake LIC clinical training within a programme known as the Comprehensive Community Clerkship (CCC) [8, 9]. The Northern Ontario School of Medicine remains the only Canadian medical school that requires all students to complete their third year clinical training this way. Beyond specialist availability, students are also limited in their OtoHNS exposure due to the limited time allotted for specialty placements in this curriculum model.

* Correspondence: gscott@laurentian.ca
[1]Laurentian University, 935 Ramsey Lake Rd, Sudbury, ON P3E 2C6, Canada
Full list of author information is available at the end of the article

Longitudinal integrated clerkships afford students the opportunity to develop meaningful therapeutic relationships with patients and trusting, collegial relationships with their preceptors [10–14]. Graduates of LIC clinical training have been shown to perform as well as their peers in traditional rotation-based programs [13, 15]. Advantages of a LIC include improved academic results, [16–18] enhanced patient-centredness, [16, 17] and more meaningful learning relationships [8, 19]. Compared to traditional rotation based clerkships in tertiary hospital settings, medical students in a LIC have increased exposure to core clinical conditions [20].

This study looks to quantify the level of OtoHNS exposure students are receiving in a LIC model, and to assess their comfort level with diagnosing and treating common otolaryngologic conditions.

Methods

Ethics approval was obtained from both Laurentian University and Lakehead University for this cross-sectional survey design study.

Subjects

Inclusion criteria were undergraduate medical students at NOSM currently enrolled in years 2–4 of the program.

Survey design

We developed a questionnaire modeled on a previous study with family medicine [21]. This questionnaire was developed for resident learners to include twenty-one OtoHNS related issues, and seventeen OtoHNS procedural skills. Though all clinical presentations and procedural skills were included in the study's questionnaire, a priori decisions were made by the authors to focus on those clinical presentations and procedural skills that would be most appropriate for undergraduate medical

Table 1 Participant characteristics

Item	Participants
Year of study (n,% total)	
2	23 (43.4)
3	14 (26.4)
4	16 (30.2)
CCC Site (n,% senior students)	
Bracebridge	1 (3.3)
Dryden[a]	1 (3.3)
Fort Frances[a]	1 (3.3)
Hearst[a]	3 (10)
Huntsville	1 (3.3)
Kapuskasing[a]	2 (6.7)
Kenora	2 (6.7)
Manitoulin Island	1 (3.3)
New Liskeard	1 (3.3)
North Bay	3 (10)
Parry Sound	2 (6.7)
Sault Ste. Marie	6 (20)
Sioux Lookout[a]	2 (6.7)
Timmins	4 (13.3)

[a]Population < 10,000

learners to understand. These focused items included the following clinical presentations: otitis media, rhinitis and sinusitis, hoarseness, dysphagia, gastroesophageal reflux, thyroid nodules, salivary gland disease, peritonsillar abscess, sensorineural hearing loss, recurrent otitis media, and sleep apnea/snoring. Of the procedural skills, the following were highlighted as being appropriate for the undergraduate medical learner: otoneurologic exam, anterior rhinoscopy/nasal exam, oral cavity exam, indirect laryngoscopy, interpretation of an audiogram,

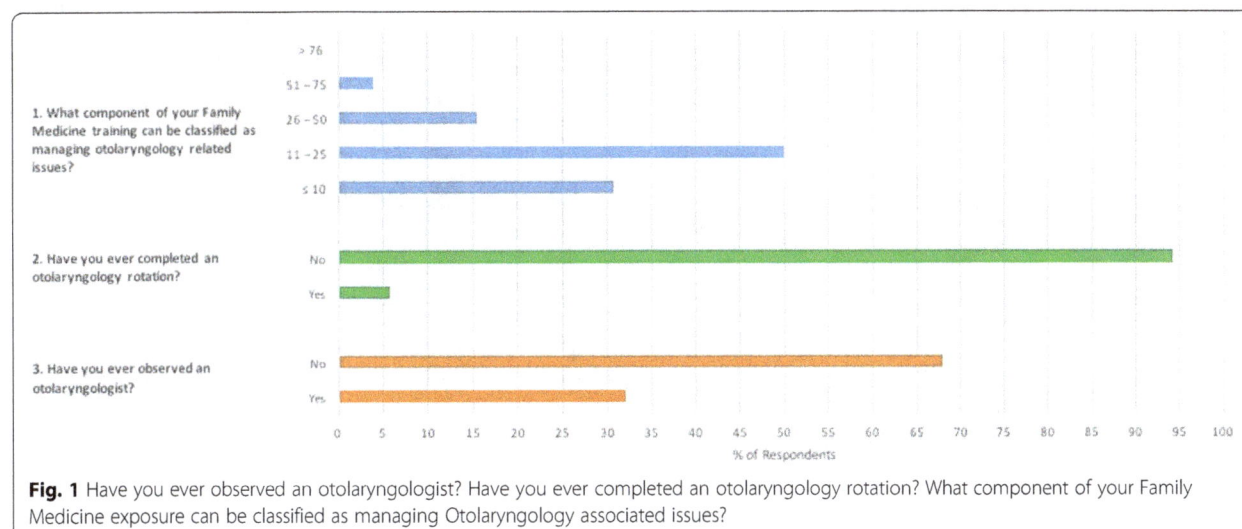

Fig. 1 Have you ever observed an otolaryngologist? Have you ever completed an otolaryngology rotation? What component of your Family Medicine exposure can be classified as managing Otolaryngology associated issues?

Table 2 Otolaryngology exposure in undergraduate medical education

Question	Answer choice	n (%)
How much classroom based ENT/ Otolaryngology instruction have you received during medical school?	Very little	48 (90.6)
	Adequate	5 (9.4)
	Very adequate	0 (0)
How much clinical ENT/Otolaryngology instruction have you received during medical school?	Very little	47 (88.7)
	Adequate	6 (11.3)
	Very adequate	0 (0)

explanation of common procedures and finally fine needle aspiration biopsy. The comprehensive survey asked medical students about: (1) their exposure to OtoHNS, (2) amount of training to date, and (3) perceived knowledge and ability to manage OtoHNS related clinical presentations. Students were also asked to identify their year of study and clinical clerkship site if they were in their clinical year of study. The survey was expected to take ten minutes to complete. A complete copy of the questionnaire can be found in Additional file 1: Appendix 1.

Survey distribution

In March 2016, an invitation to participate and link to the survey was electronically sent to all year 2–4 NOSM students by the academic class representatives. The electronic link led the students to a Survey Monkey questionnaire. The email invitation included an attached letter of information, as did the first page of the electronic survey. Survey responses were voluntary and anonymous. In order to optimize the response rate, a modified Dillman approach [22] was used. Specifically, an email reminder containing the survey link was sent to all students two-weeks and four-weeks following the initial invitation.

Data analysis

Descriptive statistics were generated using Microsoft *Excel*.

Results

In total, 53 participants completed the online survey. This afforded a response rate of 27.6% (53/192 enrolled students). Representation was gained from the three

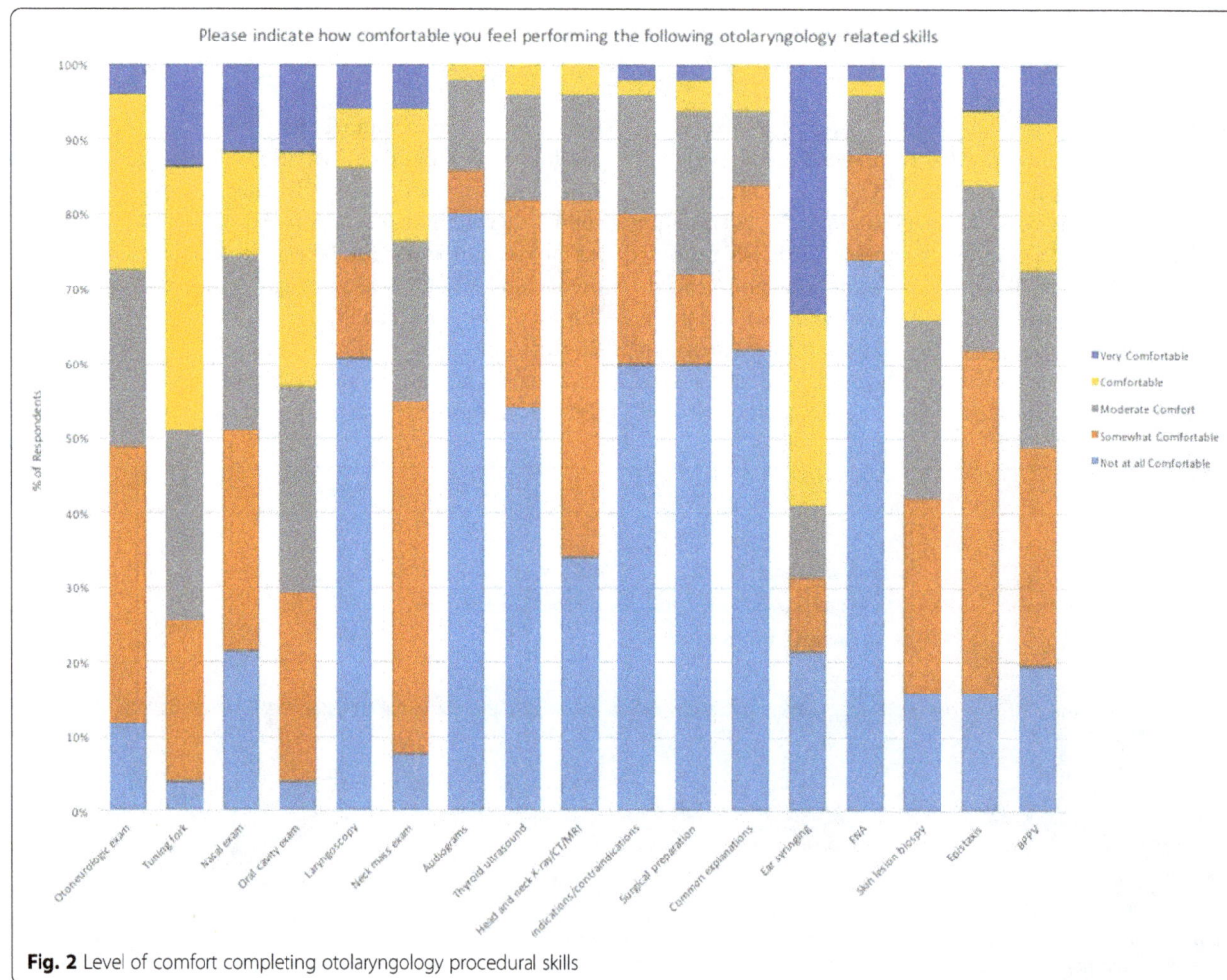

Fig. 2 Level of comfort completing otolaryngology procedural skills

years of study, as well as all 14 CCC sites (Table 1). This included 23 (43.4%) second year students, 14 (26.4%) third year students and 16 (30.2%) fourth year students. The survey did not contain a question on gender. The majority of students that responded (67.9%) had not observed an otolaryngologist and an even greater proportion (94.2%) had not completed an OtoHNS rotation (Fig. 1). In addition, 69.2% of students felt that a significant portion (≥ 11%) of their family medicine exposure included OtoHNS associated presentations (Fig. 1).

When asked how much classroom based OtoHNS instruction students received during medical school, 90.6% of participants replied 'very little'. Likewise, an overwhelming majority (88.7%) of students acknowledged receiving 'very little' clinical OtoHNS instruction. Student perspectives in OtoHNS instruction are found in Table 2.

The second section of the online survey assessed students' comfort level performing a set of OtoHNS related skills (Fig. 2) and managing/coordinating the care for a set of OtoHNS clinical presentations (Fig. 3). Of the OtoHNS related skills evaluated, the authors identified 7

skills most important for a medical students' core learning. These skills included interpretation of audiograms and tympanograms, management of epistaxis, anterior rhinoscopy/nasal examination, otoneurologic examination, ear syringing, examination of the oral cavity, and tuning fork testing. These identified skills revealed a wide range of comfort levels. When we group those respondents who selected 'not at all comfortable' and 'somewhat comfortable' together as a measure of those who were relatively uncomfortable, several trends emerge (Fig. 4). The medical learner participants felt most comfortable with tuning fork testing (25.49% felt not at all or somewhat comfortable) and least comfortable with interpretation of audiograms and tympanograms (86% felt not at all or somewhat comfortable). Of the OtoHNS clinical presentations, the authors identified 11 presentations to be important for a medical students' core learning. These clinical presentations included salivary gland diseases, sudden sensorineural hearing loss, peritonsillar abscess, hoarseness, dysphagia, thyroid nodules, recurrent otitis media, rhinitis and sinusitis, sleep

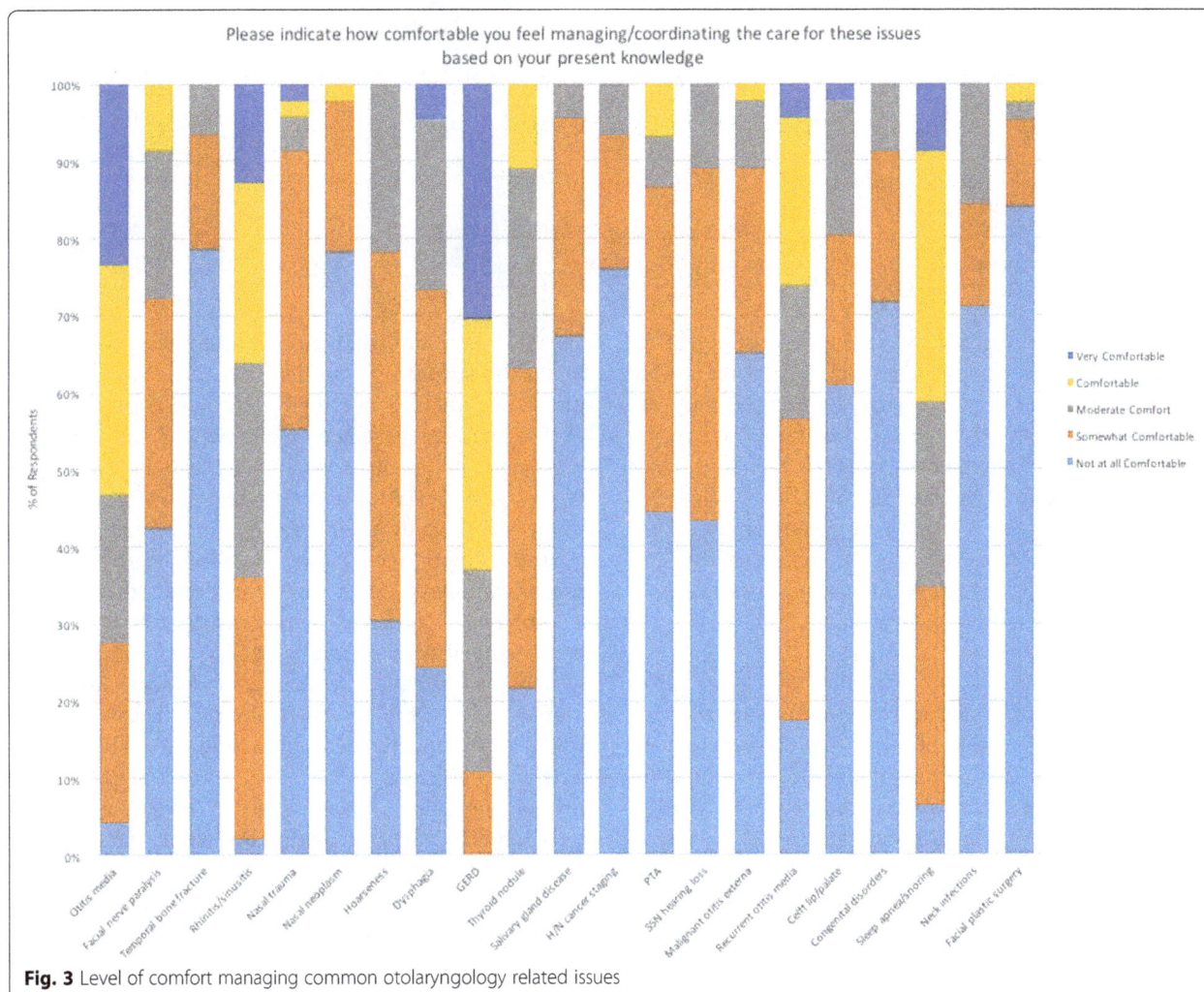

Fig. 3 Level of comfort managing common otolaryngology related issues

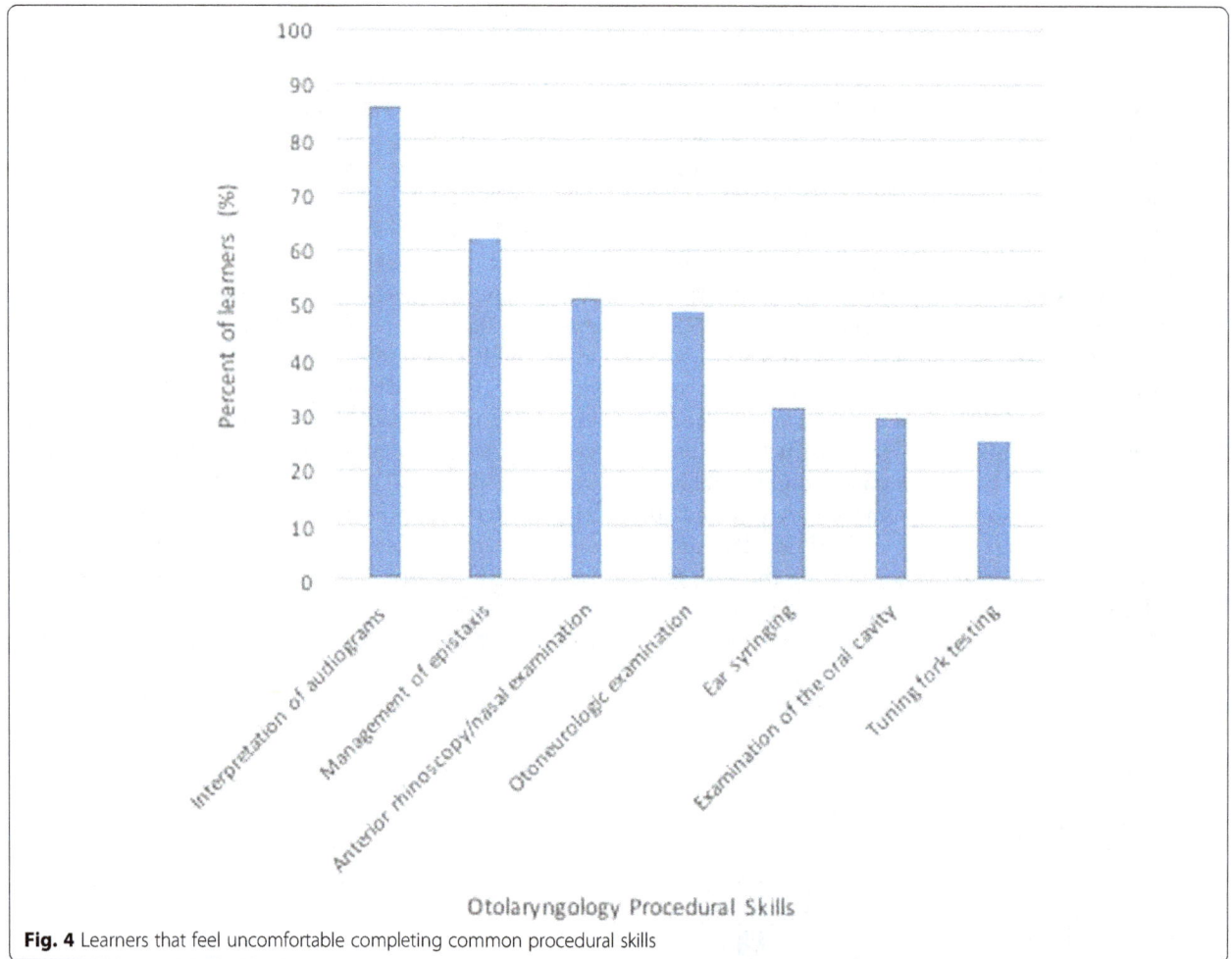

Fig. 4 Learners that feel uncomfortable completing common procedural skills

apnea and snoring, otitis media and gastroesophageal reflux disease. These clinical presentations revealed a wide range of comfort levels. Once again, we grouped those respondents who selected 'not at all comfortable' and 'somewhat comfortable' together as a measure of those who were relatively uncomfortable (Fig. 5). This revealed that learners felt most comfortable with gastroesophageal reflux disease (10.87% felt not at all or somewhat comfortable) and least comfortable with salivary gland diseases (95.65% felt not at all or somewhat comfortable).

Discussion

Our study revealed that students are receiving suboptimal exposure to OtoHNS as measured by perceived volume of training and comfort levels. A majority of students surveyed had never observed an otolaryngologist or completed an OtoHNS rotation.

These results are not unique to NOSM. Regardless of clerkship model, OtoHNS remains a challenging competency to acquire. The literature suggests that even those medical students who have completed an OtoHNS rotation reported feeling uncomfortable diagnosing and managing common and emergent conditions [23–25]. This is not surprising considering that the average clerkship time dedicated to OtoHNS in Canada was 4.6 days [7]. Specific gaps have been identified in knowledge surrounding otitis media, tonsillitis, indications for tracheostomy, and airway obstruction as well as specific skill deficits in otoscopy and nasal examination [26]. Considering the importance placed on OtoHNS by primary care practitioners [24, 27], it is imperative that training in OtoHNS be optimized and consistent at the undergraduate medical education level.

With the distributed learning model and LIC, it is essential that OtoHNS curriculum be consistent and equitable for students across teaching sites. There is the need for increased exposure to OtoHNS curriculum without burdening clinical faculty. A review of 17 published studies found students consistently rated clinic-based teaching and small group learning as effective ways to learn OtoHNS [24]. Although case-based and online learning modules are already employed in the distributed learning model at NOSM, further utilization of these learning modalities may help to bridge some of the

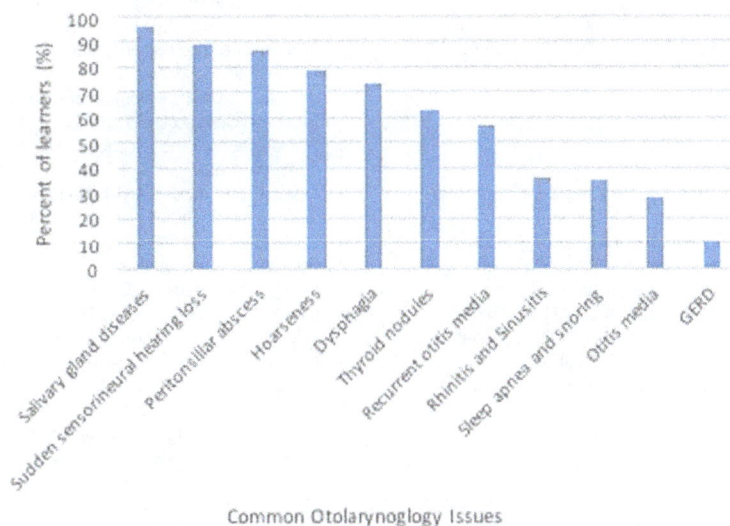

Fig. 5 Learners that feel uncomfortable managing common otolaryngology related issues

identified gaps in the OtoHNS curriculum. Simulation has also been shown to be an effective teaching modality that may prove useful in a distributed learning environment where exposure to OtoHNS pathology may vary between clerkship sites. Previous research has echoed the above sentiments by suggesting the need for increased exposure without placing additional burden on clinical faculty [24].

This study assessed OtoHNS exposure and comfort level through the lens of student perspectives. Both exposure to OtoHNS and level of comfort managing common OtoHNS conditions were assessed simultaneously, using a previously validated OtoHNS assessment tool [21]. To our knowledge, this is the first study in the literature to focus on the experience of OtoHNS instruction in a LIC model. However, the authors acknowledge several limitations do exist. The study only captured data from a single timepoint at a single Canadian medical school. Additionally, the results may be unique to NOSM as it is the only school with a comprehensive LIC model. Thus, it is conceivable that variation could exist between different medical institutions nationwide and beyond. The anonymity of the survey as well as the moderate response rate may invite concern as to whether the results reflect the perception of all medical students at NOSM. Additionally, there may be a discrepancy in level of comfort and actual knowledge, such that students who feel uncomfortable managing OtoHNS conditions may actually possess the appropriate knowledge.

Conclusions

Otolaryngology is an important specialty with relevance to family medicine, pediatrics, and general practice. Based on the volume of OtoHNS encounters in primary

care practice, there remains an underrepresentation of OtoHNS training at the undergraduate medical education level. Despite geographic distribution of students in the CCC and LIC models, the results of this study were not dissimilar to rotation based clerkship cohorts. Strategies such as standardized objectives and supplemental electronic resources may serve to solidify clinical knowledge with all undergraduate medical learners.

Abbreviations
CCC: Comprehensive Community Clerkship; LIC: Longitudinal Integrated Clerkship; NOSM: Northern Ontario School of Medicine; OtoHNS: Otolaryngology Head and Neck Surgery

Acknowledgements
Not applicable.

Funding
There are no sources of funding to declare.

Authors' contributions
GMS participated in conceptualization of experimental design, data analysis and manuscript preparation. CAEB participated in data collection and manuscript preparation. DCM participated in data analysis and manuscript preparation. All authors read and approved the final manuscript.

Authors' information
Not applicable.

Competing interests
The authors declare that they have no competing interests.

Author details

[1]Laurentian University, 935 Ramsey Lake Rd, Sudbury, ON P3E 2C6, Canada.
[2]Northern Ontario School of Medicine, 935 Ramsey Lake Rd, Sudbury, ON P3E 2C6, Canada.

References

1. Griffiths E. Incidence of ENT problems in general practice. J R Soc Med. 1979;72(10):740.
2. Doshi J, Carrie S. A survey of undergraduate otolaryngology experience at Newcastle University medical school. J Laryngol Otol. 2006;120(09):770–3.
3. Mace AD, Narula AA. Survey of current undergraduate otolaryngology training in the United Kingdom. J Laryngol Otol. 2004;118(03):217–20.
4. Steinbach WJ, Sectish TC. Pediatric resident training in the diagnosis and treatment of acute otitis media. Pediatrics. 2002;109(3):404–8.
5. Wong A, Fung K. Otolaryngology in undergraduate medical education. J Otolaryngol Head Neck Surg. 2009;38(1):38–48.
6. Ferguson GR, Bacila IA, Swamy M. Does current provision of undergraduate education prepare UK medical students in ENT? A systematic literature review. BMJ Open. 2016;6(4):e010054.
7. Campisi P, Asaria J, Brown D. Undergraduate otolaryngology education in Canadian medical schools. Laryngoscope. 2008;118(11):1941–50.
8. Strasser R, Hirsh D. commentaries. Acad Med. 2011;84:844–50.
9. Tesson G, Hudson G, Strasser R. Making of the Northern Ontario School of Medicine: A Case Study in the History of Medical Education. Montreal: McGill-Queen's Press-MQUP; 2009.
10. Hauer KE, O'Brien BC, Hansen L, Hirsh D, Ma IH, Ogur B, Teherani A. More is better: students describe successful and unsuccessful experiences with teachers differently in brief and longitudinal relationships. Acad Med. 2012;87:1389–96.
11. Hudson JN, Knight PJ, Weston KM. Patient perceptions of innovative longitudinal integrated clerkships based in regional, rural and remote primary care: a qualitative study. BMC Fam Pract. 2012;13:72.
12. Konkin J, Suddards C. Creating stories to live by: caring and professional identity formation in a longitudinal integrated clerkship. Adv Health Sci Educ Theory Pract. 2012;17:585–96.
13. Walters L, Greenhill J, Richards J, Ward H, Campbell N, Ash J, Schuwirth LWT. Outcomes of longitudinal integrated clinical placements for students, clinicians and society. Med Educ. 2012;46:1028–41.
14. Konkin DJ, Suddards CA. Who should choose a rural LIC: a qualitative study of perceptions of students who have completed a rural longitudinal integrated clerkship. Med Teach. 2015;37(11):1026–31.
15. Woloschuk W, Myhre D, Jackson W, McLaughlin K, Wright B. Comparing the performance in family medicine residencies of graduates from longitudinal integrated clerkships and rotation-based clerkships. Acad Med. 2014;89(2):296–300.
16. Ogur B, Hirsh D, Krupat E, Bor D. The Harvard Medical School-Cambridge integrated clerkship: an innovative model of clinical education. Acad Med. 2007;82(4):397–404.
17. Ogur B, Hirsh D. Learning through longitudinal patient care—narratives from the Harvard Medical School–Cambridge integrated clerkship. Acad Med. 2009;84(7):844–50.
18. Worley P, Esterman A, Prideaux D. Cohort study of examination performance of undergraduate medical students learning in community settings. BMJ. 2004;328(7433):207–9.
19. Worley P, Prideaux D, Strasser R, Magarey A, March R. Empirical evidence for symbiotic medical education: a comparative analysis of community and tertiary-based programmes. Med Educ. 2006;40(2):109–16.
20. Worley P, Strasser R, Prideaux D. Can medical students learn specialist disciplines based in rural practice: lessons from students' self reported experience and competence. Rural Remote Health. 2004;4(4):338.
21. Glicksman JT, Brandt MG, Parr J, Fung K. Needs assessment of undergraduate education in otolaryngology among family medicine residents. J Otolaryngol Head Neck Surg. 2008;37(5):668–75.
22. Dillman DA. Mail and telephone surveys: the total design method. New York: Wiley; 1978.
23. Mishra P, Deshmukh S. ENT-HNS education: what undergraduate students want? Eur Arch Otorhinolaryngol. 2013;270(11):2981–3.
24. Ishman SL, Stewart CM, Senser E, Stewart RW, Stanley J, Stierer KD, Benke JR, Kern DE. Qualitative synthesis and systematic review of otolaryngology in undergraduate medical education. Laryngoscope. 2015 Dec 1;125(12):2695–708.
25. Chawdhary G, Ho EC, Minhas SS. Undergraduate ENT education: what students want. Clin Otolaryngol. 2009;34:584–5.
26. Ganzel TM, Martinez SA. Are we teaching medical students what they need to know? Otolaryngol Head Neck Surg. 1989;100:339–44.
27. Powell J, Cooles FA, Carrie S, Paleri V. Is undergraduate medical education working for ENT surgery? A survey of UK medical school graduates. J Laryngol Otol. 2011;125:896–905.

7

Renal protective effect of a hydration supplemented with magnesium in patients receiving cisplatin for head and neck cancer

Takahiro Kimura[1,3], Taijiro Ozawa[2], Nobuhiro Hanai[3], Hitoshi Hirakawa[4], Hidenori Suzuki[3], Hiroshi Hosoi[1] and Yasuhisa Hasegawa[3*]

Abstract

Background: Our study analyzes the effect of magnesium supplementation on nephrotoxicity in patients receiving cisplatin for head and neck cancer.

Methods: We retrospectively reviewed the medical records of patients with head and neck cancer who received two doses of cisplatin (80 mg/m2) and 5-fluorouracil (800 mg/m2) 3 weeks apart from August 2008 to October 2012. The regimen prior to 2011 (crystalloid-only) involved the administration of 1000 mL of lactated Ringer's solution on the day prior to cisplatin infusion and 2000 mL of continuous infusion of saline on the day of cisplatin infusion. The regimen after 2011 (magnesium-supplemented) did not involve hydration on the day before cisplatin administration but used 1000 mL of 0.9% saline with magnesium sulfate (20 mEq) administered for 3 hours before cisplatin infusion.

Results: Sixty-five patients were treated with the crystalloid-only regimen and 56 patients with the magnesium-supplemented regimen. The mean creatinine clearance in the magnesium-supplemented group decreased by 4.9 mL/kg/min, whereas that in the crystalloid-only group decreased by 15.0 mL/kg/min after two courses. In multivariate analysis, only magnesium-supplemented hydration was an independent predictive factor for preventing cisplatin-induced nephrotoxicity (odds ratio = 0.157, 95% confidence interval 0.030–0.670, $P = 0.0124$).

Conclusion: We demonstrated that an intravenous hydration regimen supplemented with magnesium prevented cisplatin-induced nephrotoxicity in patients with head and neck cancer.

Keywords: Cisplatin, Nephrotoxicity, Magnesium, Head and neck cancer

Background

Cisplatin was first administered to a cancer patient in 1971, and it became available for general oncology practice in 1978, first in testicular cancer and then in ovarian cancer [1]. Cisplatin also exerts a potent antineoplastic effect against head and neck cancer and is still a frequently used drug in this field. However, it has various side effects, such as gastrointestinal toxicity, myelosuppression, ototoxicity and nephrotoxicity. The nephrotoxic effect of cisplatin is, in particular, the most important dose-limiting factor in chemotherapy. Cisplatin-induced nephrotoxicity can be attributed to the impairment of proximal as well as distal tubular filtration and a severe progressive decrease in the glomerular filtration rate during treatment [2]. Hypomagnesemia was initially described in 1979 as an electrolyte abnormality induced by cisplatin chemotherapy [3]. Hypomagnesemia has been repeatedly confirmed by several studies. Additionally, Vokes, et al. demonstrated a high incidence of hypomagnesemia in cisplatin-treated head and neck cancer patients and its relation to the cumulative cisplatin dose [4]. A study using rats has shown a substantial additive effect of magnesium-depletion on renal toxicity induced by cisplatin.

* Correspondence: hasegawa@aichi-cc.jp
[3]Department of Head and Neck Surgery, Aichi Cancer Center Hospital, 1-1 Kanokoden, Chikusaku, Nagoya 464-8681, Japan
Full list of author information is available at the end of the article

Therefore, attention must be paid to the aggravation of nephrotoxicity by magnesium-loss during cisplatin treatment especially in patients suffering from intense gastro-intestinal side effects [5]. Several studies have reported the prophylactic effect of magnesium supplementation on cisplatin-induced nephrotoxicity [6–8]. However, the study populations were relatively small and included patients with a history of previous treatments, surgery or chemotherapy.

To the best of our knowledge, there is no study has demonstrated the protective effect of magnesium supplementation against cisplatin-induced nephrotoxicity in patients with head and neck cancer. Here, we aimed to analyze the effect of magnesium supplementation on nephrotoxicity in patients receiving cisplatin for head and neck cancer.

Methods

We retrospectively reviewed the medical records of patients with head and neck cancer who received cisplatin and 5-fluorouracil [5-FU] as an induction chemotherapy at the Department of Head and Neck Surgery of Aichi Cancer Center Hospital, Japan from August 2008 to October 2012. We selected patients who had no history of treatment for malignant tumors including head and neck cancer. The chemotherapy regimen consisted of 5-FU [800 mg/m^2 continuous infusion from day 1 to 5] and cisplatin (80 mg/m^2 on day 6) [9]. Chemotherapy was administered for two cycles 3 weeks apart.

The crystalloid-only regimen included the administration of 1000 mL of lactated Ringer's solution on the day prior to the administration of cisplatin and 2000 mL of continuous infusion of saline on the day of cisplatin infusion. In April 2011, we changed the hydration regimen

at our institution. The magnesium-supplemented regimen did not use lactated Ringer's solution on the day before cisplatin, but instead it included 1000 mL of 0.9% saline with magnesium sulfate (20 mEq) for 3 hours before the administration of cisplatin (Fig. 1). The dose of magnesium sulfate was adopted from the cisplatin template based on the recommendations of the National Comprehensive Cancer Network. In both regimens, antiemetic agents (dexamethasone 8 mg, granisetron 1 mg) and a diuretic (furosemide 20 mg) were given, and post hydration was performed with two liters of Soldem 3A® (Na 35 mEq/L, K 20 mEq/L, L-lactate 20 mEq/L, and glucose 43.0 g/L) for 3 days after cisplatin infusion. However, while some patients in the crystalloid-only group were not given aprepitant, all patients in the magnesium-supplemented group were.

Renal damage was evaluated based on the reduction in creatinine clearance (Ccr) throughout the duration of chemotherapy. Ccr was calculated using the Cockcroft and Gault formula [10]. Nephrotoxicity was defined by a 20% reduction in Ccr after two courses of chemotherapy. Toxicities were graded using the Common Terminology Criteria for Adverse Events version 4.0.

Fisher's exact test or Student's t-test was used to compare the characteristics of patients before treatment. Student's t-test was used to evaluate the differences in Ccr reduction between the crystalloid-only regimen and the magnesium-supplemented regimen. The contingency table with patient characteristics and nephrotoxicity was analyzed using Fisher's exact test. Multivariate analyses were performed using a multiple regression model to investigate the relationship between magnesium supplementation and nephrotoxicity induced by cisplatin. The results were presented as odds ratio with 95% confidence

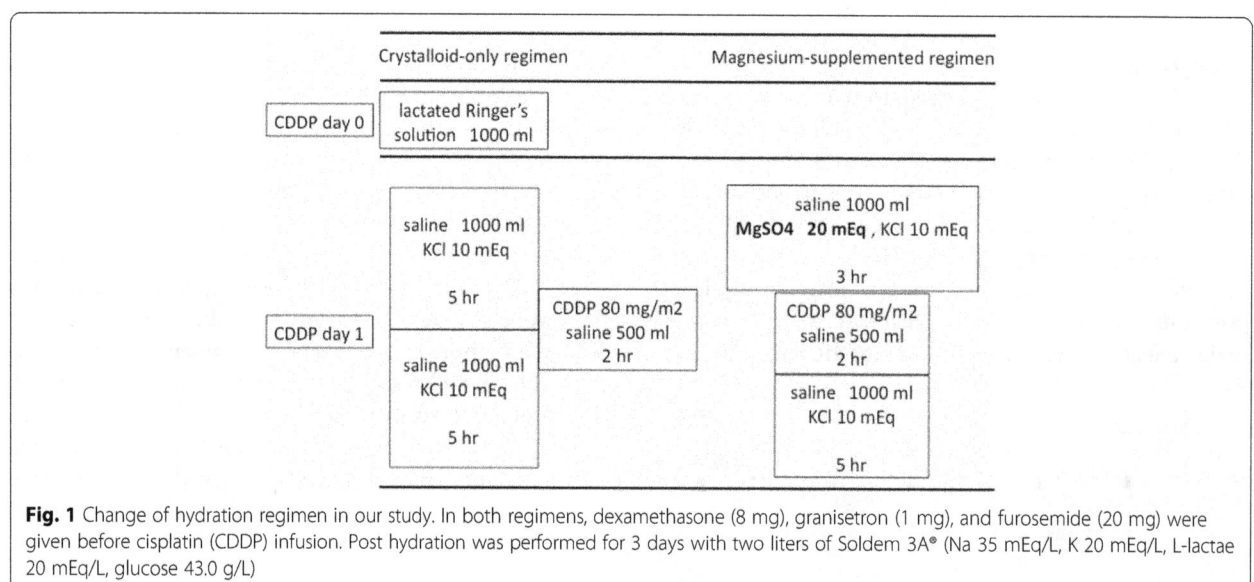

Fig. 1 Change of hydration regimen in our study. In both regimens, dexamethasone (8 mg), granisetron (1 mg), and furosemide (20 mg) were given before cisplatin (CDDP) infusion. Post hydration was performed for 3 days with two liters of Soldem 3A® (Na 35 mEq/L, K 20 mEq/L, L-lactae 20 mEq/L, glucose 43.0 g/L)

intervals. *P* values < 0.05 were considered statistically significant. Analyses were performed with using JMP® 11 (SAS Institute Inc., Cary, NC, USA).

The study design was approved by the Institutional Ethics Committee and fulfilled the guidelines of the Declaration of Helsinki regarding the ethical principles for medical research.

Results

The characteristics of all patients are shown in Table 1. There were 65 patients, 52 males and 13 females with a median age of 62 years, in the crystalloid-only group and 56 patients, 50 males and six females with a median age of 62 years, in the magnesium-supplemented group. There were no significant differences between the two groups regarding patient age, sex, performance status, body surface area (BSA), or hematocrit values. The magnesium-supplemented group had fewer cases with cancer of the nasal cavity and paranasal sinuses and oral cavity cancer and more cases of oropharyngeal cancer than the crystalloid-only group. There were no significant differences between the two groups in clinical parameters: serum levels of creatinine, albumin, and Ccr before chemotherapy. Because aprepitant was approved on October 16, 2009 in Japan, we only prescribed the antiemetic to 22 of 65 patients in the crystalloid-only

group, but it was prescribed it to all patients in the magnesium-supplemented group.

We noted significant differences in the change in Ccr (ΔCcr) between the magnesium-supplemented and crystalloid-only groups after treatment. The mean ΔCcr after two courses of chemotherapy in the crystalloid-only regimen was 15.0 mL/min (standard error (SE), 1.7), and the mean ΔCcr in the magnesium-supplemented group was 4.9 mL/min (SE, 1.4) ($p < 0.0001$). However, there was an obvious difference in the two groups regarding the administration of aprepitant, so we divided the crystalloid-only group into two groups with and without aprepitant. The incidence and severity of nausea and dehydration were worse in the group without aprepitant than in the group with aprepitant (Table 2). After one course of chemotherapy, there was no significant difference in ΔCcr between the magnesium-supplement group (4.4 mL/min) and the crystalloid-only group with aprepitant (5.4 mL/min). Renal damage in patients in the crystalloid-only group without aprepitant was significantly more severe than in patients given the magnesium-supplemented regimen (10.1 mL/min, $p < 0.0298$). However, after two courses of chemotherapy, patients in the magnesium-supplemented regimen group had lower occurrence of nephrotoxicity compared to patients in the crystalloid-only group with and without aprepitant. (4.9 vs. 14.7 and 15.1 mL/min, respectively) (Fig. 2).

Table 1 Patient characteristics

Characteristics		All (*n* = 121)	Crystalloid -only regimen (*n* = 65)	Magnesium –supplemented regimen (*n* = 56)	*P* value
Age	Median (range)	62 (28–78)	62 (28–77)	62 (42–78)	0.2943[†]
Sex	Male	102	52	50	0.1616[*]
	Female	19	13	6	
BSA (m2)	Median (range)	1.63 (1.27–2.00)	1.59 (1.33–1.96)	1.65 (1.27–2.00)	0.2542[†]
PS	0 / 1 / 2	67 / 46 / 8	38 / 22 / 5	29 / 24 / 3	0.5676[*]
Primary Site	Nasal cavity and Paranasal sinuses	15	14	1	0.0001[*]
	Oral cavity	4	4	0	
	Nasopharynx	1	0	1	
	Oropharynx	40	15	25	
	Hypopharynx	32	18	14	
	Laryynx	8	1	7	
	Cervical esophagus	13	7	6	
	Unknown	8	6	2	
Creatine (mg/dL)	Median (range)	0.71 (0.38–1.07)	0.69 (0.38–1.07)	0.73 (0.51–1.07)	0.1152[†]
Ccr (m L/min)	Median (range)	89.1 (54.5–186.7)	79.1 (54.5–156.1)	89.1 (57.0–143.6)	0.1712[†]
Albumin (g/mL)	Median (range)	4.1 (2.9–5.1)	4.1 (3.0–5.0)	4.2 (2.9–5.1)	0.1081[†]
Hematocrit (%)	Median (range)	39.7 (26.6–50.8)	39.1 (26.6–50.8)	40.4 (31.3–48.6)	0.1001[†]
Aprepitant	Administration	78	22	56	< 0.0001[†]

BSA body surface area, *Ccr* creatinine clearance
[*]Fisher's exact test; [†]Student's *t*-test

Table 2 Toxicities occurring in patients treated with cisplatin and 5-FU

	Magnesium -supplemented regimen (n = 56)	Crystalloid-only regimen with aprepitant (n = 22)	Crystalloid-only regimen without aprepitant (n = 43)	P value*
Nausea				
Grade 1–2	30 (53.6%)	7 (31.8%)	29 (67.4%)	0.010
Grade 3	2 (3.6%)	1 (2.3%)	5 (11.6%)	
Vomitting				
Grade 1–2	2 (3.6%)	2 (4.6%)	6 (14.0%)	0.175
Grade 3	0 (0%)	0 (0%)	0 (0%)	
Dehydration				
Grade 1–2	5 (8.9%)	2 (4.7%)	12 (27.9%)	0.017
Grade 3	6 (10.7%)	2 (4.7%)	9 (20.9%)	

Toxicities were graded using the Common Terminology Criteria for Adverse Event version 4.0
*Chi-square test

We examined the relationship between nephrotoxicity induced by chemotherapy and clinical characteristics and parameters by univariate and multivariate analyses. Nephrotoxicity was defined as a 20% reduction in Ccr after chemotherapy. Nephrotoxicity was more strongly correlated with Ccr before chemotherapy, administration of aprepitant and regimen by univariate analysis (Table 3).

Multivariate analyses were performed based on the results of univariate analysis. In multivariate analyses, only the magnesium-supplemented regimen of hydration was an independent predictive factor for protection against nephrotoxicity induced by cisplatin (odds ratio = 0.157, 95% confidence interval 0.030–0.670, P = 0.0124) (Table 4).

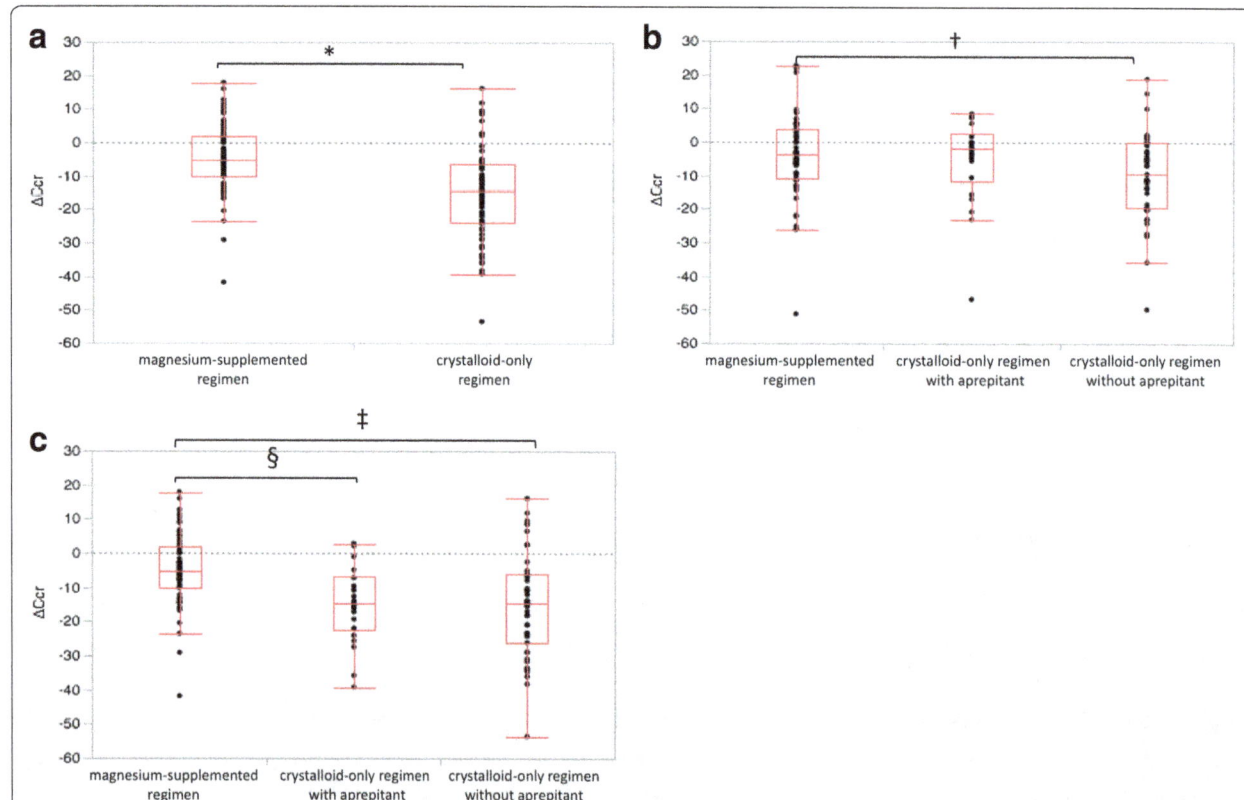

Fig. 2 a Change in creatine clearance in the regimen groups after two courses ($^*p < 0.0001$ Student's t-test). **b** The crystalloid-only regimen group was divided into with and without aprepitant groups. Change in creatine clearance in the magnesium-supplemented regimen group and crystalloid-only group with and without aprepitant after one course ($^\dagger p = 0.0298$ Student's t-test). **c** Change in creatine clearance in the three groups after two courses ($^\ddagger p < 0.0001$, $^\S p = 0.0026$ Student's t-test). ΔCcr, difference in creatine clearance between chemotherapy courses

Table 3 Characteristics of patients classified by nephrotoxicity caused by cisplatin

Characteristics		Nephrotoxicity-	Nephrotoxicity+	P value*
Age	< 65	40 (42.6)	12 (44.4)	1.0000
	≥ 65	54 (57.4)	15 (55.6)	
Sex	female	13 (13.8)	6 (22.2)	0.3671
	male	81 (86.2)	21 (77.8)	
Primary site	Hypopharynx	23 (24.5)	9 (33.3)	0.4578
	Others	71 (75.5)	18 (66.7)	
Ccr	< 120 mL/min	86 (79.3)	22 (20.4)	0.1619
	≥ 120 mL/min	8 (61.2)	5 (38.4)	
Albumin	< 4 g/mL	32 (34.4)	12 (44.4)	0.3674
	≥ 4 g/mL	62 (66)	15 (55.6)	
Aprepitant	–	25 (26.6)	18 (66.7)	0.0002
	+	69 (73.4)	9 (33.3)	
Regimen	Crystalloid-only	41 (43.6)	24 (88.9)	< 0.0001
	Magnesium-supplemented	53 (56.4)	3 (11.1)	

Nephrotoxicity+ is defined as the 20% reduction in creatinine clearance after two courses
Ccr Creatinine clearance
*Fisher's exact test

Discussion

The findings of this retrospective study showed that a magnesium-supplemented regimen of hydration reduces nephrotoxicity induced by cisplatin in patients with head and neck cancer. In univariate analysis, the characteristics of patients such as age, sex, primary tumor site and laboratory data were not associated with renal damage but change in the hydration regimen and the use of aprepitant were protective against renal dysfunction. To prevent intense gastro intestinal side effects, it is currently recommended that patients who receive cisplatin be given a three-drug combination of a 5-HT3 receptor antagonist, dexamethasone, and a neurokinin 1 receptor antagonist, such as aprepitant [11]. Patients with head and neck cancer are susceptible to dehydration, and chemotherapy-induced nausea and vomiting can aggravate dehydration. In Japan, aprepitant has been available since October 16, 2009. Administration of aprepitant prevented or reduced nausea and consequently mitigated dehydration. The patients in the magnesium-supplemented group benefited from the antiemetics more than those in the crystalloid-only group. However, in multivariate analysis, the magnesium-supplemented regimen was an independent predictive factor for protection against nephrotoxicity induced by cisplatin.

We hypothesize that supplementation with magnesium before cisplatin infusion protects against renal damage. Renal damage due to cisplatin involves a pathological change in the kidney that is characterized by focal acute tubular necrosis, primarily in the distal convoluted tubule [12]. This morphological change decreases tubular reabsorption, resulting in hypomagnesemia. It is unclear whether the depletion of serum magnesium aggravates cisplatin-induced nephrotoxicity, but previous studies have indicated some possibility of this relationship. Organic cation transporter 2, which regulates the uptake of cisplatin, is up-regulated under hypomagnesemia, and the renal accumulation of cisplatin is markedly increased [13, 14]. Several studies have reported the nephroprotective effect of magnesium supplementation during chemotherapy with cisplatin [6–8]. Willox J. C, et al. reported that all patients receiving cisplatin for testicular cancer have depleted serum levels of magnesium, indicating the protective effect of magnesium supplementation against cisplatin-induced renal tubular damage by measuring urine N-acetyl-β-D-glucosaminidase (NAG) [6] . We did not

Table 4 Multivariate analysis of protective factors against nephrotoxicity induced by cisplatin

Protective factors	OR	95% CI	P value
Ccr (≥ 120/< 120 mL/min)	0.606	0.164–2.355	0.4567
Aprepitant (+/−)	0.525	0.161–1.563	0.2515
Regimen (magnesium-supplemented/crystalloid-only)	0.157	0.030–0.670	0.0124

Ccr Creatinine clearance, *OR* Odds ratio, *CI* Confidence interval. The multivariate analyses used a multiple regression model measure serum magnesium level or urine NAG, which constitutes a limitation of this study. There was no difference in the reduction in Ccr between the magnesium-supplemented group and the crystalloid-only group with aprepitant after one course. After two courses of chemotherapy, however, Ccr significantly decreased in the crystalloid-only group with aprepitant compared to the magnesium-supplemented group. This may be because a dysfunction in magnesium reabsorption after one course promotes cisplatin-induced nephrotoxicity in the second course so that the magnesium-supplemented regimen results in significantly better outcomes after the second course.

Several studies investigating the method of supplementation of magnesium during cisplatin treatment have recommended intravenous or oral supplementation or both [15]. Approximately 50% of the infused magnesium is excreted in the urine. Plasma magnesium concentration inhibits magnesium reabsorption in the loop of Henle [16]. When magnesium is intravenously administered, an abrupt but temporary elevation in the plasma magnesium concentration partially inhibits the stimulus for magnesium reabsorption in the loop of Henle. Magnesium uptake by the cells is slow, and therefore adequate replenishment requires sustained correction of hypomagnesemia. Martin et al. assigned 41 patients into groups with no magnesium supplementation, intravenous magnesium supplementation and oral supplementation during four courses of 100 mg/m2 cisplatin treatment. The study showed that both intravenous and oral magnesium supplementation can be efficacious in the prevention of cisplatin-induced hypomagnesemia. However, two patients treated with oral magnesium developed mild gastrointestinal symptoms (emesis and diarrhea), probably from the magnesium therapy. In contrast, none of the patients with intravenous magnesium supplementation showed these symptoms [17]. Because the location of tumors can make it difficult for patients with head and neck cancer to take oral drugs, we propose that magnesium should be administered intravenously before cisplatin infusion.

In the crystalloid-only regimen, saline was administered at a slower pace and more persistently during cisplatin treatment than that in the magnesium-supplemented regimen in which one liter of saline was rapidly administered within 3 hours before the infusion of cisplatin. Saline has a high concentration of chloride ions that prevents the substitution of water for chloride ions in cisplatin, thereby reducing the formation of aquated species of cisplatin that induce necrosis in tubule cells [18]. High volume hydration with saline before and after cisplatin injection is used to lower the concentration and to shorten the period of direct cisplatin exposure [19, 20].

There are several limitations in this study, such as its retrospective design and the limited availability of some clinical data. This study could not provide evidence for the linear relationship between the grade of hypomagnesemia and increase in the risk of nephrotoxicity induced by cisplatin. However, the population in this study is larger than that in the previous studies, and it is valuable to know that none of the patients had a history of anticancer treatment before chemotherapy.

Conclusions

In conclusion, we demonstrated that an intravenous hydration regimen supplemented with magnesium has inhibitory effect on nephrotoxicity induced by cisplatin in patients with head and neck cancer.

Abbreviations

ΔCcr: Decrease in Ccr; 5-FU: 5-fluorouracil; BSA: Body surface area; Ccr: Creatinine clearance; CDDP: Cisplatin; CI: Confidence interval; OR: Odds ratio; SE: Standard error

Acknowledgements

This study was supported by a Health and Labour Sciences Research Grant for Clinical Cancer Research (H21-Gannrinshou-Ippan-016 and H24-Gannrinshou-Ippan-006) from the Ministry of Health, Labour and Welfare, Japan.

Funding

This study was supported by a Health and Labour Sciences Research Grant for Clinical Cancer Research (H24-Gannrinshou-Ippan-006) from the Ministry of Health, Labour and Welfare, Japan.

Authors' contributions

Study conception and design: YH. Acquisition of data: TO, NH, HH and HS. Analysis and interpretation of data: TK. Drafting of manuscript: TK. Critical revision: HH and YH. All authors read and approved the final manuscript.

Author details

[1]Department of Otolaryngology-Head and Neck Surgery, Nara Medical University, Kashihara, Japan. [2]Department of Oto-Rhino-Laryngology, Toyohashi Municipal Hospi-tal, Toyohashi, Japan. [3]Department of Head and Neck Surgery, Aichi Cancer Center Hospital, 1-1 Kanokoden, Chikusaku, Nagoya 464-8681, Japan. [4]Department of Otorhinolaryngology, Head and Neck Surgery, University of the Ryukyus, Nakazu, Japan.

References

1. Lebwohl D, Canetta R. Clinical development of platinum complexes in cancer therapy: an historical perspective and an update. Eur J Cancer. 1998; 34(10):1522–34.

2. Daugaard G, Abildgaard U, Holstein-Rathlou NH, Bruunshuus I, Bucher D, Leyssac PP. Renal tubular function in patients treated with high-dose cisplatin. Clin Pharmacol Ther. 1988;44(2):164–72.

3. Schilsky RL, Anderson T. Hypomagnesemia and renal magnesium wasting in patients receiving cisplatin. Ann Intern Med. 1979;90(6):929–31.

4. Vokes EE, Mick R, Vogelzang NJ, Geiser R, Douglas F. A randomised study comparing intermittent to continuous administration of magnesium aspartate hydrochloride in cisplatin-induced hypomagnesaemia. Br J Cancer. 1990;62(6):1015–7.

5. Lajer H, Kristensen M, Hansen HH, Nielsen S, Frokiaer J, Ostergaard LF, Christensen S, Daugaard G, Jonassen TE. Magnesium depletion enhances cisplatin-induced nephrotoxicity. Cancer Chemother Pharmacol. 2005;56(5):535–42.

6. Willox JC, McAllister EJ, Sangster G, Kaye SB. Effects of magnesium supplementation in testicular cancer patients receiving cis-platin: a randomised trial. Br J Cancer. 1986;54(1):19–23.

7. Bodnar L, Wcislo G, Gasowska-Bodnar A, Synowiec A, Szarlej-Wcislo K, Szczylik C. Renal protection with magnesium subcarbonate and magnesium sulphate in patients with epithelial ovarian cancer after cisplatin and paclitaxel chemotherapy: a randomised phase II study. Eur J Cancer. 2008; 44(17):2608–14.

8. Muraki K, Koyama R, Honma Y, Yagishita S, Shukuya T, Ohashi R, Takahashi F, Kido K, Iwakami S, Sasaki S, et al. Hydration with magnesium and mannitol without furosemide prevents the nephrotoxicity induced by cisplatin and pemetrexed in patients with advanced non-small cell lung cancer. J Thorac Dis. 2012;4(6):562–8.

9. Ijichi K, Adachi M, Hasegawa Y, Ogawa T, Nakamura H, Kudoh A, Yasui Y, Murakami S, Ishizaki K. Pretreatment with 5-FU enhances cisplatin cytotoxicity in head and neck squamous cell carcinoma cells. Cancer Chemother Pharmacol. 2008;62(5):745–52.

10. Cockcroft DW, Gault MH. Prediction of creatinine clearance from serum creatinine. Nephron. 1976;16(1):31–41.

11. Basch E, Prestrud AA, Hesketh PJ, Kris MG, Feyer PC, Somerfield MR, Chesney M, Clark-Snow RA, Flaherty AM, Freundlich B, et al. Antiemetics: American Society of Clinical Oncology clinical practice guideline update. J Clin Oncol. 2011;29(31):4189–98.

12. Gonzales-Vitale JC, Hayes DM, Cvitkovic E, Sternberg SS. The renal pathology in clinical trials of cis-platinum (II) diamminedichloride. Cancer. 1977;39(4): 1362–71.

13. Inui KI, Masuda S, Saito H. Cellular and molecular aspects of drug transport in the kidney. Kidney Int. 2000;58(3):944–58.

14. Yokoo K, Murakami R, Matsuzaki T, Yoshitome K, Hamada A, Saito H. Enhanced renal accumulation of cisplatin via renal organic cation transporter deteriorates acute kidney injury in hypomagnesemic rats. Clin Exp Nephrol. 2009;13(6):578–84.

15. Lajer H, Daugaard G. Cisplatin and hypomagnesemia. Cancer Treat Rev. 1999;25(1):47–58.

16. al-Ghamdi SM, Cameron EC, Sutton RA. Magnesium deficiency: pathophysiologic and clinical overview. Am J Kidney Dis. 1994;24(5):737–52.

17. Martin M, Diaz-Rubio E, Casado A, Lopez Vega JM, Sastre J, Almenarez J. Intravenous and oral magnesium supplementations in the prophylaxis of cisplatin-induced hypomagnesemia. Results of a controlled trial. Am J Clin Oncol. 1992;15(4):348–51.

18. Daley-Yates PT, McBrien DC. A study of the protective effect of chloride salts on cisplatin nephrotoxicity. Biochem Pharmacol. 1985;34(13):2363–9.

19. Faig J, Haughton M, Taylor RC, D' Agostino RB Jr, Whelen MJ, Porosnicu Rodriguez KA, Bonomi M, Murea M, Porosnicu M. Retrospective analysis of Cisplatin nephrotoxicity in patients with head and neck cancer receiving outpatient treatment with concurrent high-dose Cisplatin and radiotherapy. Am J Clin Oncol. 2016; [Epub ahead of print]

20. Hanigan MH, Deng M, Zhang L, Taylor PT Jr, Lapus MG. Stress response inhibits the nephrotoxicity of cisplatin. Am J Physiol Renal Physiol. 2005; 288(1):F125–32.

8

Peri-operative factors predisposing to pharyngocutaneous fistula after total laryngectomy: analysis of a large multi-institutional patient cohort

Nicole L. Lebo[1*], Lisa Caulley[1], Hussain Alsaffar[1], Martin J. Corsten[2] and Stephanie Johnson-Obaseki[1]

Abstract

Background: Pharyngocutaneous fistula (PCF) is a problematic complication following total laryngectomy. Disagreement remains regarding predisposing factors. This study examines perioperative factors predicting PCF following total laryngectomy using a large multicenter data registry.

Methods: Retrospective cohort analysis was performed using patients undergoing total laryngectomy in the ACS-NSQIP database for 2006–2014. Sub-analysis was performed based on reconstruction type. Outcome of interest was PCF development within 30 days.

Results: Multivariate analysis of 971 patients was performed. Three variables showed statistical significance in predicting PCF: wound classification of 3 and 4 vs. 1–2 (OR 6.42 $P < 0.0004$ and OR 8.87, $P < 0.0042$), pre-operative transfusion of > 4 units of packed red blood cells (OR 6.28, $P = 0.043$), and free flap versus no flap reconstruction (OR 2.81, $P = 0.008$).

Conclusions: This study identifies important risk factors for development of PCF following total laryngectomy in a large, multi-institutional cohort of patients, thereby identifying a subset of patients at increased risk.

Keywords: Laryngectomy, Pharyngocutaneous fistula, Predisposing factors, National surgical quality improvement program, Peri-operative

Background

Pharyngocutaneous fistula (PCF) is a common, problematic, and frustrating complication following total laryngectomy (TL) – a procedure central to the management of many laryngeal cancers. PCF is associated with longer hospital stays, delays in adjuvant therapy, discomfort, and quality of life loss for patients [1]. Rates of this complication have often been quoted as anywhere from 3 to 65% [2]; a recent meta-analysis suggests rates are within the 10–25% range [3].

Significant disagreement exists regarding predisposing factors for PCF. Most studies investigating risk factors have been relatively small and single center [4–6], which have produced conflicting results. To date, no large, multi-institutional studies using prospectively-gathered data have been published.

Three systematic reviews assessing risk factors for PCF post TL have been published [1, 2, 7]. The most consistently identified risk factors have been a post-operative hemoglobin of < 125 g/L, and a history of radiotherapy. Other factors that have been identified in at least one of the systematic reviews include prior tracheostomy, concurrent neck dissection, tumor subsite (supraglottis), positive surgical margins, advanced primary tumor (T3-T4), history of chronic obstructive pulmonary disease (COPD), receipt of blood transfusion, previous combined chemoradiotherapy, hypopharyngeal involvement, and use of catgut suture during closure [1, 2, 7].

The objective of this study is to bridge the current literature gap by examining perioperative factors predicting

* Correspondence: nlebo045@uottawa.ca
[1]Department of Otolaryngology - Head and Neck Surgery, University of Ottawa, S3, 501 Smyth Road, Ottawa, ON K1H 8L6, Canada
Full list of author information is available at the end of the article

PCF development following TL using data from a large, multi-institutional registry. The ultimate aim of this study is to assist in guiding operative planning and perioperative optimization for TL patients.

Methods

Study design

A retrospective cohort analysis was performed using data from the American College of Surgeons – National Surgical Quality Improvement Program (ACS-NSQIP) database for the years 2006 to 2014. NSQIP is a registry of prospectively-gathered demographic, comorbid, and perioperative variables collected for patients undergoing non-cardiac procedures at participating centers worldwide. The ACS-NSQIP database currently draws data from over 750 hospitals, primarily in the USA, Canada, Australia, and Middle Eastern countries [8]. Data is collected by rigorously-trained nurse reviewers, and has been well-validated [9]. Patients are routinely tracked for 30-days post-operatively. NSQIP data is de-identified, and available to all institutions complying with the ACS-NSQIP Data Use Agreement.

Population

The study population of interest – patients in the NSQIP database undergoing total laryngectomy (primary or salvage) – was isolated using Current Procedural Terminology (CPT) codes. Total laryngectomy procedures were categorized by one of two CPT codes: 31,360 and 31,365 – total laryngectomy without or with radical neck dissection, respectively. Patients undergoing partial or subtotal laryngectomy, and patients undergoing total pharyngectomy with total laryngectomy were excluded from analysis (see Table 1 for summary of relevant CPT codes). Using secondary CPT codes, patients were further divided into three sub-groups based on reconstruction type: patients were classified as having undergone (1) primary closure (i.e., no flap reconstruction), (2) free flap reconstruction, or (3) regional flap reconstruction (classification algorithm summarized in Fig. 1).

Outcome and variables

The primary outcome of interest was development of PCF within 30-days following TL. In the absence of procedure-specific variables, the NSQIP variable "wound-breakdown" was used as a proxy for PCF, recognizing that PCF will represent the majority of these occurrences, but acknowledging that this may capture patients with superficial skin dehiscence as well. The variables analyzed for prediction of PCF were: age, gender, body mass index (BMI), perioperative comorbidities (diabetes, smoking, COPD, congestive heart failure, bleeding disorder, hypertension), functional status, pre-operative wound infection, chronic

Table 1 Relevant Current Procedural Terminology (CPT) Code Definitions

CPT Code	Definition
Primary procedure	
31,360	Laryngectomy; total, without radical neck dissection
31,365	Laryngectomy; total, with radical neck dissection
31,367	Laryngectomy; subtotal supraglottic, without radical neck dissection
31,368	Laryngectomy; subtotal supraglottic, with radical neck dissection
31,370	Partial laryngectomy (hemilaryngectomy); horizontal
31,375	Partial laryngectomy (hemilaryngectomy); laterovertical
31,380	Partial laryngectomy (hemilaryngectomy); anterovertical
31,382	Partial laryngectomy (hemilaryngectomy); antero-latero-vertical
31,390	Pharyngolaryngectomy, with radical neck dissection; without reconstruction
31,395	Pharyngolaryngectomy, with radical neck dissection; with reconstruction
Flap procedure	
15,732	Muscle, myocutaneous, or fasciocutaneous flap; head and neck (eg, temporalis, masseter muscle, sternocleidomastoid, levator scapulae)
15,734	Muscle, myocutaneous, or fasciocutaneous flap; trunk
15,736	Muscle, myocutaneous, or fasciocutaneous flap; upper extremity
15,740	Flap; island pedicle requiring identification and dissection of an anatomically named axial vessel
15,750	Flap; neurovascular pedicle
15,756	Free muscle or myocutaneous flap with microvascular anastomosis
15,757	Free skin flap with microvascular anastomosis
15,758	Free fascial flap with microvascular anastomosis
Other	
31,611	Construction of tracheoesophageal fistula and subsequent insertion of an alaryngeal speech prosthesis (eg, voice button, Blom-Singer prosthesis)

CPT Current Procedural Terminology

steroid use, weight loss, perioperative blood transfusion, American Society of Anesthesia (ASA) classification, wound classification, concomitant tracheoesophageal puncture (TEP) insertion, and type of reconstruction (free flap, regional flap, primary closure). All variables were treated in either binary or categorical fashion (see Table 5 in Results section for detailed NSQIP variable definitions). Of note, the ACS-NSQIP database defines perioperative transfusions into 3 comparison groups: pre-operative transfusion of more than 4 units of pRBCs within 48 h of the operation; intra-operative pRBCs transfused in the operating suite; and postoperative transfusion of more than 4 units of PRBCs within 72 h of the operation. Wound classification was treated as a categorical variable (that is,

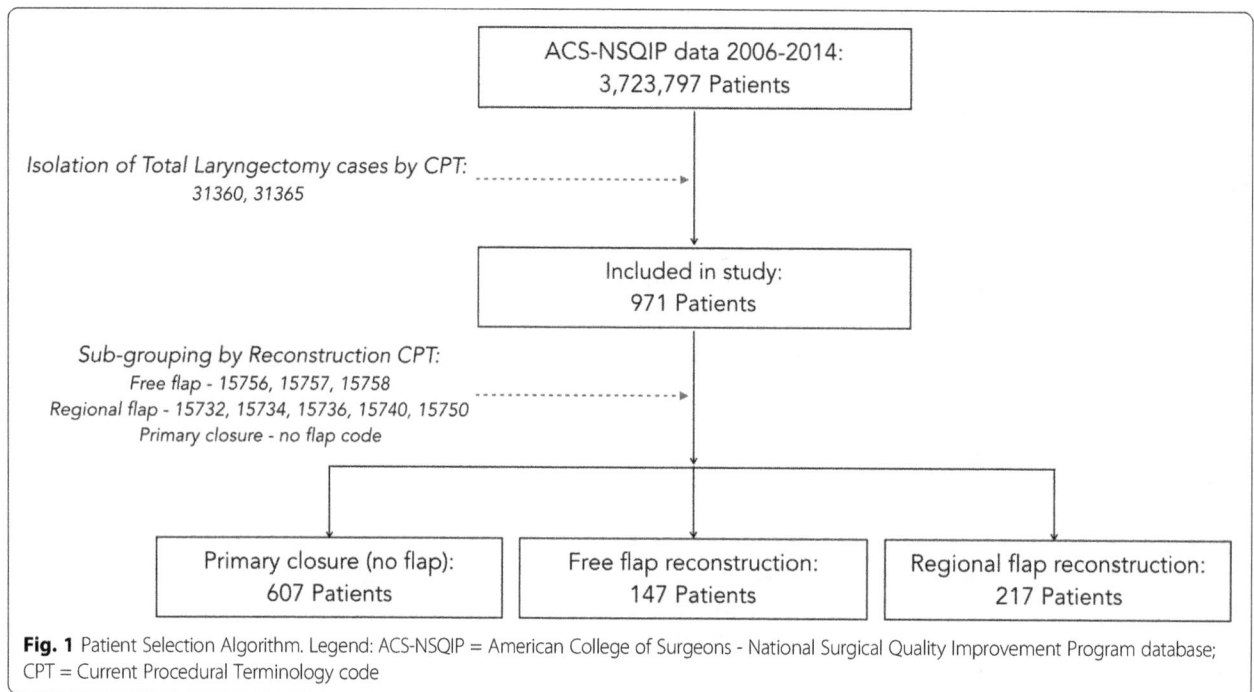

Fig. 1 Patient Selection Algorithm. Legend: ACS-NSQIP = American College of Surgeons - National Surgical Quality Improvement Program database; CPT = Current Procedural Terminology code

1–2, 3 and 4) where sufficient sample size permitted. If insufficient sample size resulted in model instability, the classifications were analyzed as a binomial variable. The variables in the regression analysis were selected because they had either been identified as risk factors for PCF in previous literature, were demographically important, or were relevant to clinical judgment.

Statistical methods
Univariate followed by multivariate logistic regression analysis assessing odds ratios for the above variables were performed for the entire cohort and within groups stratified by reconstruction type. All statistical analysis was performed using SAS 9.3 software (SAS Institute Inc., Cary, NC, USA), with significance defined as $P < 0.05$.

Results
Of the 3,723,897 patients within the ACS-NSQIP database, 971 were identified to meet the study criteria of having undergone a total laryngectomy, with or without radical neck dissection. Of these patients, 607 (62.5%) were closed primarily, 147 (15.1%) were reconstructed using a free flap, and 217 (22.3%) were reconstructed using a regional flap. Patient demographics for the reconstructive groups as well as the population as a whole are detailed in Table 2. Age distribution of patients was fairly consistent between all reconstruction groups, with the mean age of all patients being 62.8 years (SD 11.4). Male-female ratio varied somewhat between groups, with the regional flap group having the highest male-

predominance (M:F 4.95:1), and the free flap group having the lowest (M:F 2.97:1).

Of the 971 total patients, 50 developed PCF, for a rate of 5.1%. Within the subgroups, rates were 3.8% (23/607) for primary closure, 9.5% (14/147) for free-flap reconstruction, and 5.5% (12/217) for regional flap reconstruction. Rates summarized in Table 3.

For the overall group (all patients), a univariate followed by multivariate analysis was performed with each of the variables listed in the methods section; the multivariate results are displayed in Table 4. Three factors were identified through multivariate analysis to be statistically significant predictors of PCF development in the overall group. Wound class – contaminated and dirty (3 and 4) compared to clean/clean-contaminated

Table 2 Study patient demographics – overall and by reconstruction-type sub-grouping

	All patients	1° closure	Free flap	Regional flap
N	971	607	147	217
Gender				
Male	776	483	110	183
Female	195	124	37	37
M:F ratio	3.98	3.90	2.97	4.95
Age (years)				
Mean (std dev)	62.8 (11.4)	63.1 (12.0)	61.6 (10.3)	62.8 (10.7)
Maximum	90	90	83	86
Minimum	20	20	37	31

Std dev standard deviation, *M:F* male to female ratio

Table 3 Rate of pharyngocutaneous fistula development in all patients and by reconstruction type

Group	Rate of PCF development
Overall (all patients)	5.1%
Primary closure	3.8%
Free flap	9.5%
Regional flap	5.5%

PCF Pharyngocutaneous fistula

(1–2) – had the strongest correlation, with an odds ratio of 6.42 (95% CI 2.30–39.45, $P = 0.0004$) and 8.87 (95% CI 1.99–39.45, $P = 0.004$), respectively. The other factors were: transfusion of more than 4 units of packed red blood cells (PRBCs) within 72 h pre-operatively (OR 6.28, 95% CI 1.06–37.30, $P = 0.04$), and reconstruction with a free flap compared to primary closure (OR 2.81, 95% CI 1.31–5.99, $P = 0.008$). A decreased incidence of PCF in patients undergoing regional flaps compared to those with free flaps was suggested but did not reach statistical significance (OR 0.51, 95% CI 0.21–1.24, $P = 0.14$)

For the primary closure group, univariate followed by multivariate analysis was again performed using the same variables. Only variables identified in the univariate analysis as being statistically significant ($P < 0.05$) were included in the multivariate analysis. The results of the multivariate analysis are displayed in Table 5. One statistically significant risk factor was identified in this group: BMI ≥ 18.5 compared to < 18.5 (underweight) with an odds ratio of 0.28 (95% CI 0.11–0.73, $P = 0.009$) – meaning a normal or greater BMI was correlated with lower PCF rates. Of note, one variable (peri/pre-op transfusion) was omitted from the analysis for the primary closure group because of low event numbers causing model instability.

For the free flap reconstruction group, univariate analysis showed no statistically significant risk factors – possibly due to insufficient numbers (only 147 patients in this group) – thus multivariate analysis was not performed. Of note, univariate analysis could not be performed on multiple variables (functional status, history of CHF, ASA class, and peri–/post-op transfusion) because of low event numbers causing model instability.

Table 4 Multivariate regression analysis of risk factors for PCF in all patients

Variable	Comparison	Odds Ratio	95% CI	P-value
Age	Increase by 10 years	1.05	0.78–1.42	0.75
Gender	Male vs. female	0.66	0.32–1.36	0.26
BMI	≥ 18.5 vs. < 18.5 kg/m^2 (underweight)	0.67	0.30–1.51	0.33
Diabetes	Yes vs. no (Identified DM on oral agents or insulin in 30 days pre-op)	1.55	0.64–3.73	0.33
Smoking	Yes vs. no (current smoker within 1 year)	1.48	0.76–2.89	0.24
Functional Status	Dependent vs. independent (in last 30 days)	0.84	0.27–2.63	0.76
COPD history	Yes vs. no (history severe COPD)	0.72	0.31–1.67	0.44
CHF history	Yes vs. no (within last 30 days)	1.33	0.14–12.43	0.80
HTN requiring medication	Yes vs. no	0.81	0.41–1.57	0.52
Pre-op wound infection	Yes vs. no (open or infected wound at site at time of OR)	1.83	0.50–6.71	0.36
Chronic steroid use	Yes vs. no	2.39	0.80–7.20	0.12
Weight loss	> 10% loss in 6mo pre-op vs. < 10%	0.91	0.40–2.06	0.82
Bleeding disorder history	Yes vs. no identified history	1.52	0.31–7.54	0.61
Pre-op transfusion	> 4 units PRBCs vs. ≤ 4 (in 72 h pre-op)	6.28	1.06–37.30	0.04
Wound class	Contaminated vs. Clean/Clean-contaminated	6.28	2.29–17.94	0.0004
	Dirty vs. Clean/Clean-contaminated	8.87	1.99–39.45	0.004
ASA Class	3–5 vs. 1–2	0.93	0.30–2.82	0.89
Peri-op or post-op transfusion	Yes vs. no (any transfusion of PRBC or whole blood from start of OR to 72 h post-op)	0.80	0.09–6.85	0.84
TEP insertion during procedure	Yes vs. no	1.13	0.51–2.50	0.77
Reconstruction type	Free flap vs. Primary closure	2.81	1.31–5.99	0.008
	Regional flap vs. Primary closure	1.45	0.67–3.11	0.34
	Regional flap vs. Free flap	0.51	0.21–1.24	0.14

PCF Pharyngocutaneous fistula, *CI* confidence interval, *BMI* body mass index, *DM* diabetes mellitus, *COPD* chronic obstructive pulmonary disease, *CHF* congestive heart failure, *HTN* hypertension, *PRBCs* packed red blood cells, *ASA* American Society of Anesthesiologists, *TEP* tracheoesophageal puncture

Table 5 Multivariate regression analysis of risk factors for PCF in patients receiving primary closure

Variable	Comparison	Odds Ratio	95% CI	P-value
Age	Increase by 10 years	0.99	0.68–1.43	0.95
Gender	Male vs. female	0.94	0.33–2.70	0.91
BMI	≥ 18.5 vs. < 18.5 kg/m^2 (underweight)	0.28	0.11–0.73	0.009
Pre-op wound infection	Yes vs. no	5.12	0.88–29.63	0.068
Chronic steroid use	Yes vs. no	3.28	0.89–12.13	0.07
Wound class	Contaminated vs. Clean/Clean-contaminated	3.01	0.56–16.16	0.20
	Dirty vs Clean/Clean-contaminated	2.50	0.24–26.38	0.44

PCF Pharyngocutaneous fistula, *CI* confidence interval, *BMI* body mass index

For the regional flap reconstruction group, univariate analysis showed only one statistically significant risk factor: wound class – contaminated/dirty (3–4) compared to clean/clean-contaminated (1–2) – with OR 17.6 (95% CI 4.57–67.71, $P < 0.0001$). Wound class could not be analyzed as a categorical variable for this subgroup due to small sample sizes in the contaminated and dirty cohorts. Multivariate analysis was not performed. Of note, again for this group, multiple variables had to be omitted from univariate analysis because of insufficient event numbers (history of CHF, wound infection/open wound at time of operation, chronic steroid use, bleeding disorder, and pre-op transfusion).

Discussion

For head and neck surgeons and patients alike, PCF is a frustrating complication following total laryngectomy. Much effort has been expended by single institutions to investigate rates and predisposing factors for PCF [4–6] to guide potential preventative measures and identify those at high risk for such a complication. Our goal was to fill the current literature gap using a large, prospectively-gathered, multi-institutional database to study PCF risk factors, with the goal of improving understanding, and providing higher quality evidence via access to a larger study population.

Of the 917 patients included in this study, 50 (5.1%) developed PCF. This falls within the classically quoted 3–65% range in literature [2]. It is, however, lower than rates identified in recent single-institution studies, which have been in the 30–35% range [4–6]. Given the wide range of PCF rates identified between centers, it is particularly advantageous here to access and analyze a large database like NSQIP with rigorous and consistent data collection to help dilute what appears to be an institution/surgeon-dependent influence on PCF rate.

With respect to identified risk factors for PCF in all-comers, our analysis determined three factors to be of statistical significance. The first of these was wound class (contaminated or dirty, compared to clean or clean-contaminated). We observed an incremental increase in odds of PCF with progression from contaminated to

dirty wound classification (OR 6.42 vs 8.87, respectively), which lends further strength to this finding. Wound classification was not a factor identified in any of the three systematic reviews [1, 2, 7] as predisposing to PCF, although it is clinically intuitive as a risk factor for wound breakdown secondary to infection. Wound infection has been identified as a risk factor in a single institution study previously [10]. In addition, more advanced wound class may also reflect tumor involvement of the skin causing an open wound at the time of OR – a finding consistent with advanced tumor stage. Advanced tumor stage has been identified in numerous studies as an independent risk factor for PCF development [7, 11, 12]. In the same vein, existing tracheostomy at time of OR could also explain an advanced wound classification; prior tracheostomy has also been found in a number of studies to be a predictor of PCF [2, 4, 13]. Surgeons should exercise extreme vigilance in monitoring these patients in the post-operative setting given their high risk status for PCF. Neither tumor stage nor prior tracheostomy were captured in the NSQIP data, thus these factors were not assessed independently in this study. Of note, pre-operative wound infection was not found to be significant in the univariate regression analysis in our study. The reason for this finding is likely two-fold: 1) small sample size, and 2) surgeon selection bias. In our study, only 30 of 971 patients were identified with wound infection. As such, it is possible that the parameter did not reach significance in our regression model due to lack of statistical power in the cohort analysis. In addition, there is likely a component of surgeon selection bias as these patients would be treated preoperatively and only few patients would present to the OR with active wound infection. Future studies with larger sample sizes would be necessary to offer greater sensitivity for this particular covariate.

The second risk factor for PCF identified in the overall group was transfusion of more than 4 units of PRBCs within 72 h pre-operatively. This is consistent with systematic review findings that transfusion and anemia (HGB < 125 g/L) are significant risk factors [1, 2, 7]. Of note, while pre-operative transfusion was correlated with PCF in our study, peri- and post-operative transfusion were not found to be significantly so. This likely reflects different indication for transfusion in these two time periods; pre-operative transfusion is likely triggered by pre-operative anemia, which often reflects chronic disease and poor nutritional status, which are established risks for poor wound healing [14]. Peri- and post-operative transfusions, on the other hand, are likely triggered by intraoperative blood loss, which is unlikely to be related to the patient's nutritional status. These findings would emphasize the need for pre-operative management of nutritional and immune status in surgical patients. With optimization of surgical patients and close post-operative monitoring, it is possible that the rates of post-operative complications due to this subset of patients may decline.

The third factor identified in our total population was reconstruction with a free flap compared to primary closure. This is an interesting finding given previous literature suggesting that use of free flaps is protective against wound breakdown compared to wounds closed primarily [3, 4, 15]. We suspect this aberrant finding is secondary to confounding effects of a disproportionate number of patients undergoing free flap closure having had previous radiation compared to the primary closure group, since a history of local radiation is often the indication for free-tissue transfer. Previous radiotherapy has been fairly consistently identified as a risk factor for PCF in the literature [1, 2, 7, 16], however, radiation exposure is not well captured in the NSQIP database, and thus this factor could not be controlled for (NSQIP only records radiation therapy received within 30 days prior to operation; salvage laryngectomy usually occurs more than 30 days after primary radiotherapy). These findings should prompt further consideration of primary closure of the neopharynx where surgically feasible in total laryngectomies. Further studies are needed to better determine the risk of wound breakdown in previously radiated patients. Regardless, surgical patients who do require free flap reconstruction should be closely monitored for signs of PCF in the post-operative setting.

We then divided our analysis of factors predicting PCF by reconstruction-type: primary closure, regional flap closure and free tissue transfer (free flap). This particular stratified analysis was performed to control for selection bias introduced by surgeon choice in reconstruction-type. Beginning with the primary closure group, multivariate analysis identified being underweight (BMI < 18.5) at time of OR was identified as an effect modifier for PCF in this subgroup of patients. Interestingly, BMI is a unique risk factor not identified in the overall group. The correlation of low BMI with increased rates of PCF is consistent with the finding of several studies that have identified pre-operative albumin (as a proxy for pre-operative nutritional status) as a risk factor for PCF [17–19]. This is also

consistent with our earlier discussion supposing pre-operative anemia predisposes to PCF because it reflects poor pre-operative nutritional status. These findings would again support the need for pre-operative optimization of nutritional and immune status and vigilant monitoring in the post-operative setting for patients with these identified risk factors. Of note, the PCF rate for the primary closure group was quite low, at 3.8%. This may be the result of bias towards primary laryngectomy instead of salvage laryngectomy in this group, as a primary (i.e., non-radiated) field is more amenable to primary closure. Accordingly, similar to the comparison between closure types, incomplete capture of previous radiation may be influencing these results as well. Multivariate analysis could not be performed for the other two subgroups. In the regional flap group, only one statistically significant risk factor was identified with univariate analysis: wound class – contaminated/dirty (3–4) compared to clean/clean-contaminated (1–2). Low numbers precluded us from performing a multivariate analysis in this group. Similarly, in the free flap group, multivariate analysis could not be performed.

While NSQIP is a useful tool due to its size and multi-institutional nature that allows for generalizability for results, there are limitations in its use, as there are with all databases. The key limitations of this study are: (1) confounding effects from variables not captured by NSQIP, (2) low event numbers once patients divided into subgroups, (3) selection bias from surgeon selection of reconstruction type, and (4) information bias from reliance on retrospective data. With respect to the first limitation – NSQIP is a general surgical database, thus data is not captured with laryngectomy and its complications specifically in mind. As we are accessing the data retrospectively, we are limited to what is currently available in the database, which unfortunately does not capture a number of variables that are suspected to influence laryngectomy outcomes, such as: previous tracheostomy, previous radiotherapy or chemotherapy (beyond 30 days pre-operatively), tumor staging, tumor subsite, and surgical margins. Accordingly, these variables could not be controlled for in our analysis and further studies are needed to establish the impact of these variables in the rates of PCF development. As such, the risk factors that we identified in our study may not be an exhaustive list of potential predictors of post-operative PCF. With respect to the second limitation – despite the size of the NSQIP database, once divided into groups for further analysis based on reconstruction type, low event numbers within the groups limit meaningful analysis. Particularly in the free flap and regional flap groups, where either one or no variables were identified as statistically significant risk factors on univariate analysis, risk of type II error was clearly higher than in the overall group.

Only within the primary closure group, with 607 patients, were we able to perform a meaningful multivariate analysis.

An important limitation to recognize in this particular study is the bias introduced by the use of "wound-breakdown" as a proxy for PCF, in the absence of targeted documentation of PCF occurrence. As previously discussed, PCF will represent the majority of these "wound-breakdowns" and thus is a reasonable parameter to measure for this research question. However, there is a risk of positive bias due to the fact that our measured rate may represent an overestimate of PCF rate amongst our population. One would expect patients with only superficial incisional dehiscence to be included in this catchment, thereby artificially inflating the measured rate. As well, this parameter has the potential to introduce negative bias if the measured rate underestimates the risk of PCF due to misclassification of PCF by surgeons or data entry technicians. However, the rate of PCF was found to be 5.1%, which falls within the classically quoted 3–65% range in literature [2]. This allowed for reassurance that this parameter was still able to represent the outcome of interest with measured accuracy.

Despite these limitations, our study does derive strength from the high quality of the NSQIP database, which draws information from hundreds of centers to provide large samples sizes, has rigorous data collection methods with trained data collectors, and is prospectively gathered. In addition, the fact that the database draws from many centers worldwide improves the generalizability of our results.

Conclusion

In summary, this is the largest multi-center study evaluating the risk factors for PCF using prospectively-gathered data to date. Identified statistically significant risk factors of PCF for all-comers were: wound class, pre-operative transfusion, and free-flap reconstruction compared to primary closure. These factors should prompt surgeons to consider close monitoring in the post-operative setting for PCF, given the higher risk in these selected patients. As the NSQIP data set continues to evolve, particularly to include more patients and procedure-targeted data, more in-depth and nuanced analysis will become possible.

Abbreviations
ACS-NSQIP: American college of surgeons national surgical quality improvement program; ASA: American society of anaesthesia; BMI: Body mass index; CHF: Congestive heart failure; CI: Confidence interval; COPD: Chronic obstructive pulmonary disease; CPT: Current procedural terminology; DM: Diabetes mellitus; HGB: Hemoglobin; HTN: Hypertension; PCF: Pharyngocutaneous fistula; PRBCs: Packed red blood cells; TEP: Tracheoesophageal puncture; TL: Total laryngectomy

Acknowledgements
None.

Funding
No funding to declare.

Authors' contributions
NLL was involved in study design, data interpretation, and was the primary contributor to the manuscript. LC was involved in data analysis and interpretation, as well as drafting of the manuscript. HA was involved in study design, data interpretation, and drafting of the manuscript. MJC was involved in study design and drafting of the manuscript. SJO was involved in study design, data interpretation, and drafting of the manuscript. All authors read and approved the final manuscript.

Competing interests
The authors declare that they have no competing interests.

Author details
[1]Department of Otolaryngology - Head and Neck Surgery, University of Ottawa, S3, 501 Smyth Road, Ottawa, ON K1H 8L6, Canada. [2]Department of Otolaryngology, Aurora Health Care, Aurora St. Luke's Hospital, Milwaukee, WI, USA.

References
1. Liang J, Li Z, Li S, Fang F, Zhao Y, Li Y. Pharyngocutaneous fistula after total laryngectomy : a systematic review and meta-analysis of risk factors. Auris Nasus Larynx. 2015;42(5):353–9.
2. Paydarfar JA, Birkmeyer NJ. Complications in head and neck surgery. Arch Otolaryngol Head Neck Surg. 2015;132:67–72.
3. Sayles M, Grant DG. Preventing Pharyngo-Cutaneous fistula in Total Laryngectomy : a systematic review and meta-analysis. Laryngoscope. 2014; 124(May):1150–63.
4. Benson EM, Hirata RM, Thompson CB, et al. Pharyngocutaneous fistula after total laryngectomy: a single-institution experience, 2001-2012. Am J Otolaryngol Head Neck Med Surg. 2015;36(1):24–31.
5. Cavalot AL, Gervasio CF, Nazionale G, et al. Pharyngocutaneous fistula as a complication of total laryngectomy: review of the literature and analysis of case records. Otolaryngol Head Neck Surg. 2000;123(5):587–92.
6. Mäkitie AA, Niemensivu R, Hero M, et al. Pharyngocutaneous fistula following total laryngectomy: a single institution's 10-year experience. Eur Arch Otorhinolaryngol. 2006;263(12):1127–30.
7. Dedivitis A, Aires FT, Cernea CR, Brand LG. Pharyngocutaneous fistula after total laryngectomy : systematic review of risk factors. Head Neck. 2015:1691–7.
8. American College of Surgeons. ACS National Surgical Quality Improvement Program® (ACS NSQIP®). https://www.facs.org/quality-programs/acs-nsqip (2016). Accessed October 1, 2016.
9. Khuri SF, Daley J, Henderson W, et al. The Department of Veterans Affairs' NSQIP: the first national, validated, outcome-based, risk-adjusted, and peer-controlled program for the measurement and enhancement of the quality of surgical care. National VA surgical quality improvement program. Ann Surg. 1998;228(4):491–507.
10. Markou KD, Vlachtsis KC, Nikolaou AC, Petridis DG, Kouloulas AI, Daniilidis IC. Incidence and predisposing factors of pharyngocutaneous fistula formation after total laryngectomy. Is there a relationship with tumor recurrence? Eur Arch Otorhinolaryngol. 2004;261(2):61–7.
11. Grau C, Johansen LV, Hansen HS, et al. Salvage laryngectomy and pharyngocutaneous fistulae after primary radiotherapy for head and neck cancer: a national survey from Dahanca. Head Neck. 2003;25(9):711–6.
12. Soylu L, Kiroğlu M, Aydoğan B, et al. Pharyngocutaneous fistula following laryngectomy. Head Neck. 1998;20(1):22–5.
13. Dedivitis RA, Ribeiro KCB, Castro MAF, Nascimento PC. Pharyngocutaneous fistula following total laryngectomy. Acta Otorhinolaryngol Ital. 2007;27(1):2–5.
14. Barbul A, Efron DT, Kavalaukas SL. Wound Healing. In: Brunicardi FC, Anderson DK, Billiard TR, et al. Schwartz's Principles of Surgery, 10th Edition. Chapter 9. New York: McGraw-Hill Education; 2015:

15. Patel UA, Moore BA, Wax M, et al. Impact of pharyngeal closure technique on fistula after salvage laryngectomy. JAMA Otolaryngol Head Neck Surg. 2013;139(11):1156–62.

16. Dirven R, Swinson BD, Gao K, Clark JR. The assessment of pharyngocutaneous fistula rate in patients treated primarily with definitive radiotherapy followed by salvage surgery of the larynx and hypopharynx. Laryngoscope. 2009;119(9):1691–5.

17. Kong H, Wang Y, Zheng J. Analysis of predisposing factor for pharyngocutaneous fistula in laryngeal carcinoma patients. Otolaryngol - Head Neck Surg (U S). 2014;151(1 SUPPL. 1):P156.

18. Boscolo-Rizzo P, De Cillis G, Marchiori C, Carpenè S, Da Mosto MC. Multivariate analysis of risk factors for pharyngocutaneous fistula after total laryngectomy. Eur Arch Otorhinolaryngol. 2008;265:929–36.

19. Pinar E, Oncel S, Colli C, Guclu E, Tatar B. Pharyngocutaneous fistula after total laryngectomy: emphasis on lymph node metastases as a new predisposing factor. J Otolaryngol - Head Neck Surg. 2008;37(3):312–8.

9

Treatment of early stage Supraglottic squamous cell carcinoma: meta-analysis comparing primary surgery versus primary radiotherapy

Krupal B. Patel, Anthony C. Nichols, Kevin Fung, John Yoo and S. Danielle MacNeil*

Abstract

Objectives: For early stage supraglottic squamous cell carcinoma (SCC), single modality treatment either in the form of primary organ preservation surgery alone or radiation alone is recommended. Thus, a definite treatment strategy for early stage supraglottic SCC remains undefined. The primary objective of this study was to conduct a systematic review and meta-analysis comparing the oncologic outcomes of surgery and radiotherapy in early stage (Stage I and II) T1 N0 and T2 N0 supraglottic SCC.

Methods: Systematic methods were used to identify published and unpublished data. Two reviewers independently screened all titles, abstracts and articles for relevance using predefined criteria. Pooled odds ratios (ORs) and 95% confidence intervals (CIs) were calculated.

Results: Five studies met the inclusion criteria for disease specific mortality with a total of 2864 pooled patients. 5-year disease specific mortality was lower in the surgery group (ORs 0.43, 95% CI 0.31–0.60). Four studies met the inclusion criteria for 5-year overall mortality with a total of 2790 pooled patients. Five-year overall mortality was lower in surgery group (ORs 0.40, 95% CI 0.29–0.55).

Conclusions: This is the first study to examine the management of early stage supraglottic SCC using meta-analytic methodology. Our results suggest that primary surgery may result in decreased disease specific and overall mortality compared to primary radiotherapy.

Keywords: Early stage, Supraglottic squamous cell carcinoma, Supraglottic SCC, Outcomes, Meta-analysis

Background

Early stage supraglottic squamous cell carcinoma (SSCC) is defined as T1 (tumor limited to one subsite of supraglottis with normal vocal cord mobility) or T2 (tumor invading more than one adjacent subsite of supraglottis or glottis or region outside of supraglottis), with no regional nodal spread [1]. In a large review of nearly 160,000 cases of laryngeal SCC in the United States, the incidence of SSCC was noted to be 33% [2]. National Comprehensive Cancer Network (NCCN) guidelines for treatment of early stage SSCC suggest either organ

preservation strategy – surgery with/without neck dissection or definitive radiation (RT) [3]. Early stage SSCC are small, however the 5-year survival of early stage SSCC is 64% [4, 5]. This is thought to be due to rich lymphatic supply of the area making it more likely to have occult regional and distant metastasis. Over the last 30 years, the oncologic outcomes for SSCC have not improved [2, 5, 6]. In fact, a review of National Cancer Database found that 5-year relative survival from SSCC decreased 52.2% (1985–1987) to 47.3% (1994–1996). The greatest decline in survival was in early stage SSCC patients with T1 N0 and T2 N0 disease.

Despite the poor survival of patients with early stage SSCC, there are a limited number of studies that have directly compared the survival outcomes of surgery

* Correspondence: Danielle.MacNeil@lhsc.on.ca
Department of Otolaryngology – Head & Neck Surgery, Schulich Medicine & Dentistry, London Health Sciences Centre, Western University, Victoria Hospital, London, ON, Canada

versus radiation for early stage SSCC [7–16]. There are no prospective clinical trials, and the majority of the studies reported are small and retrospective. To date no meta-analysis comparing the survival outcomes for early stage SSCC comparing radiation and surgery has been reported. Our objectives were to, systematically review the literature to find all the relevant studies directly comparing surgery with radiation for early stage SSSC, synthesize the results and perform meta-analysis when possible of overall survival, disease specific survival and loco-regional control.

Methods

A systematic review protocol was developed a priori to ensure the objectives and aims were outlined from the outset. This was approved by PROSPERO in November 2015 (CRD42015026590).

Randomized controlled trials, head-to-head comparative studies, observational studies, case series (greater than 3 patients) were assessed. Studies comparing surgery (open organ preservation (OPS), transoral endoscopic laser microsurgery (TLM) or transoral robotic surgery(TORS)) with/without neck dissection to definitive radiotherapy (RT) were included. Single arm studies that reported results of open surgery, transoral surgery alone or radiotherapy alone were not considered., due to the inherent selection biases and lack of ability to compare results between different modalities of treatment. The study population was limited to patients aged 18 and older and diagnosed with early stage supraglottic SCC (Tis, T1 N0, T2 N0).

Included studies were assessed for the following oncologic outcomes: 5-year overall mortality (OM); 5-year disease-specific mortality (DSM); 5-year local control (LC); 5-year laryngectomy free survival (LFS); and functional outcomes (quality of life, swallowing and voice quality).

Computerized bibliographic databases: Medline, EMBASE and Cochrane Central Register of Controlled Trials were searched to identify studies. English language records were included from January 1990 to May 2015. Search strategy was designed by two authors (K.B.P and S.D.M.) and an experienced librarian.

Two authors (K.B.P and S.D.M.) reviewed the titles, abstracts and full texts of the studies independently, with disagreements resolved by consensus. Interobserver agreement was analyzed with quadratic-weighted kappa. Titles were screened for the keywords: "squamous cell carcinoma" and "supraglottic", or "supraglottis", or "glottic", or "glottis", or "larynx", or "laryngeal". All abstracts of the studies that met the eligibility criteria were then screened. The full text of studies that met the criteria were then included. Newcastle-Ottawa quality assessment scale for cohort studies was used determine the quality of the studies [17]. The relevant data on outcome

measures were extracted with the use of standardized data extraction forms. Not all studies contained data on all of the outcome measures.

Statistical Analysis was performed by Review Manager 5.3. Dichotomous outcomes were compared using odds ratios (OR) or weighted mean differences and 95% confidence intervals (CI). Heterogeneity across the studies was evaluated by the chi-square statistic and significance was set at $p < 0.1$. The I2 test was used to measure the extent of inconsistency among results. Fixed effects model was used given the assumption that included studies are only representative samples of all potentially available studies. The Z statistic was used to test for overall pooled effect and significance was set at $p < 0.05$.

Results

The search strategy produced 5867 records. After removing 2026 duplicate records, the final number of unique records was 3841. After reviewing 3841 titles, 1098 studies were selected for reviewing the abstracts. Sixty-two abstracts were deemed appropriate for inclusion. After reviewing abstracts, 16 studies were deemed appropriate for inclusion and the full text was reviewed. Only 7 studies met the final inclusion criteria after reviewing the full text. Figure 1 illustrates the PRISMA (Preferred Reporting Items for Systematic Reviews and Meta-Analyses) flow chart to identify the appropriate studies. Kappa statistic for the agreement at the abstract screening stage was 0.57 (CI 0.46–0.67).

Study characteristics and methodologic quality

No randomized controlled trials were found that compared the oncologic and functional outcomes of primary surgery versus RT. Of the seven studies included in the analysis, seven were retrospective and none were prospective in design. The total number of patients was 418 in the surgical arm, with patients undergoing organ preservation surgery with or without neck dissections. There were 2397 patients in the RT arm. Characteristics of the included studies are summarized in Table 1. Table 2 summarizes number of patients in each treatment group. Table 3 summarizes the quality of the included studies.

Oncologic outcomes

Of the seven studies included that were head-to-head studies, all seven contained data on oncologic outcome. Among them, data on overall survival were reported in four studies, data on disease specific survival were reported in five studies, data on local control were reported in one study.

Median age of the patients in the included studies was similar across the different studies. There were similar number of T1 and T2 patients within the RT

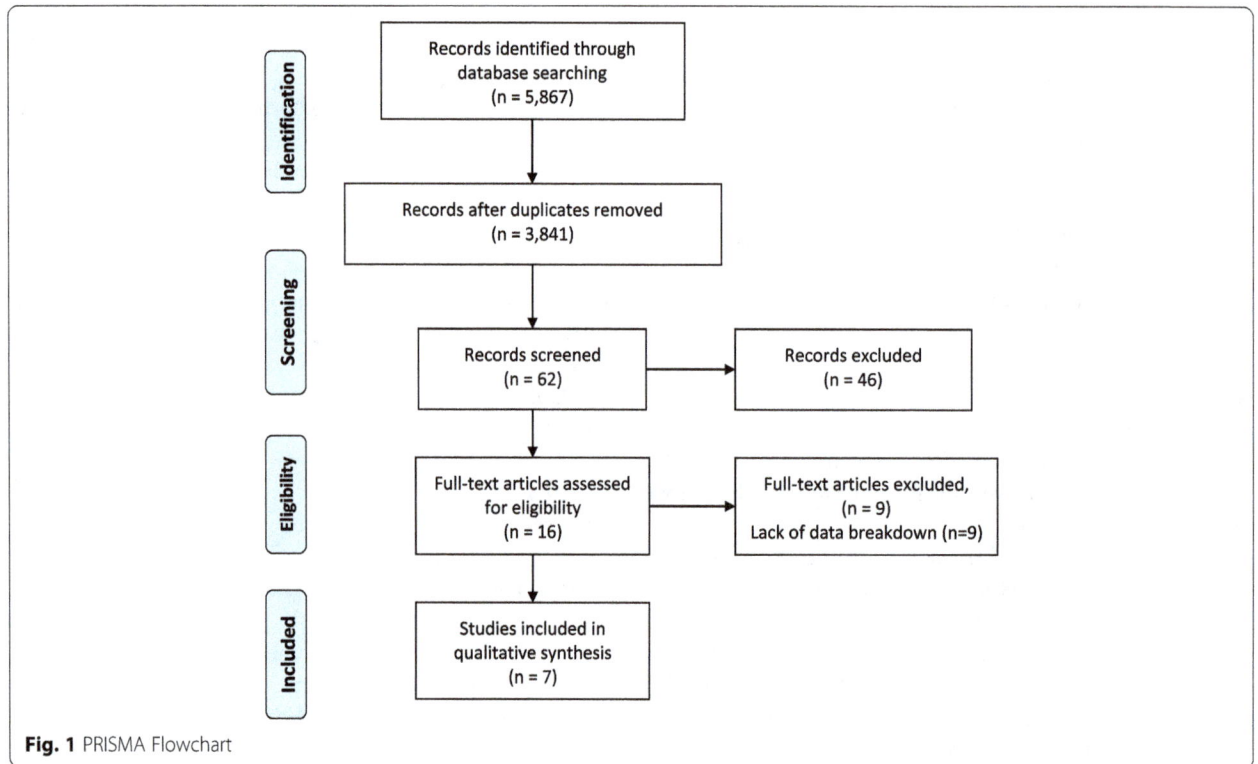

Fig. 1 PRISMA Flowchart

and OPS groups for each study. There were higher number of patients in the RT group compared to the OPS +/− ND group.

5-year overall mortality (OM)

With respect to 5-year OM, in the head-to-head studies, there were 403 patients in the OPS with/without arm and 2387 patients in the RT arm in four studies. The results of pooled effect showed that the OR was 0.4 with 95% CI 0.29–0.55 favoring OPS with/without ND (Fig. 2).

5-year disease-specific mortality (DSM)

With respect to 5-year DSM, in the head-to-head studies, there were 310 patients in the OPS with/without ND arm and 2554 patients in the RT arm in five studies. The

results of pooled effect showed that the OR was 0.43 with 95% CI 0.31–0.59 favoring OPS with/without ND (Fig. 3).

5-year local control (LC)

With respect to 5-year LC, in the head-to-head studies, there were 25 patients in the OPS arm and 90 patients in the RT arm in one study. The results of pooled effect showed that the OR was 0.71 with 95% CI 0.22–2.32 (Fig. 4).

5-year larynx preservation

No head-to-head studies were identified that compared the laryngeal preservation after surgery and radiotherapy.

Table 1 Demographic characteristics of studies comparing survival outcomes between Surgery and Radiotherapy

Study	Median Age (years)		Gender (M/F)		Median Follow up (years)	
	RT	OPS	RT	OPS	RT	OPS
Arshad 2014 [7]	63	58	1476/802	119/48	NR	NR
Jones 2004 [10]	63[a]	61[a]	NR	NR	8.5	9.6
Orus 2000 [12]	63.5[a]	58.1[a]	NR	NR	1.5	
Santos 1998 [13]	56		NR	NR	NR	
Sessions 2005 [14]	N/A	N/A	NR	NR	> 5	
Spector 1995 [15]	61.3		41/12		NR	NR
Spriano 1997 [16]	62		141/16		5	

[a]numbers represent means Abbreviations: *RT* Radiotherapy, *OPS* Organ Preservation Surgery, *NR* Not Reported

Table 2 Staging characteristics of studies comparing survival outcomes between Surgery and Radiotherapy

Study	RT		OPS +/− ND	
	T1	T2	T1	T2
Arshad 2014 [7]	1043	1235	92	75
Jones 2004[a] [10]	90		41	
Orus 2000[b] [12]	27	63	11	14
Santos 1998[c] [13]	3	6	3	6
Sessions 2005 [14]	5	5	90	102
Spector 1995[d] [15]	4	1	1	2
Spriano 1997[a] [16]	91		66	

RT Radiotherapy, *OPS* Organ Preservation Surgery, *ND* Neck Dissection
[a]T1 and T2 reported together, [b]All OPS patients received ND, 7 patients received post-operative RT, [c]Patients received post-operative RT, [d]Only Aryepiglottic fold

Functional outcomes
No head-to-head studies were identified that compared the functional outcomes after surgery and radiotherapy.

Discussion
To our knowledge, this is the first meta-analysis comparing the survival outcomes of surgery versus radiotherapy for early-stage SSCC. Pooled analysis for 5-year OM favors OPS with/without ND over RT with OR of 0.4 (95% CI 0.29–0.55). These results however do need to be interpreted with caution as the heterogeneity was high amongst the studies with a significant *p*-value for the heterogeneity. Pooled analysis for 5-year DSM favors OPS with/without ND over RT with OR of 0.43 (95% CI 0.31–0.59). In this case the heterogeneity was low amongst the studies with a non-significant p-value for

the heterogeneity, thus suggesting that these results are valid. Additionally, a jack-knife analysis was done to determine the validity of the results and to ensure that excessive contribution by one of the studies was not skewing the conclusions. The results of the jack-knife analysis produced similar results which were statistically significant and favoring OPS with/without ND. Only one study examined rate of local control which also showed better outcomes with OPS. Unfortunately, functional comparisons could not be made due to paucity of studies in the literature.

Strengths
This review has several strengths. The review was designed, conducted and reported in accordance with published guidelines (PRISMA) and our protocol and search strategy was published a priori. To our knowledge, this is the first comprehensive review of all available literature comparing surgery versus radiation for patients with early stage SSCC. A comprehensive search strategy was undertaken and led to the review of 3841 unique citations of which seven studies met our inclusion criteria. This resulted in the analysis of 3086 patients with early stage SSCC.

Limitations
There were no head-to-head studies that compared TLM or TORS to RT in oncologic or functional outcomes for early stage supraglottic cancer. As with all meta-analyses, the strength of the conclusions that can be drawn from this study depend on the quality of the primary studies. Although, we only included studies published from 1990 and onwards, some of the studies in our review included patients treated

Table 3 Quality of the studies reporting survival outcomes between Surgery and Radiotherapy (Newcastle-Ottawa Scale)[†]

Study	Selection				Comparability	Outcome			Score[*]
	Representativeness of exposed cohort	Selection of non exposed cohort	Ascertainment of exposure	Outcome not present at outset of study		Assessment	F/U Length	Adequacy of F/U	
Arshad 2014 [7]	*	*	*	*	**	*	*	*	9
Jones 2004 [10]	*	*	*	*	**	*	*	*	9
Orus 2000 [12]	*	*	*	*		*	*	*	7
Santos 1998 [13]	*	*	*	*	*	*	*		7
Sessions 2005 [14]	*	*	*	*		*	*	*	7
Spector 1995 [15]	*	*	*	*	**	*	*	*	9
Spriano 1997 [16]	*	*	*	*	*	*	*	*	8

[*]Maximum total score that a study can get is 9
[†]A study can receive a maximum of 1 asterisk for each numbered item within the selection and outcome categories. A maximum of 2 asterisks can be given for comparability

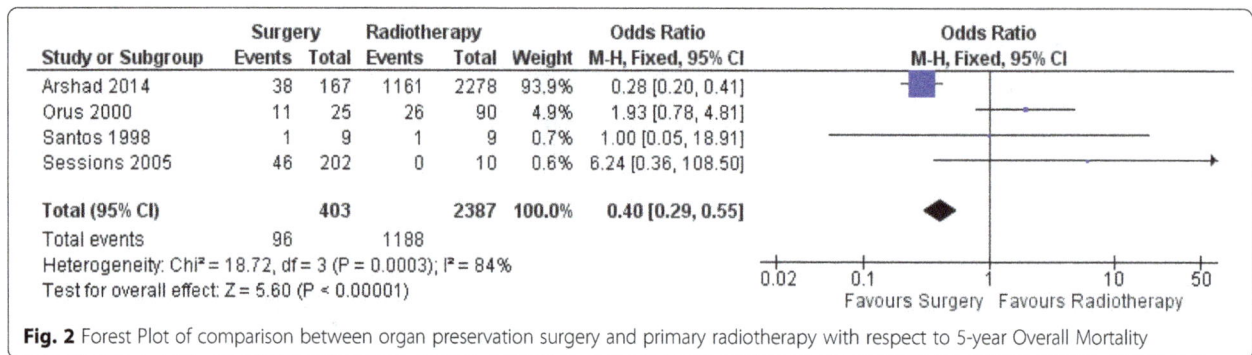

Fig. 2 Forest Plot of comparison between organ preservation surgery and primary radiotherapy with respect to 5-year Overall Mortality

well before that time period. Due to poor quality of CT scanners before 1990, some patients may have had regional nodal disease (thus advanced stage disease) which was not apparent on a poor quality scan. Additionally, many of the contemporary modalities of treatment such intensity modulated radiotherapy (IMRT), Chemo-radiotherapy, TLM and TORS were not in clinical practice prior to 1990. All seven studies that met the inclusion criteria were retrospective, there were no randomized controlled trials. Retrospective studies have their inherent biases including selection biases, wherein patients with other health comorbidities would have been poor surgical candidates and would have likely received radiotherapy. Significant heterogeneity was noted between the studies. Not all studies included the type of radiation and the radiotherapy protocol used to treat these SSCC, the recruitment period for the patients was different which may have resulted in different radiotherapy protocols being used for the patients. In the surgical group, not all patients may have received the same extent of surgery including elective neck dissections. With regards to weight of the individual studies, Arshad et al. had the majority of the patients that were included in our analysis and thus their study was weighted proportionally larger skewing the results [7]. We only considered English

language studies for our meta-analysis; this did limit the number of titles screened and studies included however, the effect of this would likely be small. OR were used for our statistical analysis as time to event (Hazard Ratios) could not be used given the lack of consistency in reporting the outcomes in the included studies.

Surgery and radiotherapy for early stage SSCC

There are several advantages of RT. Although we did not find any head-to-head comparison studies assessing functional outcomes of RT in SSCC, it has been reported to have better functional outcomes in glottic cancers. Additionally, RT can be used in patients who are not candidates for OPS due to their underlying medical conditions. Risks of using RT in treating early stage SSCC is that this patient population does have a higher risk of developing a second primary malignancy in the aerodigestive tract [4, 5, 18]. If radiation is used as the primary treatment modality, most patients can only be salvaged with surgery and in the case of recurrent or new laryngeal cancer the treatment is almost always total laryngectomy.

Surgical approaches include open surgery or transoral surgical approaches, including laser (TLM) and robotic (TORS) and has several advantages over RT. As mentioned, patients with SSCC have a reasonable 5-year overall survival rates with a risk of developing

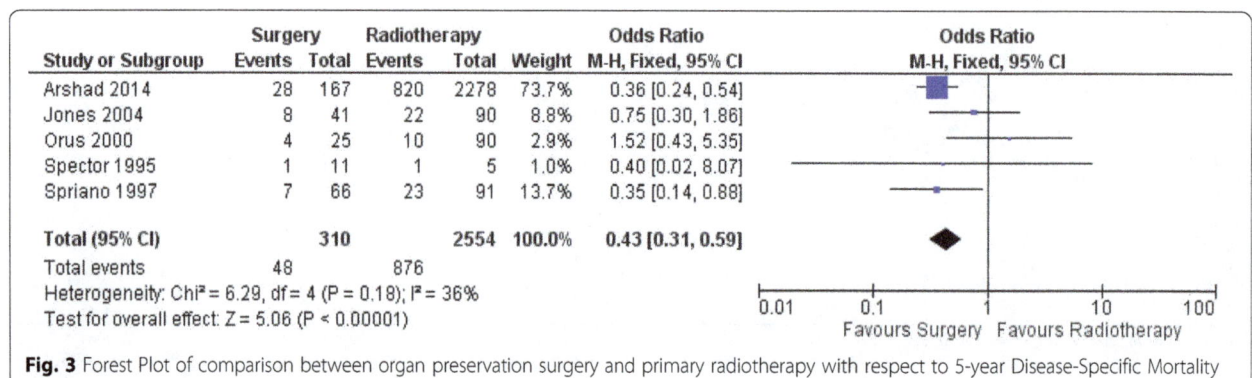

Fig. 3 Forest Plot of comparison between organ preservation surgery and primary radiotherapy with respect to 5-year Disease-Specific Mortality

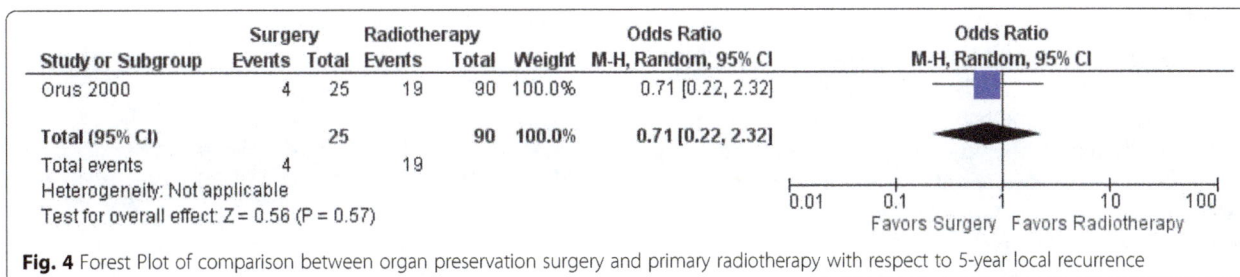

Study or Subgroup	Surgery Events	Total	Radiotherapy Events	Total	Weight	Odds Ratio M-H, Random, 95% CI
Orus 2000	4	25	19	90	100.0%	0.71 [0.22, 2.32]
Total (95% CI)		25		90	100.0%	0.71 [0.22, 2.32]
Total events	4		19			
Heterogeneity: Not applicable						
Test for overall effect: Z = 0.56 (P = 0.57)						

Fig. 4 Forest Plot of comparison between organ preservation surgery and primary radiotherapy with respect to 5-year local recurrence

second primary aerodigestive tract malignancy [4, 5, 18]. Surgery can thus be utilized as the first line and if there is failure, radiation can be used for salvage. Another advantage of surgery is the cost benefit of surgical intervention over radiotherapy. Cost analysis of open supraglottic laryngectomy, TLM and TORS by Dombree et al. in a Belgian model suggests that open supraglottic laryngectomy is almost equal to TLM in upfront surgical costs and TORS tends to be more expensive primarily due to purchase and maintenance costs [19]. This cost-analysis did not account for in-hospital costs such as length of admission, complications or readmission rates. Cost analysis comparing radiotherapy and TLM in a Canadian model for treatment of glottic cancers showed TLM to be a better cost saving modality [20].

One of the advantage of OPS with neck dissection is to identify patients with occult nodal metastasis in the neck. This is an important consideration given that up to 30% patients with SSCC may have occult nodal metastasis [21]. Thus, although these patients were early stage at the time of recruitment, the discovery of positive nodal metastasis after elective neck dissection results in the patients being upstaged and adjuvant radiotherapy is usually recommended. Some of the patients included in our study who underwent an elective neck dissection received adjuvant radiotherapy for positive nodal disease [12, 13]. This may in part be one of the reasons why patients in our study in the surgical arm had improved oncologic outcomes. Results from Arshad et al. corroborate this, as patients who underwent OPS with neck dissections fared better than those who only underwent RT or OPS without neck dissections [7].

Disadvantages of surgery include risk of general anesthetic, especially in patients with significant comorbidities, bleeding, infection, pharyngocutaneous fistula, dysphagia and tracheostomy. Additionally, one of the main criticisms of OPS are the associated poor functional outcomes [22]. However, TLM and TORS have gained popularity recently, due to several advantages of transoral surgery over open surgery and RT. TLM was first introduced by Strong and

Jako for laryngeal surgery [23]. Since then several reports have been published investigating the role of TLM for supraglottic laryngectomy [23–36]. Long-term oncologic outcomes comparing TLM and open surgery suggest that oncologic outcomes are similar. Cabanillas et al. compared TLM versus open laryngeal preservation surgery in a total of fifty-two patients, who also underwent concurrent bilateral neck dissections, and found that 5-year DSS was 80% in the TLM group versus 72% in the open surgical group and 5-year local control rate was 70% in both groups [34]. Transoral laser surgery, when compared to open surgery, resulted in reduced incidence of permanent gastrostomies and tracheostomies [37]. Importantly, the survival outcomes were no different between the two groups.

TORS was first described by Weinstein and colleagues, and since then there have been several reports assessing its oncologic and functional outcomes, the majority of the studies report on all stages of supraglottic SCC [32, 38–49]. Although, long-term oncology outcomes have not been reported, initial results with mean follow up ranging from 6.8 to 28.1 months, indicate that locoregional control is the same as RT [38, 41, 44]. Additionally, long-term tracheostomy and gastric feeding tube rates range from 0 to 20% in patients treated with TORS [38, 41, 44].

Given the paucity of high level evidence guiding the optimal management of early stage supraglottic cancer and potential biases of retrospective studies, a head to head comparison between newer modalities such as TLM and/or TORS with RT is crucial in determining the therapeutic algorithm that can yield better oncologic and functional outcomes in early stage SSCC patient. Although studies comparing surgery and radiation have been challenging to accrue to, ongoing efforts comparing OPS to RT for oropharyngeal cancer are underway and actively accruing [50, 51]. This high level of evidence will ultimately be necessary to guide the guide treatment of these patients with early stage disease that have a surprisingly poor prognosis.

Conclusions

To our knowledge, this is the first meta-analysis comparing RT and OPS for early stage SSCC. Patients who underwent OPS had better survival outcomes compared to primary radiation therapy. Five studies met the inclusion criteria for disease specific mortality with a total of 2864 pooled patients. 5-year disease specific mortality was lower in the surgery group (ORs 0.43, 95% CI 0.31–0.60). Four studies met the inclusion criteria for 5-year overall mortality with 5-year overall mortality being lower in surgery group (ORs 0.40, 95% CI 0.29–0.55). We were unable to compare the functional outcomes. Given the paucity of studies in the literature comparing open surgery, TLM, TORS and radiotherapy evaluating both oncologic and functions outcomes, future studies and research should include well designed randomized controlled trials.

Abbreviations

CI: Confidence Intervals; DSM: Disease Specific Mortality; LC: Local Control; NCCN: National Comprehensive Cancer Network; ND: Neck Dissection; NR: Not Reported; OM: Overall Mortality; OPS: Organ Preservation Surgery; OR: Odds Ratios; PRISMA: Preferred Reporting Items for Systematic Reviews and Meta-Analyses; RT: Radiation Therapy; SSCC: Supraglottic squamous cell carcinoma; TLM: Transoral endoscopic laser microsurgery; TORS: Transoral robotic surgery

Acknowledgements

The authors would like to acknowledge Alla Iansavitchene at London Health Sciences for her help with designing the search strategy for literature review.

Meeting Presentation.

Poliquin Podium Presentation – 2nd Place Clinical Category at Canadian Society of Otolaryngologists in Charlottetown, PEI in Jun 2016.

Funding

No funding was required or made available. The study was presented at the Canadian Society of Otolaryngology Meeting in Charlottetown, PEI and won 2nd prize in the Poliquin Competition.

Author's contributions

KBP and SDM – Designed study design, search strategy, title screen, abstract screen, data extraction, data analysis, review and writing of the manuscript. ACN, KF, JY – review and writing of the manuscript. All authors read and approved the final manuscript.

Authors' information

KBP – PGY 5 Resident, Otolaryngology – Head and Neck Surgery, Western University, London, Ontario.
ACN – Associate Professor, Otolaryngology – Head and Neck Surgery, Western University, London, Ontario.
KF – Professor, Otolaryngology – Head and Neck Surgery, Western University, London, Ontario.
JY – Professor, Otolaryngology – Head and Neck Surgery, Western University, London, Ontario.
SDM – Assistant Professor, Otolaryngology – Head and Neck Surgery, Western University, London, Ontario.

Competing interests

The authors declare that they have no competing interests.

References

1. Edge SBD, Compton C, Fritz A, Greene F, Trotti AAJCC. Cancer staging handbook. New York: Springer-Verlag; 2010.
2. Hoffman HT, Porter K, Karnell LH, et al. Laryngeal cancer in the United States: changes in demographics, patterns of care, and survival. Laryngoscope. 2006:116:1–13.
3. NCCN clinical practice guidelines in oncology in Head and Neck Cancers (version 1.2015). http://www.nccn.org/professionals/physician_gls/pdf/head-and-neck.pdf (2015). Accessed 10 Nov 2015.
4. Piccirillo F. Cancer of the larynx in SEER survival monograph: cancer survival among adults: U.S. SEER Program 1988–2001, Patient and Tumor Characteristics. National Cancer Insitutite, SEER Program. NIH Pub. No, 07-6215, Bethesda, MD, 2007.
5. Cosetti M, Yu GP, Schantz SP. Five-year survival rates and time trends of laryngeal cancer in the US population. Arch Otolaryngol. 2008;134:370–9.
6. Chen AY, Fedewa S, Zhu J. Temporal trends in the treatment of early- and advanced-stage laryngeal cancer in the United States, 1985-2007. Arch Otolaryngol. 2011;137:1017–24.
7. Arshad H, Jayaprakash V, Gupta V, et al. Survival differences between organ preservation surgery and definitive radiotherapy in early supraglottic squamous cell carcinoma. Otolaryngol Head Neck Surg. 2014;150:237–44.
8. Bron LP, Soldati D, Zouhair A, et al. Treatment of early stage squamous-cell carcinoma of the glottic larynx: endoscopic surgery or cricohyoidoepiglottopexy versus radiotherapy. Head Neck. 2001;23:823–9.
9. Chun JY, Kim YH, Choi EC, Byeon HK, Jung J, Kim SH. The oncologic safety and functional preservation of supraglottic partial laryngectomy. Am J Otolaryngol. 2010;31:246–51.
10. Jones AS, Fish B, Fenton JE, Husband DJ. The treatment of early laryngeal cancers (T1-T2 N0): surgery or irradiation? Head Neck. 2004;26:127–35.
11. Laccourreye O, Weinstein G, Chabardes E, Housset M, Laccourreye H, Brasnu D. T1 squamous cell carcinoma of the arytenoid. Laryngoscope. 1992;102:896–900.
12. Orus C, Leon X, Vega M, Quer M. Initial treatment of the early stages (I, II) of supraglottic squamous cell carcinoma: partial laryngectomy versus radiotherapy. Eur Arch Otorhinolaryngol. 2000;257:512–6.
13. Santos CR, Kowalski LP, Magrin J, et al. Prognostic factors in supraglottic carcinoma patients treated by surgery or radiotherapy. Ann Otol Rhinol Laryngol. 1998;107:697–702.
14. Sessions DG, Lenox J, Spector GJ. Supraglottic laryngeal cancer: analysis of treatment results. Laryngoscope. 2005;115:1402–10.
15. Spector JG, Sessions DG, Emami B, Simpson J, Haughey B, Fredrickson JM. Squamous cell carcinomas of the aryepiglottic fold: therapeutic results and long-term follow-up. Laryngoscope. 1995;105:734–46.
16. Spriano G, Antognoni P, Piantanida R, et al. Conservative management of T1-T2N0 supraglottic cancer: a retrospective study. Am J Otolaryngol. 1997; 18:299–305.
17. Newcastle-Ottawa Scale [type]. Updated http://www.ohri.ca/programs/clinical_epidemiology/oxford.htm. Accessed 10 Nov 2015.
18. Vaamonde P, Martin C, del Rio M, LaBella T. Second primary malignancies in patients with cancer of the head and neck. Otolaryngol Head Neck Surg. 2003;129:65–70.
19. Dombree M, Crott R, Lawson G, Janne P, Castiaux A, Krug B. Cost comparison of open approach, transoral laser microsurgery and transoral robotic surgery for partial and total laryngectomies. Eur Arch Otorhinolaryngol. 2014;271:2825–34.
20. Phillips TJ, Sader C, Brown T, et al. Transoral laser microsurgery versus radiation therapy for early glottic cancer in Canada: cost analysis. J Otolaryngol Head Neck Surg. 2009;38:619–23.
21. Byers RM, Wolf PF, Rationale BAJ. For elective modified neck dissection. Head Neck Surg. 1988;10:160–7.
22. Lewin JS, Hutcheson KA, Barringer DA, et al. Functional analysis of swallowing outcomes after supracricoid partial laryngectomy. Head Neck. 2008;30:559–66.
23. Strong MS, Jako GJ. Laser surgery in the larynx. Early clinical experience with continuous CO 2 laser. Ann Otol Rhinol Laryngol. 1972;81:791–8.

24. Breda E, Catarino R, Monteiro E. Transoral laser microsurgery for laryngeal carcinoma: survival analysis in a hospital-based population. Head Neck. 2015;37:1181–6.

25. Bussu F, Almadori G, De Corso E, et al. Endoscopic horizontal partial laryngectomy by CO(2) laser in the management of supraglottic squamous cell carcinoma. Head Neck. 2009;31:1196–206.

26. Canis M, Martin A, Ihler F, et al. Results of transoral laser microsurgery for supraglottic carcinoma in 277 patients. Eur Arch Otorhinolaryngol. 2013;270:2315–26.

27. Csanady M, Czigner J, Vass G, Jori J. Transoral CO2 laser management for selected supraglottic tumors and neck dissection. Eur Arch Otorhinolaryngol. 2011;268:1181–6.

28. Davis RK, Kriskovich MD, Galloway EB 3rd, Buntin CS, Jepsen MC. Endoscopic supraglottic laryngectomy with postoperative irradiation. Ann Otol Rhinol Laryngol. 2004;113:132–8.

29. Grant DG, Salassa JR, Hinni ML, Pearson BW, Hayden RE, Perry WC. Transoral laser microsurgery for carcinoma of the supraglottic larynx. Otolaryngol Head Neck Surg. 2007;136(6):900.

30. Iro H, Waldfahrer F, Altendorf-Hofmann A, Weidenbecher M, Sauer R, Steiner W. Transoral laser surgery of supraglottic cancer: follow-up of 141 patients. Arch Otolaryngol Head Neck Surg. 1998;124:1245–50.

31. Peretti G, Piazza C, Ansarin M, et al. Transoral CO2 laser microsurgery for tis-T3 supraglottic squamous cell carcinomas. Eur Arch Otorhinolaryngol. 2010;267:1735–42.

32. Solares CA, Strome M. Transoral robot-assisted CO2 laser supraglottic laryngectomy: experimental and clinical data. Laryngoscope. 2007;117:817–20.

33. Vilaseca I, Blanch JL, Berenguer J, et al. Transoral laser microsurgery for locally advanced (T3-T4a) supraglottic squamous cell carcinoma: sixteen years of experience. Head Neck. 2016;38(7):1050.

34. Cabanillas R, Rodrigo JP, Llorente JL, Suarez C. Oncologic outcomes of transoral laser surgery of supraglottic carcinoma compared with a transcervical approach. Head Neck. 2008;30:750–5.

35. Cabanillas R, Rodrigo JP, Llorente JL, Suarez V, Ortega P, Suarez C. Functional outcomes of transoral laser surgery of supraglottic carcinoma compared with a transcervical approach. Head Neck. 2004;26:653–9.

36. Kollisch M, Werner JA, Lippert BM, Functional RH. Results following partial supraglottic resection. Comparison of conventional surgery vs. transoral laser microsurgery. Adv Otorhinolaryngol. 1995;49:237–40.

37. Karatzanis AD, Psychogios G, Zenk J, et al. Evaluation of available surgical management options for early supraglottic cancer. Head Neck. 2010;32:1048–55.

38. Razafindranaly V, Lallemant B, Aubry K, et al. Clinical outcomes with transoral robotic surgery for supraglottic squamous cell carcinoma: experience of a French evaluation cooperative subgroup of GETTEC. Head Neck. 2016;38:E1097–101.

39. Weinstein GS, O'Malley BW Jr, Snyder W, Hockstein NG. Transoral robotic surgery: supraglottic partial laryngectomy. Ann Otol Rhinol Laryngol. 2007;116:19–23.

40. Durmus K, Gokozan HN, Ozer E. Transoral robotic supraglottic laryngectomy: surgical considerations. Head Neck. 2015;37:125–6.

41. Ozer E, Alvarez B, Kakarala K, Durmus K, Teknos TN, Carrau RL. Clinical outcomes of transoral robotic supraglottic laryngectomy. Head Neck. 2013;35:1158–61.

42. Park YM, Byeon HK, Chung HP, Choi EC, Kim SH. Comparison of treatment outcomes after transoral robotic surgery and supraglottic partial laryngectomy: our experience with seventeen and seventeen patients respectively. Clin Otolaryngol. 2013;38:270–4.

43. Park YM, Lee WJ, Lee JG, et al. Transoral robotic surgery (TORS) in laryngeal and hypopharyngeal cancer. J Laparoendosc Adv S. 2009;19:361–8.

44. Dowthwaite S, Nichols AC, Yoo J, et al. Transoral robotic total laryngectomy: report of 3 cases. Head Neck. 2013;35:E338–42.

45. Mendelsohn AH, Remacle M. Transoral robotic surgery for laryngeal cancer. Curr Opin Otolaryngol Head Neck Surg. 2015;23:148–52.

46. Mendelsohn AH, Remacle M, Van Der Vorst S, Bachy V, Lawson G. Outcomes following transoral robotic surgery: supraglottic laryngectomy. Laryngoscope. 2013;123:208–14.

47. Olsen SM, Moore EJ, Koch CA, Price DL, Kasperbauer JL, Olsen KD. Transoral robotic surgery for supraglottic squamous cell carcinoma. Am J Otolaryngol. 2012;33:379–84.

48. Rodrigo JP, Suarez C, Silver CE, et al. Transoral laser surgery for supraglottic cancer. Head Neck. 2008;30:658–66.

49. More YI, Tsue TT, Girod DA, et al. Functional swallowing outcomes following transoral robotic surgery vs primary chemoradiotherapy in patients with advanced-stage oropharynx and supraglottis cancers. JAMA Otolaryngol Head Neck Surg. 2013;139:43–8.

50. Nichols AC, Yoo J, Hammond JA, et al. Early-stage squamous cell carcinoma of the oropharynx: radiotherapy vs. trans-oral robotic surgery (ORATOR)–study protocol for a randomized phase II trial. BMC Cancer. 2013;13:133.

51. EORTC 1420-HNCG-ROG "The best of" trial. http://www.eortc.org/research-groups/head-and-neck-cancer-group/ongoing-projects/. Accessed 10 Nov 2015.

10

Rheopheresis in treatment of idiopathic sensorineural sudden hearing loss

Milan Kostal[1]*[ID], Jakub Drsata[2], Milan Bláha[1], Miriam Lánská[1] and Viktor Chrobok[2]

Abstract

Backround: Only few therapeutic options exist for patients with refractory sudden idiopathic sensorineural hearing loss (SISHL). Little is known about the efficacy of second-line therapies. Rheopheresis seems to be an effective therapeutic possibility.

Methods: Between 2012 and 2015, 106 patients with SISHL were enrolled in the study, of whom 52 were refractory to initial treatment. As salvage therapy, these patients were offered either 3 sessions of rheopheresis (33 pts) or intratympanic steroid treatment through MicroWick application (19 pts). Pure tone audiometry was performed at diagnosis, at the 1st month and the 1st year during the follow-up.

Results: Patients in the rheopheretic arm had higher hearing loss than in the MicroWick arm (81% vs. 52%, $p = 0.04$). In spite of this, there was a significant improvement for patients in the rheopheretic arm (27% of hearing loss reduction, $p < 0.001$) after the 1st month and this remained unchanged during the 1st year, while no improvement was seen in the MicroWick arm (0% of hearing loss reduction, $p = 0.424$). We found no predictive factor for steroid-failure in first-line therapy. Older age ($p = 0.003$), presence of vertigo ($p = 0.006$) and more profound initial hearing loss ($p < 0.001$) were identified as negative prognostic markers.

Conclusion: Rheopheresis can be used as a potentially effective and safe salvage therapy for patients with cortico-refractory SISHL.

Keywords: Rheopheresis, Sudden idiopathic hearing loss, MicroWick

Background

Sudden hearing loss is defined as a hearing loss of over 30 dB with an acute onset (i.e. within a 72-h period), in at least 3 consecutive frequencies in one or both ears [1]. It has a global incidence rate of 5–20 cases in 100,000 people per year. This number may be underestimated because of diffuse diagnostic criteria and spontaneous remissions, which produces a case drop-off for statistical purposes [2]. Sudden hearing loss can be associated with specific causes, such as inflammatory, mechanic, chemical or acoustic damage of the cochlea, Ménière's disease, vestibular schwannoma and others [3]. However about 90% of cases remain idiopathic [4].

Four major hypotheses have been proposed for these cases – traumatic, vascular, autoimmune and infectious [5]. The fact that the labyrinthine artery is a functional end artery (very vulnerable to vascular events) [6, 7] is in favor of the vascular hypothesis. The main underlying cause is atherosclerosis and its risk factors, such as abdominal obesity, arterial hypertension, hyperglycemia, hypertriglyceridemia, low HDL cholesterol or high BMI [8]. Other risk factors include thrombophilias and hyperviscosity syndrome [7].

The cochlear blood flow can be impaired by several synergistic factors causing vessel injury and elevating blood viscosity. Among them, a high level of cholesterol and fibrinogen (major factors of blood hyperviscosity) are a possible target for treatment with fibrinogen–LDL-apheresis, covering some of the currently established methods of lipidapheresis/rheopheresis [9, 10]. Rheopheresis simultaneously eliminates an exactly defined spectrum of high-molecular weight rheologically relevant

* Correspondence: kosmil@seznam.cz
[1]4th Department of Internal Medicine, University Hospital Hradec Kralove Charles University, Faculty of Medicine in Hradec Kralove, Hradec Králové, Czech Republic
Full list of author information is available at the end of the article

plasma proteins (i.e. alpha-2-macroglobulin, fibrinogen, LDL cholesterol, von Willebrand factor (vWF), IgM, fibronectin, putatively multimeric vitronectin), thus lowering full blood and plasma viscosity [11]. These procedures have pleiotropic effects, including favorable modifications of cytokine and adhesive molecule levels, increased production of endothelial NO, improved erythrocyte deformability and reduced aggregability of both erythrocytes and platelets [7, 12]. Improvement of perfusion in inner ear microcirculation as a result of lower blood viscosity is a possible therapeutic approach in patients with SISHL.

Study objective and methods

The primary objective of the study is to prove the efficacy of rheopheresis and MicroWick in patients with SISHL, for whom the first-line corticosteroid therapy has failed. We conducted an open-label observational prospective study with rheopheresis and MicroWick in steroid-refractory patients between 2012 and 2015 in a university-based tertiary care hospital. Institutional Review Board approval was obtained before proceeding with the study.

Patients meeting SISHL criteria (hearing loss of over 30 dB, in at least 3 consecutive frequencies in one or both ears within a 72-h period) were enrolled after signing informed consent. To exclude known causes of hearing loss, a complete history and physical examination, audiological and vestibular tests, laboratory workup and imaging study (MRI or CT, if indicated) were undertaken. All patients received corticosteroid therapy, consisting of 250 mg of solumedrol administered on 3 consecutive days (total of 750 mg of corticosteroid); then the assessment was performed (Days 3–5). Patients with a response of less than 50% improvement in PTA (pure tone average) were considered as partial or non-responders to the treatment [13]. These were offered a continuation of the therapy with MicroWick (intratympanic application of 7.5 mg dexamethasone in total) or rheopheresis. We collected demographic data (age, sex, time to treatment – TTT, BMI). A pure-tone audiogram and the Fowler percentage of hearing loss was performed before the treatment and during follow-up at the 1st and 12th months (final outcome) after treatment. PTA was calculated as the dB average of the thresholds at 0.5, 1, 2, and 4 kHz. The Fowler percentage of hearing loss was calculated according to the AMA (American medical association) standards, which has been proven as the optimal method for percentage evaluation of hearing loss in Czech language [14]. The presence of tinnitus or vertigo was noted. Adverse events were scored, using Common Terminology Criteria for Adverse Events (CTCAE v. 4.0, 7/2010).

We used rheohemapheresis (formally known as rheopheresis), which is our modification of double plasma filtration performed in the Hematological Department, University Hospital in Hradec Králové. Plasma is obtained not by filtration but by centrifugal separators. Blood is collected from a peripheral vein. Plasma is obtained by high-speed centrifugation (Cobe-Spectra or Optia blood cell separators, Terumo, Lakewood, Co, USA) and, in the second grade, is pumped through a high-molecular filter (Evaflux 4A, Kawasumi, Tokyo, Japan). This filter is made of ethylene-vinyl-alcohol hollow fibers with 0.03 mm sized holes, which captures a sizeable amount of LDL cholesterol, lipoprotein(a), fibrinogen, α_2-macroglobulin and immunoglobulins (IgM in particular). After crossing the filter, plasma is returned, together with the formed elements of the blood, to the patient's bloodstream. The filter is placed and controlled by the CF 100 instrument (Infomed, Geneva, Switzerland). In the case of increased pressure in the filter capillaries, the filter is automatically rinsed with a physiological solution, which is then discarded with the eliminated particles into the waste bag. The flow of plasma is continual; anticoagulation is ensured with heparin and ACD-A (Baxter, Munich, Germany); the amount of processed plasma: one and a half of body volume - is calculated by the blood cell separator computer. Duration of the procedure is approximately 2 h, which depends on influx of blood (status of peripheral veins). We prefer a peripheral venous access and only if they are insufficient do we use venous access via v. subclavia or v. femoralis. Contraindications of rheopheresis are identical to the general contraindications of hemapheresis - uncontrolled metabolic conditions (diabetes), cardiovascular disorders (unstable hypertension or coronary artery disease), malignancies, acute infections and cerebral insufficiency. Some other details have previously been described elsewhere [12, 15]. Patients with acute hearing loss underwent 3 procedures within one week.

Patients treated in the MicroWick arm were operated on in the standard conditions of an operating theater. With the patient in the supine position, the ear canal and eardrum of the impaired ear were cleaned of earwax and topically anesthetized using 10% lidocaine. On the cleaned ear canal and under microscopic control, the postero-inferior ear drum quadrant was incised by a sickle knife. The malleus handle was used as a landmark for localizing the round window membrane. A Silverstein MicroWick system was then smoothly inserted, and the wick was congested with dexamethasone solution (4 mg/mL). The patient was instructed to administer two drops of dexamethasone solution 4 times daily to the external ear canal of the hearing-impaired ear for a period of one month.

Statistics

Descriptive statistics for demographic and baseline characteristics were summarized for all randomized

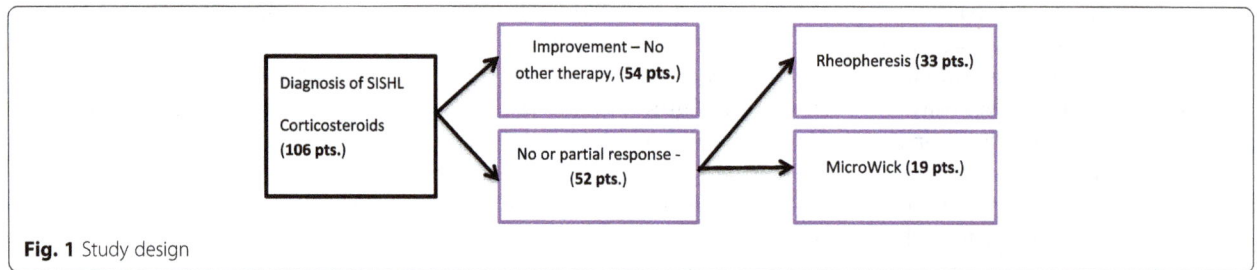

Fig. 1 Study design

patients. For treatment outcomes, the Fowler percentage of hearing loss on the affected ear was analyzed before and after treatment with the paired T-test or Wilcoxon test for non-parametric data. For comparison of independent groups, the T-test, non-parametric Mann—Whitney rank sum or one-way ANOVA test was used. For associations between factors, we used the Pearson Product Moment Correlation. Data are presented as mean ($\pm$SD) or median (lower, upper quartile). The significance level was set at $p < 0.05$. The statistical analyses were performed with SigmaPlot for Windows, version 11.0 (Systat Software, California, USA).

Results

We examined 157 patients with SISHL, 110 of whom met the inclusion criteria, signed consent and entered into the study. One patient was rejected before the start of treatment for spontaneous remission. In the study group, 2 patients were lost to follow-up for personal reasons after completing corticosteroid-arm therapy and their final audiograms were missing. One patient was lost in the MicroWick arm for the same reason. The final number of 106 patients met the inclusion and exclusion criteria, were followed up for 12 months after treatment and enrolled in the statistical analysis.

After initial corticosteroid therapy, 54 patients showed significant improvement - partial or complete recovery according to the guidelines [13] and required no other treatment (Standard arm). The rest - 52 patients chose either rheopheresis (33 patients) or MicroWick (19 patients) as shown in Fig. 1. The demographics and

baseline audiological data of the patients are summarized in Table 1, which shows that there was no significant difference between the groups. Patients started steroid treatment after 4 days from onset of symptoms. Patients who failed steroid treatment entered rheopheresis after 9 days from onset symptoms, or the MicroWick arm after 10 days after onset of symptoms. There was no statistical difference in time to treatment between the MicroWick and rheopheresis arm ($p = 0,279$). Patients with more profound hearing loss were more likely to choose rheopheresis rather than MicroWick (81% (54, 98) vs. 52% (30, 92), $p = 0.04$) as is shown in Table 2.

We found age ($p = 0.001$), BMI ($p = 0.0371$) and vertigo ($p = 0,041$) to be positively correlated with the initial level of PTA. Sex ($p = 0.285$) and the presence of tinnitus ($p = 0.567$) were independent of initial hearing loss. Data from follow-up visits are shown in Figs. 2, 3 and 4. Hearing loss was significantly improved during the first month after the initial treatment in the steroid arm ($p < 0.001$) and in the rheopheresis arm ($p < 0.001$), and remained unchanged during the first year, as is shown in Table 2. Steroid-refractory patients in the MicroWick arm reached only mild, non-significant improvement within the first month ($p = 0.940$) after the treatment, and no further improvement was observed ($p = 0.359$). We observed a similar outcome in final absolute hearing loss levels in both arms after 1 month ($p = 0.682$). We found a positive correlation between final hearing loss and age ($p = 0,003$), and initial hearing loss ($p < 0.001$). Also patients with vertigo had higher final hearing loss ($p = 0.006$). Other

Table 1 Demographic data

	Steroid therapy only (No. = 54)	Rheopheresis (No. = 33)	MicroWick (No. = 19)	
Age (median)	53 (38,65)	58 (44,66)	54 (29,61)	$p = 0.234$
Sex male/female	29/25	21/12	7/12	$p = 0.175$
Vertigo (%)	19	15	26	$p = 0.609$
Tinnitus (%)	74	79	74	$p = 0.867$
Time to treatment (days, median)	4 (1,7)	10 (8,15)	9 (6,14)	$p < 0.001$
BMI (median)	25.7 (23,29)	26.6 (24,29)	24.1 (23,29)	$p = 0.653$

No. number of patients

Table 2 Comparison of hearing losses at time of follow-up (median in % of Fowler scale, (lower, upper quartile))

	Day 0/1 month		1 month/1 year	
Steroid therapy	54 (18,87)/13 (4, 50)	$p < 0.001$	13 (4,50)/11 (4, 29)	$p = 0.224$
Rheopheresis	81(54, 98)/54 (19, 74)	$p < 0.001$	54 (19, 74)/53 (25, 78)	$p = 0.963$
MicroWick	52 (30, 92)/52 (16, 83)	$p = 0.940$	52 (16, 83)/77 (14, 100)	$p = 0.359$

factors showed no correlation with results (BMI ($p = 0.23$), tinnitus ($p = 0.30$) and sex ($p = 0.878$)).

There were 6 mild adverse events during steroid therapy: 4x decompensation of diabetes and 2x local complications after catheter insertion. Rheopheresis was complicated with 6 adverse events: 5x mild (short nausea during procedure) and 1x moderate (hypotension requiring saline infusion). In the MicroWick arm, we observed 7 adverse events: 2 mild – lasting perforation of tympanic membrane 1 year after procedure; in 3 other cases there was a need for operative occlusion (myringoplasty), classified as moderate according to CTCAE. In 2 other cases, there was progression to deafness on the treatment, which we classified as a serious adverse event.

Discussion
Success of the treatment of any disorder depends on a full understanding of the underlying pathophysiological characteristics. Glucocorticoids exert a variety of immunosuppressive, anti-inflammatory, and anti-allergic effects on primary and secondary immune cells and tissues. Systemic steroid treatment is one of the few treatment options that has data showing efficacy and is recommended as first-line therapy in SHL according to 2012 guidelines [13, 16]. As a second-line treatment for non-responding patients (salvage therapy), several possibilities have been proposed: hyperbaric oxygen therapy, intratympanic steroid application, antiviral therapies, vasoactive agents, anticoagulants, rheopheresis and other [13]. Only some of these therapeutic options were proven effective in clinical trials.

We conducted a prospective, observational clinical trial of setting efficacy of rheopheresis and intratympanic steroid application (MicroWick system) in the treatment of systemic-steroid refractory SISHL. Efficacy of rheopheresis as the first-line therapy in comparison to corticosteroids was proven in other studies [7, 10, 17]. The superiority of rheopheresis over established first-line standard treatment could not be shown in general. Rheopheresis seems to be especially effective in patients with high fibrinogen or cholesterol [18]. Only few retrospective data are available [19] for refractory SISHL.

Efficacy of rheopheresis is based on the vascular theory of SISHL. Vascular compromise and associated cochlear ischemia are thought to be contributory to SISHL in some cases, or could be a final common pathway to hearing loss. And indeed atherosclerotic and rheological risk factors (hypercholesterolemia [20–22], hyperfibrinogenemia [23], age [24], BMI [22], metabolic syndrome [25] or hyperhomocysteinemia [26]) have recently been proven to be important in the etiology and prognosis of SISHL, although not all studies support such evidence

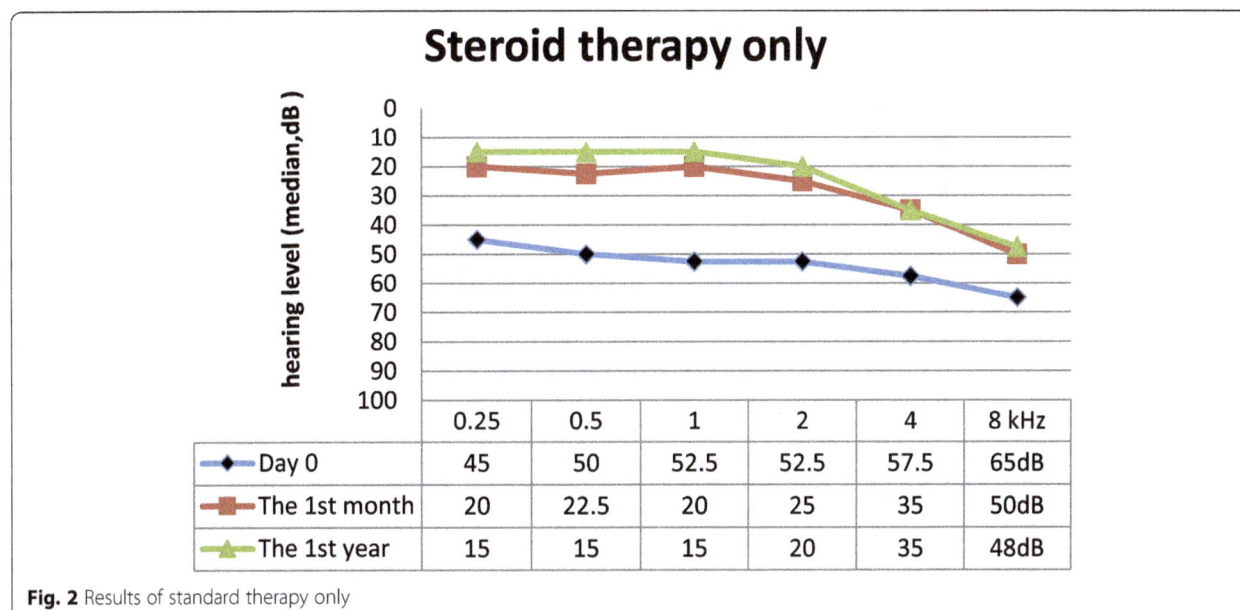

Steroid therapy only

	0.25	0.5	1	2	4	8 kHz
Day 0	45	50	52.5	52.5	57.5	65dB
The 1st month	20	22.5	20	25	35	50dB
The 1st year	15	15	15	20	35	48dB

Fig. 2 Results of standard therapy only

Rheopheresis

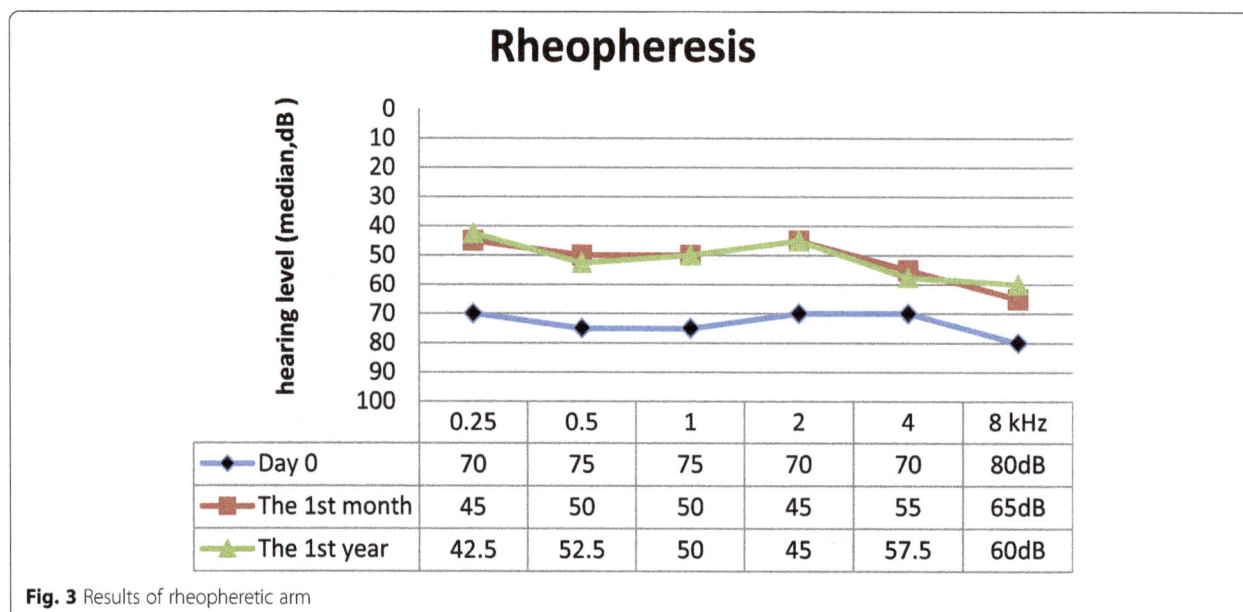

	0.25	0.5	1	2	4	8 kHz
Day 0	70	75	75	70	70	80dB
The 1st month	45	50	50	45	55	65dB
The 1st year	42.5	52.5	50	45	57.5	60dB

Fig. 3 Results of rheopheretic arm

[27, 28]. When analyzing our data, we cannot confirm an elevated baseline level of LDL-cholesterol, fibrinogen or viscosity in SISHL patients. However, after rheopheresis the level was significantly reduced in the case of some high molecular substances, such as cholesterol, immunoglobulin M, fibrinogen and others which have a significant influence on blood viscosity (Table 3.). This improves blood microcirculation and may be the main pathophysiological reason why rheopheresis is effective in the treatment of SISHL. During one procedure, the level of fibrinogen is reduced by 56%, similar to the other rheological important factors which we published

elsewhere [12]. One procedure reduce total blood viscosity by 15.6%. We maintained reduced blood viscosity by repeating the procedures 3 times [12].

As a secondary outcome, we searched for possible factors predicting steroid failure in the first-line therapy. All obtainable factors at the time of diagnosis (age, sex, vertigo, tinnitus, BMI,) failed to be predictive for steroid failure.

We used these factors for another analysis to learn whether these factors could serve as possible prognostic factors. Age ($p = 0.003$), vertigo ($p = 0.006$), and initial hearing loss ($p < 0.001$) were positively correlated with

MicroWick

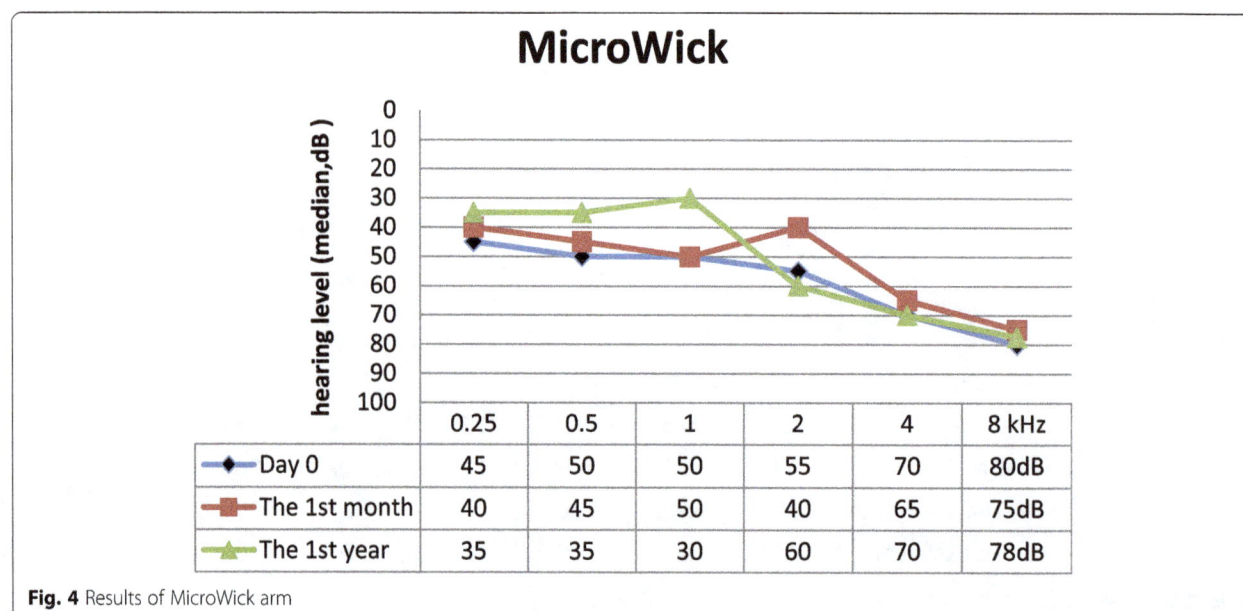

	0.25	0.5	1	2	4	8 kHz
Day 0	45	50	50	55	70	80dB
The 1st month	40	45	50	40	65	75dB
The 1st year	35	35	30	60	70	78dB

Fig. 4 Results of MicroWick arm

Table 3 Change in selected blood parameters (data available for 56 procedures)

	Before (± SD)	After(± SD)	p	Difference (%)
Fibrinogen (g/l)	3.22 (0.82)	1.43 (0.43)	<0.0001	−55.6
Plasma viscosity (mPa.sec)	2.11 (0.25)	1.82 (0.24)	<0.0001	−13.7
Blood viscosity (mPa.sec)	6.83 (1.6)	5.77 (1.07)	<0.0001	−15.6
Total cholesterol (mmol/L)	4.75 (1.01)	2.29 (0.54)	<0.0001	−51.8

final outcome, while BMI ($p = 0.23$), tinnitus ($p = 0.30$) and sex ($p = 0.878$) were not. Other data (severity of hearing loss, time to treatment, BMI, vertigo) were identified as negative prognostic factors of SISHL in other trials [22–25]. When we performed the same analysis adjusted for therapeutic benefit (difference between initial and final hearing loss), only patients with higher initial hearing loss showed a significant positive correlation with hearing improvement ($p < 0.001$). The rest of the factors showed no prognostic relevance.

Safety evaluations included assessment of adverse events, clinically significant abnormal laboratory findings (i.e. blood chemistry, hematology, urinalysis), vital signs, and physical examination findings. Both procedures are safe, with more adverse events in the MicroWick arm. Two patients showed progression to deafness (evaluated as serious adverse events), which is a relatively high incidence. The cause was a long-lasting perforation of the eardrum - the prolonged open middle ear caused irritation of the middle ear and a series of complications (inflammatory and infectious) which could not be managed by therapy, so they progressed to complete deafness.

Our study has some important limitations. Out of the original 110 patients entering the study, 52 showed no improvement after steroid therapy and required other treatment. An optimal design with blind randomization into three arms (MicroWick, Rheopheresis and Placebo) was not possible due to the low number of patients and for ethical reasons (performing no therapy is impossible in patients requiring therapy). We could not even blindly randomize patients into two arms (patient's refusal to undergo the invasive MicroWick system, contraindications for operation, patient's wish, clinician's opinion, etc.). From the results, it is evident that MicroWick and rheopheresis patients have different hearing losses - more severe cases of refractory SISHL were recruited into the rheopheretic arm (median loss 81% vs. 52%, $p = 0.04$, Table 2). In spite of the fact that such patients have significantly inferior prognoses, rheopheresis was able to significantly improve hearing loss to approximately the same level as was observed in the MicroWick arm. On the other hand, it is possible that in patients with more severe hearing loss, there is simply more room for recovery, which can explain the only mild-nonsignificant effect of the MicroWick system ($p = 0.940$, Table 2).

Conclusions

The question of therapy for patients currently remains under discussion and a considerable number of patients are not improving spontaneously or following corticotherapy. Rheopheresis can be used as a potentially effective and safe salvage therapy for patients with steroid-refractory SISHL.

Funding
Supported by a grant of the Czech Ministry of Health, MH CZ - DRO (UHHK, 00179906).

Authors' contributions
MK 50%, JD 30%, MB 10%. ML 5%, VC 5%. All authors read and approved the final manuscript.

Competing interests
ALL authors have no conflicts of interest.

Author details
[1]4th Department of Internal Medicine, University Hospital Hradec Kralove Charles University, Faculty of Medicine in Hradec Kralove, Hradec Králové, Czech Republic. [2]Department of Otorhinolaryngology and Head and Neck Surgery, University Hospital Hradec Kralove Charles University, Faculty of Medicine in Hradec Kralove, Hradec Králové, Czech Republic.

References
1. Schwartz J, Winters JL, Padmanabhan A, et al. Guidelines on the use of therapeutic apheresis in clinical practice-evidence-based approach from the writing committee of the American society for apheresis: the sixth special issue. J Clin Apher. 2013;28:145–284.
2. Klemm E, Deutscher A, Mosges R. A present investigation of the epidemiology in idiopathic sudden sensorineural hearing loss. Laryngorhinootologie. 2009;88:524–7.
3. Atay G, Kayahan B, Cinar BC, Sarac S, Sennaroglu L. Prognostic factors in sudden sensorineural hearing loss. Balkan Med J. 2016;33:87–93.
4. Zarandy M, Rutka J. Diseases of the inner ear. Berlin Heidelberg: Springer Verlag; 2010.
5. Lazarini PR, Camargo AC. Idiopathic sudden sensorineural hearing loss: etiopathogenic aspects. Braz J Otorhinolaryngol. 2006;72:554–61.
6. Selmani Z, Pyykko I, Ishizaki H, Marttila TI. Cochlear blood flow measurement in patients with Meniere's disease and other inner ear disorders. Acta Otolaryngol Suppl. 2001;545:10–3.
7. Mosges R, Koberlein J, Heibges A, Erdtracht B, Klingel R, Lehmacher W. Rheopheresis for idiopathic sudden hearing loss: results from a large prospective, multicenter, randomized, controlled clinical trial. Eur Arch Otorhinolaryngol. 2009;266:943–53.
8. Schillaci G, Pirro M, Vaudo G, et al. Prognostic value of the metabolic syndrome in essential hypertension. J Am Coll Cardiol. 2004;43:1817–22.
9. Ohinata Y, Makimoto K, Kawakami M, Haginomori S, Araki M, Takahashi H.

Blood viscosity and plasma viscosity in patients with sudden deafness. Acta Otolaryngol. 1994;114:601–7.

10. Suckfull M. Fibrinogen and LDL apheresis in treatment of sudden hearing loss: a randomised multicentre trial. Lancet (London, England). 2002;360:1811–7.

11. Klingel R, Fassbender C, Fassbender T, Erdtracht B, Berrouschot J. Rheopheresis: rheologic, functional, and structural aspects. Ther Apher. 2000;4:348–57.

12. Blaha M, Andrys C, Langrova H, et al. Changes of the complement system and rheological indicators after therapy with rheohemapheresis. Atheroscler Suppl. 2015;18:140–5.

13. Stachler RJ, Chandrasekhar SS, Archer SM, et al. Clinical practice guideline: sudden hearing loss. Otolaryngol Head Neck Surg. 2012;146:S1–35.

14. Novotny Z, Novak M. Correlation of speech audiometry with the Fowler and Sabin method of hearing loss evaluation. Ceskoslovenska otolaryngologie. 1990;39:146–53.

15. Blaha M, Rencova E, Langrova H, et al. Rheohaemapheresis in the treatment of nonvascular age-related macular degeneration. Atheroscler Suppl. 2013;14:179–84.

16. Eftekharian A, Amizadeh M. Pulse steroid therapy in idiopathic sudden sensorineural hearing loss: a randomized controlled clinical trial. Laryngoscope. 2016;126:150–5.

17. Ullrich H, Kleinjung T, Steffens T, Jacob P, Schmitz G, Strutz J. Improved treatment of sudden hearing loss by specific fibrinogen aphaeresis. J Clin Apher. 2004;19:71–8.

18. Bianchin G, Russi G, Romano N, Fioravanti P. Treatment with HELP-apheresis in patients suffering from sudden sensorineural hearing loss: a prospective, randomized, controlled study. Laryngoscope. 2010;120:800–7.

19. Uygun-Kiehne S, Straube R, Heibges A, Klingel R, Davids H. Rheopheresis for recurrent sudden hearing loss : therapeutic options for patients refractory to infusion therapy. HNO. 2010;58:445–51.

20. Chang SL, Hsieh CC, Tseng KS, Weng SF, Lin YS. Hypercholesterolemia is correlated with an increased risk of idiopathic sudden sensorineural hearing loss: a historical prospective cohort study. Ear Hear. 2014;35:256–61.

21. Quaranta N, Squeo V, Sangineto M, Graziano G, Sabba C. High total cholesterol in peripheral blood correlates with poorer hearing recovery in idiopathic sudden sensorineural hearing loss. PLoS One. 2015;10:e0133300.

22. Lee JS, Kim DH, Lee HJ, et al. Lipid profiles and obesity as potential risk factors of sudden sensorineural hearing loss. PLoS One. 2015;10:e0122496.

23. Wittig J, Wittekindt C, Kiehntopf M, Guntinas-Lichius O. Prognostic impact of standard laboratory values on outcome in patients with sudden sensorineural hearing loss. BMC Ear Nose Throat Disord. 2014;14:6.

24. Zhao H, Zhang TY, Jing JH, Fu YY, Luo JN. Prognostic factors for patients with the idiopathic sudden sensorineural hearing loss. Zhonghua Er Bi Yan Hou Ke Za Zhi. 2008;43:660–4.

25. Chien CY, Tai SY, Wang LF, et al. Metabolic syndrome increases the risk of sudden sensorineural hearing loss in Taiwan: a case–control study. Otolaryngol Head Neck Surg. 2015;153:105–11.

26. Fusconi M, Chistolini A, de Virgilio A, et al. Sudden sensorineural hearing loss: a vascular cause? Analysis of prothrombotic risk factors in head and neck. Int J Audiol. 2012;51:800–5.

27. Chang IJ, Kang CJ, Yueh CY, Fang KH, Yeh RM, Tsai YT. The relationship between serum lipids and sudden sensorineural hearing loss: a systematic review and meta-analysis. PLoS One. 2015;10:e0121025.

28. Ciorba A, Hatzopoulos S, Bianchini C, et al. Idiopathic sudden sensorineural hearing loss: cardiovascular risk factors do not influence hearing threshold recovery. Acta Otorhinolaryngol Ital. 2015;35:103–9.

11

Maxillofacial prosthodontics practice profile: a survey of non-United States prosthodontists

Nina Ariani[1,2], Harry Reintsema[3], Kathleen Ward[4], Cortino Sukotjo[5] and Alvin G. Wee[6,7]*

Abstract

Background: This study surveyed non-United States maxillofacial prosthodontists (MFP) to determine their practice profile and rationale for pursuing an MFP career.

Methods: Email addresses for the MFP were obtained from the International Society for Maxillofacial Rehabilitation, American Academy of Maxillofacial Prosthetics, and International Academy for Oral Facial Rehabilitation. Emails with a link to the electronic survey program were sent to each participant. Chi-square and Mann–Whitney-U tests were used to investigate the influence of formal MFP training on professional activities and type of treatments provided.

Results: One hundred twelve respondents (response rate 39%) from 33 nationalities returned the survey. The top three reasons for pursuing an MFP career were personal satisfaction, prosthodontics residency exposure, and mentorship. The predominant employment setting was affiliation with a university (77%). There were significant differences between respondents with and without formal MFP training regarding provision of surgical treatments ($P = 0.021$) and dental oncology ($P = 0.017$). Most treatments were done together with otolaryngology, oral surgery (68%) and head and neck surgery (61%). Practitioners not affiliated with a university spent significantly more time in clinical practice ($P = 0.002$), whereas respondents affiliated with universities spent significantly more time in teaching/training ($P = 0.008$) and funded research ($P = 0.015$).

Conclusions: Personal satisfaction is the most important factor in a decision to choose an MFP career. Most of the MFPs work at a university and within a multidisciplinary setting. There were differences regarding type of treatments provided by respondents with and without formal MFP training.

Keywords: Prosthodontics, Oral oncology, Rehabilitation, Career decision

Background

Maxillofacial prosthetics is a subspecialty of prosthodontics that deals with rehabilitation of patients with defects or disabilities caused by trauma, tumor, or congenital disorders [1]. Prostheses are made to replace teeth, lost bone, or soft tissue to restore oral function and esthetics. Prosthetic devices also are fabricated to shield and protect the facial structure during radiotherapy. Sometime, facial or body prosthesis is fabricated for psychosocial reasons. Given the vast services provided to patients as illustrated above, maxillofacial prosthodontists (MFP) are trained to work in a multidisciplinary setting together with oral surgeons; ear, nose, and throat surgeons; plastic surgeons; speech pathologists; etc. [2].

There are a number of professional organizations dealing with maxillofacial prosthodontics. The mission of the International Society for Maxillofacial Rehabilitation (ISMR) is to advance interdisciplinary maxillofacial rehabilitation through education, patient care, outreach and research. The International Academy for Oral Facial Rehabilitation (IAOFR) is a small international group of surgeons and prosthodontists (fewer than 50 fellows) with particular interest in optimizing treatment outcomes of surgical-prosthetic interventions. In the United States, the American Academy of Maxillofacial Prosthetics (AAMP)

* Correspondence: alvingwee@gmail.com
[6]Department of Prosthodontics, Creighton University School of Dentistry, Omaha, NE, USA
[7]Department of Surgery, Dental Service, Veterans Affairs Nebraska-Western Iowa Healthcare System, 4101 Woolworth Ave, Omaha, NE 68105, USA
Full list of author information is available at the end of the article

is an association of prosthodontists who are engaged in the art and science of maxillofacial prosthetics. The academy has approximately 300 fellows devoted to the study and practice of methods used to habilitate the esthetics and function of patients with acquired, congenital, and developmental defects of the head and neck. Methods used to maintain the oral health of patients exposed to cancercidal doses of radiation or cytotoxic drugs is also of interest to this association.

In the United States, training for prosthodontists in this area of maxillofacial prosthetic rehabilitation is unique in that most who are interested in this area have one year of additional training in maxillofacial prosthodontics, which is recognized by the Commission on Dental Accreditation [3, 4]. In a survey of dental schools worldwide, an average of 62 h with a range of 10–200 h were provided for maxillofacial prosthodontics instruction at the graduate level. However, 7% of dental schools presented the topics as lectures only, 62% had courses with lectures and clinical and laboratory exposure, while 28% had lecture/clinical courses with no laboratory component [5]. Training and recognition of MFP is not uniform globally.

To our knowledge, there is no published information regarding the number of MFP providing their services to society. Furthermore, there is only one known publication on the practice of MFPs in the UK, but this study is limited to maxillofacial technicians' practice of silicone maxillofacial prostheses [1]. No published data is available on the characteristics of the practice of MFPs, such as what services individuals trained in maxillofacial prosthodontics provide to their patients, whether they are practicing their specialty, and how much they practice compared to general prosthodontics. Since US and non-US training is different for maxillofacial prosthodontics, this study focuses on the non-US practice profile. This information, along with background information, such as why they enter the specialty, is investigated in this study to understand more about trends in maxillofacial prosthodontic practices outside the United States. The aim was to map the availability of these services for patients and reveal the need for educational facilities around the globe.

The purpose of the study was to characterize non-US MFP practice profiles and their rationale for the decision to pursue maxillofacial prosthodontics training.

Methods
Questionnaire
A 28-items questionnaire was developed specifically for this study. The first part covered personal information: gender, age, country, affiliation, salary, and professional background. The second part covered the decision to pursue a career in MFP. The third part consisted of questions about maxillofacial prosthodontics treatment provided and multidisciplinary care.

The MFPs' email addresses were obtained from the 2014 membership directories of ISMR, AAMP, and IAOFR. Since dentists, prosthodontists and anaplastologists members provide MFP services as well (e.g. specifically facial prostheses), they were included in the survey. An email with a link to the BlueQ electronic survey program from Creighton University was sent to each participant. The survey delivery protocol followed the Dillman Total Design Survey methodology [6]. A total of four emails were sent to the respondents. One week after the first email, the same email was sent again. Three and seven weeks from the initial email, the email containing the survey link was again sent only to participants who had not responded.

Analysis
The data on the questionnaires were entered into an Excel spreadsheet (Microsoft Corporation, Redmond, WA). Blank or unclear responses were considered as missing. Descriptive statistics were given as percentages (%). The data was not normally distributed, and thus Chi-square and Mann–Whitney-U Tests (SPSS IBM, New York, NY) were used to investigate the influence of formal maxillofacial prosthodontics training on professional activities and type of treatments provided. One-way repeated measures ANOVA was considered a robust test against the normality assumption and therefore used for the most important factors for pursuing maxillofacial prosthodontics career.

Results
Response rate
Surveys were initially sent out to a sub total of 316 potential individuals, including to anaplastologists as they are part of workforce that provides MFP services. Forty entries were eliminated from the 316 potential individuals, resulting in 276 individuals who were surveyed. Of the 40 that were eliminated, 28 were duplicates, nine could not be contacted as their emails bounced, one was US maxillofacial prosthodontist and two were physical therapists. Total number of responses was 115 for a response rate of 41.6% (115/276). Five individuals who were not DDS, prosthodontists nor anaplastologists and three responses that provide no answers at all were excluded for a 39% response rate (107/276).

Respondents could provide information as they wished and were not required to complete all items. Therefore, the sample size of individual items varies. Non-response was regarded as missing.

Demographic data
Thirty-three nationalities working in 32 different countries across five continents participated in the study: Australia ($n = 8$), Africa ($n = 4$), America excluding USA ($n = 20$), Asia ($n = 37$) and Europe ($n = 38$). The following

are the countries where the participants work: Australia, Brazil, Canada, Chile, Colombia, Cyprus, Egypt, France, Germany, Greece, India, Iraq, Israel, Italy, Japan, Kenya, Libya, Malaysia, Mexico, Nepal, Netherlands, New Zealand, Peru, Saudi Arabia, Serbia, Singapore, South Africa, Spain, Sweden, Switzerland, Turkey, and United Kingdom. The three countries with the highest percentage of respondents were India (18, 17%), the Netherlands (15, 14%), and Canada (10, 9%). The majority of respondents were male (77%). The age of the respondents ranged from 26–71 years old (mean = 46 ± 11).

Respondents were asked to provide their education level and allowed to mark all that apply. Seventy-four responded with DDS/DMD/BDS, 62 held Master degree, 31 respondents were PhD and 35 respondents had certifications such as prosthodontics and fellow in MFP.

Maxillofacial training and professional organizations

Seventy-one percent of respondents had formal maxillofacial prosthetics training. The training could either be part of or separate from prosthodontics specialty training. Eleven percent of those with formal maxillofacial training stated they did the training in an institution in the United States or Canada. They were not required to specify from which of those two countries they graduated.

When asked about professional background, 81% responded with maxillofacial prosthodontist, 2% were anaplastologists, 3% were prosthodontists, 1% were oral surgeons with formal maxillofacial prosthodontics training, 13% were other. The 13% who responded with 'other' stated they received formal MFP training or having at least a DDS/DMD/BDS degree and attend to patients. Thirty-two percent learned maxillofacial prosthodontics from colleagues, 30% from continuing education, and 38% either from an undergraduate/graduate program, observation program, the internet, textbooks, seminars, or experience.

A one-way repeated measures ANOVA was conducted to compare factors deemed important for an individual's decision to pursue a career in maxillofacial prosthodontics. The results showed a statistically significant difference in the various factors ($p < 0.0001$). Multiple pairwise comparisons were carried out between factors, with adjusted $\alpha = 0.05/45 = 0.001$ after Bonferroni correction for multiple comparisons. Table 1 reveals the means

Table 1 Factors important for decision to pursue maxillofacial prosthodontics career ($N = 29$)

Factor	Mean	SD
Personal satisfaction	4.66	0.67
Prosthodontics residency exposure	4.03	0.87
Mentorship	3.97	0.98
Involvement in national prosthodontics society	2.90	1.20
Other*	2.79	1.42
AAMP conference	2.59	1.32
Family history	2.41	1.52
The American College of Prosthodontists maxillofacial prosthodontics session	2.28	1.28
Potential salary	2.24	1.09
Media exposure	2.07	1.19

Based on a Likert scale where 1 = not important, 2 = less important, 3 = indifferent, 4 = important, 5 = very important.

Vertical lines denotes non-significant difference (P > 0.05)

* Other: academic request, lack of this kind of service in one's country, quality of the training, do something meaningful for oncologic patients

(standard deviation) and also which factors are significantly different from each other. There were differences in scores across the different factors ($P < 0.05$). Personal satisfaction was the most important factor for the decision.

Training facilities in the various countries were rated rather low by respondents, with 51% unsatisfied, 43% satisfied, and 6% very satisfied with training facilities available in their country. However, only 23.7% of respondents were not satisfied with their own maxillofacial prosthodontics training. For the remaining respondents, 44.7% were satisfied and 31.6% were very satisfied with their training.

There were no statistically significant differences between respondents with or without formal maxillofacial prosthodontics training regarding academic ranking at school ($P = 0.101$), salary ($P = 0.103$), involvement in national prosthodontics organizations ($P = 0.713$) and national MFP organizations ($P = 0.516$), and satisfaction working as maxillofacial prosthodontics ($P = 0.636$) (Table 2).

Table 2 Profiles of practitioners with vs without formal MFP training

	Formal MFP training (%)	Without formal MFP training (%)	P
Academic rank			
Top 5%	50	27	0.101
6–10%	11	27	
11–25%	0	18	
26–50%	14	9	
Not known	25	18	
Salary (in USD)			
≤ $ 50.000	24	7	0.103
$ 50.001–100.000	28	38	
$100.001–200.000	25	17	
≥ $200.001	23	38	
Fellow/member of national prosthodontics organizations			
Yes	82	83	0.713
No	7	10	
Organization does not exist	11	7	
Fellow/member of national MFP organizations			
Yes	38	31	0.516
No	7	14	
Organization does not exist	55	55	
Satisfaction working as MFP			
Unsatisfied	14	28	0.636
Satisfied	32	28	
Very satisfied	54	46	

Maxillofacial prosthodontics practice and multidisciplinary care

There were no statistically significant difference in affiliations (Fig. 1) between those with formal and non-formal training ($P = 0.302$). The predominant employment setting for respondents with formal and non-formal training was related to universities (77%).

The percentage of respondents providing various types of treatment is presented in Table 3. Included in standard prosthodontics treatment are complete dentures, removable partial dentures, fixed partial dentures, and restoring implants. There were significant differences between respondents with and without formal MFP training regarding provision of surgical treatments ($P = 0.021$) and dental oncology ($P = 0.017$).

The multidisciplinary nature of MFP treatment is reflected in Table 4. The respondents were asked to indicate all disciplines with which they work when treating patients. Most treatments were done in conjunction with otolaryngology (68%) and oral surgery (68%) followed by head and neck surgery (61%).

There were significant differences between practitioners affiliated and not affiliated with a university regarding percentage of time for professional activities (Table 5). Practitioners not affiliated with a university spent a significantly higher percentage of time in clinical practice ($P = 0.002$), whereas respondents affiliated with universities spent significantly more time in teaching/training ($P = 0.008$) and working on funded research ($P = 0.015$).

There was no statistically significant difference in the satisfaction of working as maxillofacial prosthodontists ($P = 0.636$) between respondents with and without formal maxillofacial prosthodontics training. Ninety-eight percent would recommend the MFP profession to other colleagues.

Discussion

The response rate of this study was 39%. There have been some variations in the response rates of surveys of maxillofacial prosthodontists. In 1992, a survey among members of the AAMP, ACP, and American Anaplastology Association had a response rate of 26% [7]. A survey in 2010 yielded a usable response rate of 22% [1], and another survey on MFPs reported a 16% response rate [8]. The response rate of this study gave a reasonable sampling for this population; future studies should include strategies to improve MFP response rates [9].

MFPs from 32 countries participated in this study. The majority of the respondents were male, indicating that either MFP is more popular among males or more males are active in the professional organization, as the respondents of this study were from the ISMR, AAMP, and IAOFR 2014 membership directories. It is also possible

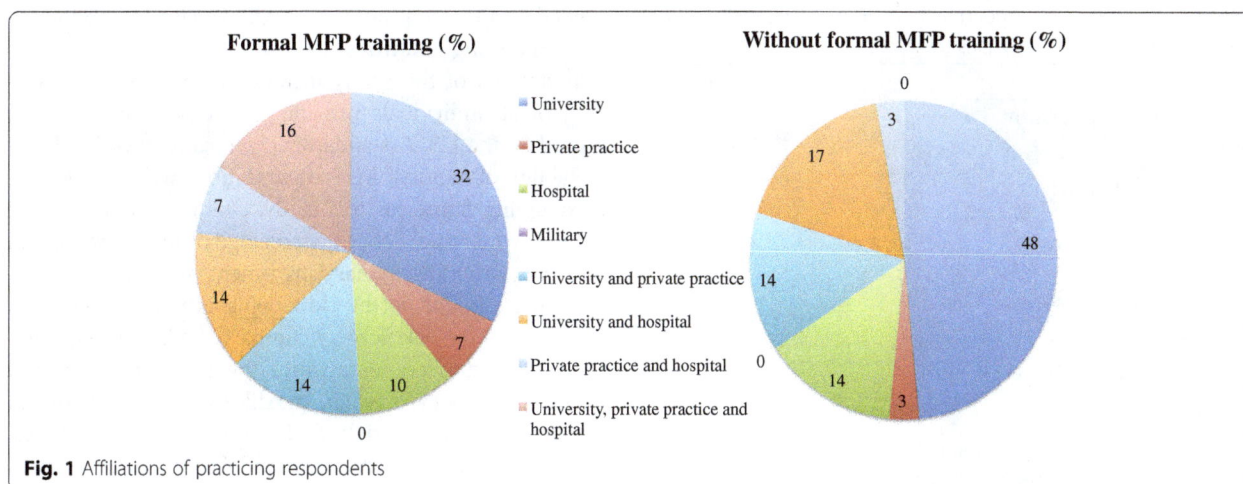

Fig. 1 Affiliations of practicing respondents

that a higher percentage of females chose not to respond to the survey.

Despite 51% of the respondents being unsatisfied with the training facilities in their home countries, when asked further about their own training 77% of respondents were either satisfied or very satisfied regardless of the quality of the training facilities. Eleven percent of respondents completed MFP training in the United States or Canada institution. There are also some prominent MFP centers available in Asia, Europe, North America, and South Africa that providing MFP trainings [10, 11].

The decision to pursue training abroad at an institution with better training facilities may be the cause of the MFP training satisfaction.

The most important factor in the decision to pursue MFP as a career is personal satisfaction, followed by prosthodontics residency exposure. Net earnings have been described as one of major determinants of choosing advanced education [12]. However, the potential salary ranked low as a factor important for the decision to pursue MFP career. Mentoring, interest among dental students, literature concerning the need for the profession in the future, and

Table 3 Types of treatment provided

	Formal MFP training (%)		Without formal MFP training (%)		P
	Mean	Median	Mean	Median	
Types of treatment provided					
•Standard prosthodontics treatment	34 ± 33.6	30	39 ± 33.8	40	0.672
•General dentistry	22 ± 25.9	10	21 ± 22.7	11	0.828
•Maxillofacial prosthodontics	36 ± 27.8	23	37 ± 27.9	38	0.815
•Surgical	8 ± 11.0	5	3 ± 9.5	0	0.021*
Types of maxillofacial treatment provided					
•Trauma	8 ± 8.6	5	4 ± 5.2	0	0.182
•Mandibular resection	12 ± 11.3	10	22 ± 14.9	28	0.068
•Obturation	26 ± 17.5	20	38 ± 26.0	40	0.268
•Maxillofacial implant cases	12 ± 15.8	7.5	7 ± 12.5	0	0.115
•Facial prosthetics	13 ± 17.9	5	6 ± 8.3	0	0.169
•Dental oncology	12 ± 14.1	7.5	2 ± 4.2	0	0.017*
•Speech aid	3 ± 4.5	1	2 ± 3.4	0	0.144
•Palatal drop	2 ± 2.7	0	1 ± 1.6	0	0.079
•Palatal lift	3 ± 4.6	0	2 ± 3.4	0	0.227
•Naso-alveolar moulding	1 ± 3.3	0	1 ± 3.0	0	0.477
•Prosthetic treatment of cleft	5 ± 5.4	5	7 ± 9.5	0	0.862
•Radiation intra oral devices	4 ± 10.0	0	1 ± 1.6	0	0.068

*Statistically significant difference (P ≤ 0.05)

Table 4 Percentage of respondents practising multidisciplinary treatment with other disciplines (N = 107)

Disciplines	Percent
No multidisciplinary treatment	5
Otolaryngology	68
Head and Neck Surgery	61
Oral Surgery	68
Plastic surgery	45
Oral Pathology / Oral Medicine	40
Radiation Oncology	50
Medical Oncology	26
Sleep Medicine	16
Other disciplines: psychiatry, dermatology, rheumatology, nephrology, speech therapy, neurosurgery	18

marketing of the profession as a career are identified as factors impacting the increase in the applicant pool for prosthodontics training [13]. These could fit into the MFP profession as well. Putting emphasis on prosthodontics residency exposure might ignite interest in the profession and help overcome this problem, since prosthodontics training is more readily available around the globe. Prosthodontics residency exposure may also be of high importance because, in some countries, maxillofacial prosthodontics is part of prosthodontics training [5]. Therefore, prosthodontics residents might receive enough exposure and training in the field to pursue an MFP career.

The results of this study can be used to attract more individuals into the profession, as factors important in the decision to purse an MFP career are described here. This survey also adds to the literature available on the practice profile of MFPs around the world. Included in the highlights of this study are the fact that some practitioners find a lack of maxillofacial prosthodontics service, and that more than 50% of respondents said that no maxillofacial prosthodontics organization exists in their country. This indicates there might be differences

in need and development of maxillofacial prosthodontics services among countries.

Limitations of this study include non-randomized sampling of all individuals providing MFP services in world other than the US. A standardized recognition of MFP and availability of national MFP organizations will provide better sampling frame for this study. Due to certain practice cultures, when asked about percentage of respondents who practicing multidisciplinary treatment with other disciplines there might not be clear demarcation of individuals with Head and Neck Surgery compared to Otolaryngology.

Future studies could tap into the need, demand, and profile differences between maxillofacial prosthodontics services in resource-rich and resource-poor countries. The needs and demands for maxillofacial prosthodontics services and education around the globe are not well-documented, with the most current worldwide study dating back to the 1987 [10]. Center-specific studies were conducted in the 1986 [14] and 2001 [15]. There might be need and demand differences between more resource-rich and resource-poor countries, and cultural differences may play a role. By understanding the characteristics of a particular country, maxillofacial prosthodontics services could be maximized for that particular society. An international training criteria for MFP is needed to set the minimum standard for MFP training. Realizing the multidisciplinary nature of MFP, multidisciplinary professional organizations have the advantage to define the blueprint of such comprehensive MFP training.

The results of this study can only be extrapolated for MFPs with demographics similar to the respondents of this survey. Other limitations of this study include the variety in the number of responses to each item in the survey, as well as no detailed information available on the types of treatment provided or the reason training facilities in countries were rated unsatisfactory by respondents. Having a complete set of responses and more detailed information would provide a better picture of the population.

Table 5 Time for professional activities

	Affiliated to university		Not affiliated to university		P
	Mean	Median	Mean	Median	
Hours/week seeing patients	29 ± 14.9	30	31 ± 14.8	40	0.251
Percentage of time for professional activities					
Clinical practice	44 ± 23.4	40	69 ± 14.6	70	0.002*
Teaching or training	26 ± 17.7	30	9 ± 7.3	10	0.008*
Funded research	6 ± 10	0	0 ± 0	0	0.015*
Non-funded research	7 ± 8	5	3 ± 6.0	0	0.192
Supervision of personnel	5 ± 4.6	5	6 ± 11.8	0	0488
Non-clinical administration work	9 ± 9.1	10	12 ± 11.1	10	0.347

*Statistically significant difference (P ≤ 0.05)

Conclusions

It was found that personal satisfaction is the most important factor in the decision to choose MFP career. A university and multidisciplinary approach describe the work settings of the majority of the MFPs. There were statistically significant differences regarding the type of treatments provided by respondents with and without formal MFP training that may appeal to individuals considering pursuing this sub-specialty training.

Abbreviations
AAMP: American academy of maxillofacial prosthetics; ACP: American college of prosthodontists; IAOFR: International academy for oral facial rehabilitation; ISMR: International society for maxillofacial rehabilitation; MFP: maxillofacial prosthodontists

Acknowledgements
The work was performed as part of the International Society of Maxillofacial Rehabilitation's External Relations Committee. The authors thank Ms. Barbara Bittner, Creighton University Office of Sponsored Programs Administration, for her editorial help. The material was presented in part at the International Society of Maxillofacial Rehabilitation meeting in Belgrade, Serbia from May 3-8, 2016.

Funding
Supported in part by grant from the Health Future Foundation Faculty Development Grant (#240046).

Authors' contributions
NA, CS and AGW made substantial contribution to conception and design of the study. NA, HR, KW and AGW made substantial contribution to acquisition of data, or analysis and interpretation of data. NA, HR, KW, CS and AGW were involved in drafting the manuscript or revising it critically for important intellectual content.

Competing interests
The authors declare that they have no competing interests.

Author details
[1]Department of Prosthodontics, Faculty of Dentistry, Universitas Indonesia, Jakarta, Indonesia. [2]Division of Preventive Dentistry, Niigata University Graduate School of Medical and Dental Sciences, Niigata, Japan. [3]Department of Oral and Maxillofacial Surgery, University of Groningen, University Medical Center Groningen, Groningen, The Netherlands. [4]Creighton University School of Dentistry, Omaha, NE, USA. [5]Department of Restorative Dentistry, University of Illinois at Chicago, College of Dentistry, Chicago, IL, USA. [6]Department of Prosthodontics, Creighton University School of Dentistry, Omaha, NE, USA. [7]Department of Surgery, Dental Service, Veterans Affairs Nebraska-Western Iowa Healthcare System, 4101 Woolworth Ave, Omaha, NE 68105, USA.

References
1. Hatamleh MM, Haylock C, Watson J, Watts DC. Maxillofacial prosthetic rehabilitation in the UK: a survey of maxillofacial prosthetists' and technologists' attitudes and opinions. Int J Oral Maxillofac Surg. 2010;39: 1186–92.
2. Salinas TJ. Prosthetic rehabilitation of defects of the head and neck. Semin Plast Surg. 2010;24:299–308.
3. Desjardins RP. Maxillofacial prosthetics: demand and responsibility. J Prosthet Dent. 1986;56:473–7.
4. Wolfaardt JF. Maxillofacial prosthetics–an international perspective of the British status quo. J Oral Rehabil. 1992;19:1–11.
5. Polyzois GL. Teaching maxillofacial prosthetics: a survey of dental curricula. Int J Prosthodont. 1988;1:308–11.
6. Hoddinott SN, Bass MJ. The dillman total design survey method. Can Fam Physician. 1986;32:2366–8.
7. Andres CJ, Haug SP, Brown DT, Bernal G. Effects of environmental factors on maxillofacial elastomers: Part II–Report of survey. J Prosthet Dent. 1992;68:519–22.
8. Montgomery PC, Kiat-Amnuay S. Survey of currently used materials for fabrication of extraoral maxillofacial prostheses in North America, Europe, Asia, and Australia. J Prosthodont. 2010;19:482–90.
9. Locker D. Response and nonresponse bias in oral health surveys. J Public Health Dent. 2000;60:72–81.
10. Polyzois GL. Educational status of maxillofacial prosthetics in Europe. J Dental Educ. 1987;51:489–91.
11. Firtell DN, Curtis TA. Maxillofacial prosthetics in the dental school curriculum. J Prosthet Dent. 1982;48:336–9.
12. Nash KD, Pfeifer DL. Private practice and the economic rate of return for residency training as a prosthodontist. J Am Dent Assoc. 2005;136:1154–62.
13. Munoz DM, Kinnunen T, Chang BM, Wright RF. Ten-year survey of program directors: trends, challenges, and mentoring in prosthodontics. Part 1. J Prosthodont. 2011;20:587–92.
14. Bonner EM, Wolfaardt JF, Cleaton-Jones P. The need for and value of a maxillofacial prosthodontic service in the Witwatersrand-Vaal area: Part I: A survey of the disciplines requiring a maxillofacial prosthodontic service. J Dent Assoc S Africa. 1986;41:177–80.
15. Sykes LM, Essop AR, Sukha AK. An 8-year assessment of maxillofacial prosthetic patients treated in a Department of Prosthetic Dentistry. SADJ. 2001;56:198–202.

12

Systematic review of ototoxic pre-surgical antiseptic preparations – what is the evidence?

Shubhi Singh*[ID] and Brian Blakley

Abstract

Objective: There is uncertainty regarding the safety of surgical antiseptic preparations in the ear. A systematic review of the literature was conducted to assess the evidence regarding ototoxicity of surgical antiseptic preparations.

Methods: A literature search was conducted using the PRISMA methods. Key words included "ototoxicity" "hearing loss", "antiseptic", "surgical preparation", "tympanoplasty", "vestibular dysfunction", "chlorhexidine", "iodine", "povidone", "ethanol", and "hydrogen peroxide" using Medline, Embase, Cochrane Library, Scopus and Web of Science. We included peer-reviewed papers that 1) objectively measured ototoxicity in humans or animals through hearing, vestibular function or histologic examination, 2) studied topically applied surgical antiseptic preparations, 3) were either in English or had an English abstract. We excluded papers that were 1) in vitro studies, 2) ear trauma studies, 3) studies of ototoxic ear drops intended for therapy, or 4) case reports. Studies included in the final review were screened using the PRISMA method.
Current systematic review registration number pending: 83,675.

Results: Fifty-six papers were identified as using PRISMA criteria. After applying our exclusion criteria, 13 papers met overall study criteria. Of these, six papers reported ototoxicity of iodine based solutions, five papers reported ototoxicity of chlorhexidine and ethanol and two papers assessed hydrogen peroxide. All papers reviewed were animal studies. Iodine based solutions show least harm overall, while chlorhexidine and high concentrations of alcohol based solutions showed most harm. The evidence on hydrogen based solutions was inconclusive.

Conclusions: The overall evidence for anyone antiseptic solution is weak. There is some evidence that iodine, chlorhexidine, hydrogen peroxide and alcohol based antiseptics have ototoxicity. Conclusive evidence for human ototoxicity from any solution is not strong.

Keywords: ototoxicity, hearing loss, antiseptic, vestibular dysfunction, chlorhexidine, iodine, povidone, ethanol, hydrogen peroxide

Background

Antiseptic cleaning of skin prior to surgical intervention is the standard of care globally. Pre-surgical antiseptic preparation has been known to reduce the number of wound infections when used adequately [1]. However some standard antiseptic preparations have been shown to cause toxicity to the eyes and ears when used in head and neck surgery [2]. Currently, in otologic surgery, there remains uncertainty regarding the safety of surgical antiseptic preparations in the ear. This has been a long standing area of concern as described in a case series conducted by Bicknell et al. in the early 1960s. Bicknell et al. describe varying degrees of morbidity following tympanoplasty surgery, ranging from high frequency hearing loss to "dead ears" with the main commonality between patients being pre-surgical preparation of the ear with chlorhexidine [3]. The purpose of this study was to conduct a systematic review of the literature to

* Correspondence: shubhi.singh@dal.ca
Division of Otolaryngology-Head and Neck Surgery, University of Manitoba, Health Sciences Centre GB421, 820 Sherbrook Street University of Manitoba, Winnipeg, MB R3T 2N2, Canada

assess the evidence regarding ototoxicity of standard surgical antiseptic preparations. The focus of this study was to review ototoxicity of povidone-iodine, chlorhexidine gluconate, ethanol and hydrogen peroxide.

Methods

A systematic literature review was conducted using various combinations of the following key words: "ototoxicity", "hearing loss", "antiseptic", "surgical preparation", "tympanoplasty", "vestibular dysfunction", "chlorhexidine", "iodine", "povidone", "ethanol", and "hydrogen peroxide" using the databases: Medline, Embase, Cochrane Library, Scopus and Web of Science through September 2016. Further studies were obtained through screening references from relevant articles and the authors' own databases and grey literature including legal proceedings. Criteria for inclusion of a published article in this review were applied to the collected studies by two independent reviewers.

Studies included were peer-reviewed papers that 1) objectively measured ototoxicity in humans or animals through hearing, vestibular function or histologic examination, 2) studied topically applied surgical antiseptic preparations, 3) were either in English or had an English abstract. Excluded studies were 1) in vitro studies, 2) ear trauma studies, 3) studies of ototoxic ear drops intended for therapy and 4) case reports. Studies included in the final review were screened using the PRISMA method [4].

Each paper identified through PRISMA criteria was reviewed for the following data items including: experimental subjects, solutions and concentrations tested and objective measure of ototoxicity. Objective measure of ototoxicity was defined as having any of the following: audiological or vestibular testing done before and after exposure to the solution, histological examinations or gross pathologic examinations. Due to the broad variation in objective measures of ototoxicity, no direct meta-analysis of the data was conducted between studies. However, the data obtained from the final results of studies meeting the set criteria in all studies are summarized in Tables 1, 2 and 3. Sources of error for these studies are further assessed in the discussion section.

Results

Fifty-six studies were identified through database searches and searches of relevant article references. Using pre-set criteria as mentioned above, 43 articles were eliminated as outlined in Fig. 1. Of the final 13 articles included in this review; six pertained to iodine based solutions, five to chlorhexidine and ethanol and two papers to hydrogen peroxide. All papers identified were animal studies.

Of the papers assessing the ototoxicity of povidone-iodine, Aursnes et al. found that povidone-iodine solutions in 70% alcohol with greater then 10 min of middle ear exposure to the solution caused an increase in cochlear damage [5]. Ichibangase et al. assessed ototoxicity of povidone-iodine 10% solution in guinea pigs of varying ages [6]. They found that those animals deemed to be infant or young had increased cochlear toxicity compared to adult guinea pigs. One reason they suggested for this finding was increased permeability of the round window membrane in infant versus adult guinea pigs as the membrane thickens with age [6]. Of the studies pertaining to povidone-iodine scrubs that contain detergents, all studies found that scrubs caused higher ototoxicity than povidone-iodine solutions, suggesting that detergent facilitates entry of the scrub into the inner ear [6–8].

In studies assessing chlorhexidine gluconate solutions, Igarashi et al. found that a concentration of 0.05% caused no change in Auditory Brainstem Response (ABR) from baseline after three applications of solution to the middle ear [9]. Perez showed that after three applications of 0.5% chlorhexidine gluconate to the middle ear of sand rats, no ABR were present in previously normal hearing animals [10]. Finally, three applications of chlorhexidine solution at 2.0% concentration caused destruction of outer hair cells on histological examination of the cochlea. Concentrations of 0.05 and 2.0% were shown to cause thick serous middle ear discharge on gross pathological examination. Similarly,. Perez et al. found that 70% Ethyl Alcohol caused gross pathological changes to the middle ear space including erythema and edema. In some animals oedema of the external ear canal was so severe that testing of hearing was not possible [10]. Morizono et al. tested several strengths of ethanol ranging from 0.1 to 100% pure ethanol in the middle ear cavities of chinchillas [11]. They concluded that there was evidence of ototoxicity for ethanol concentrations greater than 10% using cochlear microphonics [11].

Finally, Perez et al. and Nader et al. assessed the ototoxicity of 3% hydrogen peroxide solutions [12]. While Nader et al. found no difference in ABR from baseline after a 5 min exposure of 3% hydrogen peroxide to the middle ear of chinchillas, Perez et al. found the majority of sand rats tested had an increase in threshold from an average of 55 dB to 108 dB after 5 applications of 3% hydrogen peroxide [12, 13].

Discussion

In this review, we identified 13 studies showing the ototoxicity of povidone-iodine, chlorhexidine gluconate, ethanol/ ethyl alcohol and hydrogen peroxide in controlled non-trauma settings. All studies were

Table 1 Results for iodine-based antiseptic preparations

Author, Year	Population	Intervention	Control	Outcome
J Aursnes, 1982 [5]	28 Guinea Pigs. Baseline Preyer's reflex measured in all study animals.	Solutions tested: a) Iodine in 70% alcohol b) Iodophor in 70% alcohol c) Iodine in aqua dest. d) Iodophor in aqua dest. Exposure time 10, 30 or 60 minuets. Histopathology assessed after 2 weeks	Contralateral ear to experimental ear	a) Gross examination of the ear showed no mucosal changes after 10 mins of exposure for Iodine or Iodophor in aqua dest. b) Middle ear mucosal damage worst for solutions in 70% alcohol. c) Cochlear damage with exposure time of 60 min with Iodophor in 70% alcohol. d) Vestibular damage seen with Iodophor in 70% with exposure times of 30-60min
T Morizono, 1982 [7]	30 Chinchilla	Solutions tested: a) Povidone-iodine Solution at 1:10 dilution (1.0% available iodine) b) Povidone-iodine Scrub* at 1:10 dilution (0.75% available iodine) c) Povidone-iodine Scrub at 1:100 dilution Exposure time 10mins Effect on Compound Action potential (CAP) tested 2 hours, 24 hours post exposure *Scrub contains detergent	Contralateral ear to experimental ear	a) Povidone-iodine Scrub more toxic to cochlear function then solution b) Evoked action potential measure at round window, no change 2 hours after exposure with 1:10 dilution of Iodine Solution c) Evoked action potential measure at round window 2 hours after exposure with 1:10 dilution of Iodine Scrub caused severe depression at all tested frequencies (2, 4, 8, 12kHz) d) Increased toxicity with increased concentrations for both solution and scrub
T Morizono, 1983 [8]	30 Chinchilla	Solutions at different dilutions d) Povidone-iodine Solution at 1:10 dilution (1.0% available iodine) e) Povidone-iodine Scrub* at 1:10 dilution (0.75% available iodine) f) Povidone-iodine Scrub at 1:100 dilution Duration of exposure time 10mins Effect on Compound Action potential (CAP) tested 2 hours, 24 hours post exposure *Scrub contains detergent	Contralateral ear to experimental ear	a) High frequency losses (8 and 12kHz) after 10, 30 and 120min exposure to iodine scrub at 1:100 dilution
T. Inchibangase, 2011 [6]	70 Guinea Pigs – Divided into groups based on age (infant, young and adult)	Solution tested a) Povidone-iodine 10% solution b) Povidone-iodine scrub Effect on Compound Action potential (CAP) tested at 24h, 7days and 28days	Contralateral ear to experimental ear	a) No action potential at 24hours after application of Povidoneiodine scrub b) 24 hours after exposure to povidone-iodine solution, significant ototoxicity measured in infant group, less in young and least in adult c) 8 fold dilution of povidoneiodine solution showed no hearing loss in adults, loss for young at 2 and 4kHz d) Showed aged related variation associated with ototoxicity in guinea pigs
M. Ozkiris [16]	24 Sprague-Dawley Rats	Solution tested a) 5, 7.5, 10% Povidone-iodine solutions No exposure time given. Otoacoustic emissions measured at 1 and 10 days after exposure	Contralateral ear to experimental ear	a) At 5% concentration some statistically significant decreased hearing at day 1 but resolved by day 10 b) At 7.5% and 10%, day 10 results showed decreased in hearing in frequencies ranging from 1.5-12kHz
R. Yagiz, 2003 [17]	7 adult guinea pigs	Solution Tested a) Povidone-iodine 10% solution No exposure time given. Hearing tested at 10 days and 4 weeks after exposure	a) Saline as a negative control in the contralateral ear to experimental ear in 4 animals b) Gentamycin as a positive control the contralateral ear of 3 experimental animals	a) 4 animals could not be tested due to severe oedema of the external auditory canal b) No Otoacustic emissions present 10days or 4 weeks after exposure

Table 2 Results for chlorhexidine and ethanol-based antiseptic preparations

Author, Year	Population	Intervention	Control	Outcomes
R. Perez, 2000 [10]	25 Sand Rats	Solutions tested a) Povidone-iodine 10% solution b) Chlorhexidine Gluconate 0.5% solution c) Ethyl alcohol in 70% aqueous solution Exposure time 3 days ABR and vestibular evoked potentials (VsEP) testing 8 days after initial exposure	a) Saline as negative control b) Gentamycin as positive control	a) ABR not present after Chlorhexidine Gluconate 0.5% solution b) ABR present at baseline after application of Povidone-iodine 10% solution, VsEP present in all test animals c) No ABR or VsEP recorded in 2/5 animals after Ethyl alcohol 70% solution, 3/5 had elevated thresholds (70-80 dB) d) Erythema and oedema noted in 5/5 middle ear cavities after application of ethyl alcohol
Y. Igarashi, 1985 [9]	12 Cats	Solutions tested a) Chlorhexidine Gluconate 2.0% b) Chlorhexidine Gluconate 0.05% Exposure time every 2 days × 3 applications. Histologic examination at 7 days and 4 weeks	Contralateral ear to the experimental ear	a) Gross examination of middle ear space showed thick serous fluid retention in12/12 animals b) Histological examination showed loss of outer hair less in lower cochlear turns, with 85% loss near the round window after application of Chlorhexidine gluconate 2% solutions c) Little to no damage to the outer hair cells seen with Chlorhexidine 0.05% solution
J. Aursnes, 1981 [14]	48 Guinea Pigs	Solutions tested a) Chlorhexidine 0.1% in 70% alcohol b) Chlorhexidine 0.1% in aqua. Solution c) Chlorhexidine 0.5% in 70% alcohol d) Chlorhexidine 0.5% in aqua. Solution Exposure time 10, 30 and 60 mins. Histological examination done after 2, 3, 4 or 10 weeks post exposure	Contralateral ear to experimental ear	a) Gross examination showed extensive fibrotic tissue after 60 min exposure time b) Greater degree of fibrosis with 0.5% solution compared to 0.1% solution c) Total destruction of outer hair cells seen 3 weeks after exposure with Chlorhexidine 0.5% in 70% alcohol
H. G. Galle, 1986 [18]	2 Guinea Pigs	Solution tested a) Savlon™* in 1:100 dilution Cochlear microphonics, histologic examination and behaviour measured at 24 h and 48 h after exposure * Composed of 1.5% Chlorhexidine Gluconate and 0.15% cetrimide (quaternary ammonium compound)	Contralateral ear to experimental ear	a) Severe vestibular dysfunction based on behaviour but effects diminished after 24 h and again after 48 h b) Hearing thresholds increased from baseline of 35 dB to 70 dB SPL
T. Morizono, 1981 [11]	23 Chinchillas	Solutions tested a) Ethanol in contractions of 0.1, 1, 3, 10, 25, 50, 70 and 100% Exposure time was 10mins, 24 h. Cochlear mircophonics and endocochlear Action potentials tested	Contralateral ear to experimental ear	a) Variable outcomes with some animals showing decrease in all frequencies tested with cochlear microphonics with 3% solutions while others showed no deficits with 50% solution

animal studies and no direct human correlation can be drawn given the differences in anatomy of the middle ear space, dosing of antiseptic preparations and in some cases the duration of exposure being in the order of several weeks. However, some solutions showed high ototoxicity in relatively low concentrations and short exposure times. This includes povidone-iodine scrub which contains detergent,

Table 3 Results for hydrogen peroxide-based antiseptic preparations

Author, Year	Population	Intervention	Control	Outcome
R. Perez, 2003 [13]	22 Sand Rats	a) Hydrogen peroxide 3% solution Exposure time 5 days. ABR and VsEP tested on day 8 after initial exposure	a) Saline as negative control b) Gentamicin as positive control	a) ABR could not be tested in 3/12 animals. All remaining animals had elevated base line from 55 dB to 108 dB b) VsEP could not be recorded in 5/12 animals. All remaining animals had a increased from baseline of mean latency time
ME Nader, 2007 [12]	18 Chinchillas	Solution tested a) Hydrogen peroxide 3% solution Exposure time 5 min ABR performed 1 day after exposure	Contralateral ear to experimental ear	b) No difference of ABR from baseline recording prior to instillation of hydrogen peroxide.

povidone-iodine in 70% alcohol, and chlorhexidine gluconate in 70% alcohol [5–7, 14]. However for other solutions there is no consensus from the studies identified. (Tables 1, 2 and 3).

There are several limitations of this current review. The methods and objective measures are inconsistent.

All the studies identified in this review were animal studies so we are cautious about drawing conclusions from different species using different methods on the potential of the solutions to cause damage in human subjects. In studies conducted on guinea pigs and chinchillas the main hypothesized method of inner ear penetration for solutions is through the round window. The Chinchilla round window membrane is 1/6 of the thickness of that of humans therefore this model is likely over estimating ototoxicity in humans [15].

There are also several challenges differentiating conductive hearing loss from sensorineural hearing loss in animal subjects. The time period over which animals were assessed may not have been adequate [7].

Conclusion

Given the findings of this review, the evidence of human ototoxicity of currently used antiseptic preparations is not strong. Iodine based, non-alcoholic, non-detergent solutions may be the least ototoxic but all should be used with caution.

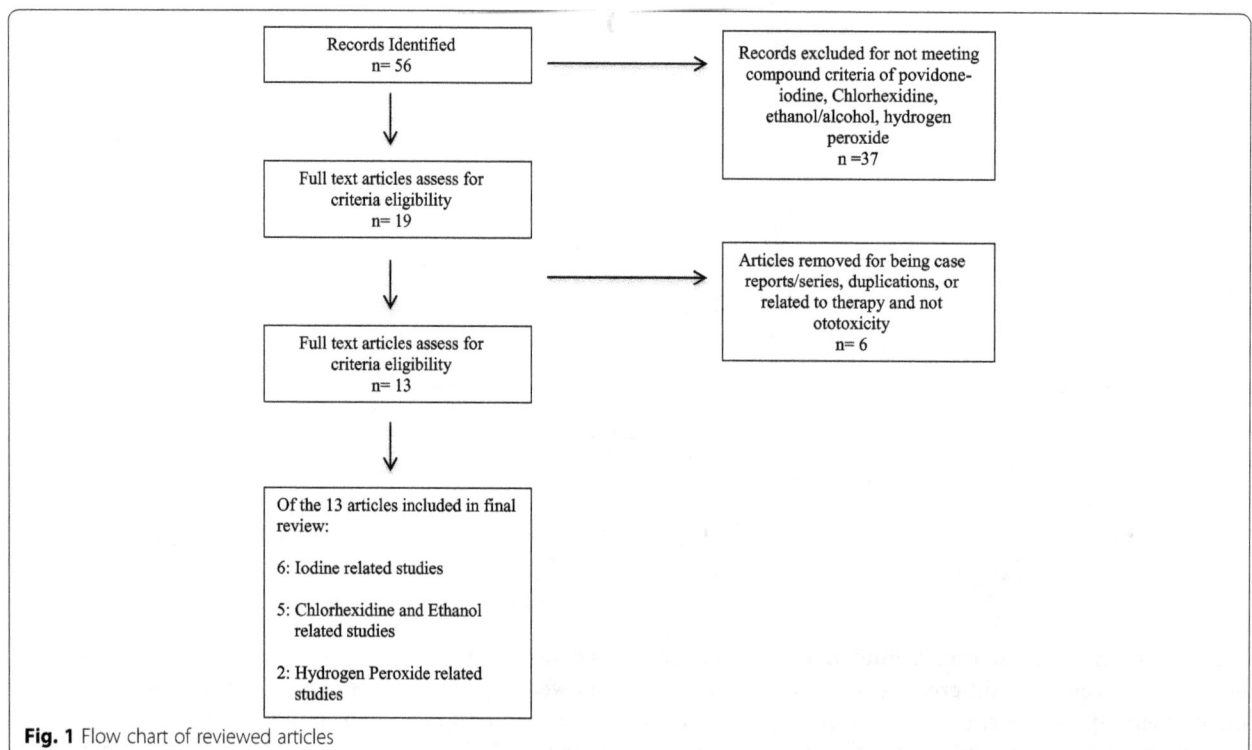

Fig. 1 Flow chart of reviewed articles

Systematic review of ototoxic pre-surgical antiseptic preparations – what is the...

83

Abbreviations
ABR: Auditory Brainstem Response; CAP: Compound Action Potential; PRISMA: Preferred Reporting Items for Systematic Reviews and Meta-Analysis; SPL: Sound Pressure Level; VsEP: Vestibular Evoked Potential

Funding
No funding was obtained for preparation of this manuscript.

Authors' contributions
Both authors of this paper were responsible for screening articles obtained through databases researches for inclusion in the final paper. Dr. SS was responsible for setting database search criteria and database searches, review inclusion criteria and preparation of the final manuscript. All authors read and approved the final manuscript.

Competing interests
The authors declare that they have no competing interests.

References
1. Mangram AJ, Horan TC, Pearson ML, Silver LC, Jarvis WR, Committee HICPA. Guideline for prevention of surgical site infection, 1999. Am J Infect Control. 1999;27:97–134.
2. Steinsapir KD, Woodward JA. Chlorhexidine Keratitis: Safety of Chlorhexidine as a Facial Antiseptic. Dermatologic Surgery 2016.
3. Bicknell P. Sensorineural deafness following myringoplasty operations. J Laryngol Otol. 1971;85:957–62.
4. Liberati A, Altman DG, Tetzlaff J, et al. The PRISMA statement for reporting systematic reviews and meta-analyses of studies that evaluate health care interventions: explanation and elaboration. PLoS Med. 2009;6:e1000100.
5. Aursnes J. Ototoxic effect of iodine disinfectants. Acta Otolaryngol. 1982;93:219–26.
6. Ichibangase T, Yamano T, Miyagi M, Nakagawa T, Morizono T. Ototoxicity of Povidone-Iodine applied to the middle ear cavity of guinea pigs. Int J Pediatr Otorhinolaryngol. 2011;75:1078–81.
7. Morizono T, Sikora MA. The ototoxicity of topically applied povidone-iodine preparations. Arch Otolaryngol. 1982;108:210–3.
8. Morizono T, Sikora MA. Compound action potential input-output decruitment: effect of topically applied antiseptics. Arch Otolaryngol. 1983; 109:677–81.
9. Igarashi Y, Suzuki J-I. Cochlear ototoxicity of chlorhexidine gluconate in cats. Arch Otorhinolaryngol. 1985;242:167–76.
10. Perez R, Freeman S, Sohmer H, Sichel JY. Vestibular and cochlear ototoxicity of topical antiseptics assessed by evoked potentials. Laryngoscope. 2000; 110:1522–7.
11. Morizono T, Sikora MA. Ototoxicity of ethanol in the tympanic cleft in animals. Acta Otolaryngol. 1981;92:33–40.
12. Nader ME, Kourelis M, Daniel SJ. Hydrogen peroxide ototoxicity in unblocking ventilation tubes: a chinchilla pilot study. Otolaryngol Head Neck Surg. 2007;136:216–20.
13. Perez R, Freeman S, Cohen D, Sichel JY, Sohmer H. The effect of hydrogen peroxide applied to the middle ear on inner ear function. Laryngoscope. 2003;113:2042–6.
14. Aursnes J. Cochlear damage from chlorhexidine in guinea pigs. Acta Otolaryngol. 1981;92:259–71.
15. Rauch S. Membrane problems of the inner ear and their significance. J Laryngol Otol 1966; 80:1144–155.
16. Özkiriş M, Kapusuz Z, Saydam L.Ototoxicity of different concentrations povidone-iodine solution applied to the middle ear cavity of rats. Indian Journal of Otolaryngology and Head & Neck Surgery. 2013;65:168–72.
17. Yagiz R, Tas A, Uzun C, Adali MK, Koten M, Karasalihoglu AR. Effect of topically applied povidone-iodine on transient evoked otoacoustic emissions in guinea pigs. J Laryngol Otol. 2003;117:700–3.
18. Galle H, Haagen AVV. Ototoxicity of the antiseptic combination. Vet Q 1986; 8:56–60.

13

Morphoproteomics, E6/E7 in-situ hybridization, and biomedical analytics define the etiopathogenesis of HPV-associated oropharyngeal carcinoma and provide targeted therapeutic options

Robert E. Brown[1*], Syed Naqvi[2], Mary F. McGuire[1], Jamie Buryanek[1] and Ron J. Karni[2]

Abstract

Background: Human papillomavirus (HPV) has been identified as an etiopathogenetic factor in oropharyngeal squamous cell carcinoma. The HPV *E6* and *E7* oncogenes are instrumental in promoting proliferation and blocking differentiation leading to tumorigenesis. Although surgical intervention can remove such tumors, the potential for an etiologic field effect with recurrent disease is real. A downstream effector of E7 oncoprotein, enhancer of zeste homolog 2 (EZH2), is known to promote proliferation and to pose a block in differentiation and in turn, could lead to HPV-induced malignant transformation. However, the EZH2 pathway is amenable to low toxicity therapies designed to promote differentiation to a more benign state and prevent recurrent disease by inhibiting the incorporation of HPV into the genome. This is the first study using clinical specimens to demonstrate EZH2 protein expression in oropharyngeal carcinoma (OPC).

Methods: The study included eight patients with oropharyngeal carcinoma, confirmed p16INK4a- positive by immunohistochemistry (IHC). The tissue expression of E6/E7 messenger RNA (mRNA) was measured by *RNAscope®* in-situ hybridization technology. Expression of EZH2, Ki-67, and mitotic indices were assessed by morphoproteomic analysis. Biomedical analytics expanded the results with data from Ingenuity Pathway Analysis (IPA) and KEGG databases to construct a molecular network pathway for further insights.

Results: Expression of *E6* and *E7* oncogenes in p16INK4a- positive oropharyngeal carcinoma was confirmed. EZH2 and its correlates, including elevated proliferation index (Ki-67) and mitotic progression were also present. Biomedical analytics validated the relationship between HPV- E6 and E7 and the expression of the EZH2 pathway.

Conclusion: There is morphoproteomic and mRNA evidence of the association of p16INK4a-HPV infection with the *E6* and *E7* oncogenes and the expression of EZH2, Ki-67 and mitotic progression in oropharyngeal carcinoma. The molecular network biology was confirmed by biomedical analytics as consistent with published literature. This is significant because the biology lends itself to targeted therapeutic options using metformin, curcumin, celecoxib and sulforaphane as therapeutic strategies to prevent progression or recurrence of disease.

Keywords: HPV-associated oropharyngeal carcinoma, E6/E7 in-situ hybridization, Morphoproteomics, Biomedical analytics, Biology, EZH2, Therapeutic options

* Correspondence: robert.brown@uth.tmc.edu
[1]Department of Pathology and Laboratory Medicine, at UT Health McGovern Medical School, Houston, TX, USA
Full list of author information is available at the end of the article

Background

HPV-associated oropharyngeal carcinoma (OPC) has been reported to account for up to 60% of this subtype of head and neck cancer cases [1]. The E7 oncoprotein of HPV has been linked with the upregulation of p16INK4a protein, which serves as a surrogate marker of HPV-associated oropharyngeal carcinoma [1]. Although the prognosis of HPV-associated oropharyngeal carcinoma has been associated with a 58% reduction in mortality risk vis-à-vis the HPV-negative cases [1, 2], there is still the risk of recurrent disease and an opportunity for therapeutic intervention. Relatedly, high EZH2 expression in patients with head and neck squamous cell carcinoma was associated with advanced T stage and portended a poor survival outcome [3]. A possible connection is that E7 oncoprotein in cervical squamous cell carcinoma has been associated with the activation of EZH2 expression by HPV16 E7 at the transcriptional level [4]. However, no reports of the association of E7 in HPV-associated OPC and EZH2 pathway expression in clinical specimens from patients with OPC are currently cited in the National Library of Medicine's MEDLINE Database (https://www.ncbi.nlm.nih.gov/pubmedhealth/).

The purpose of this report is to address gaps in the knowledge of EZH2 expression in OPC patient specimens by: 1. providing morphoproteomic and mRNA evidence of the association of p16INK4a-HPVinfection with the *E6* and *E7* oncogenes in oropharyngeal carcinoma; 2. documenting and correlating both the expression of E6 mRNA in such cases with cell cycle progression and the expression of E7 mRNA with p16INK4a, EZH2 and Ki-67 and mitotic progression; 3. confirming the biology of HPV-associated oropharyngeal carcinoma with biomedical analytics; and 4. investigating targeted therapeutic options based on biomedical analytics and preclinical data.

Methods

Patient population

Eight adult patients (7 males and 1 female) ranging in age from 51 to 72 years were included in this study. The anatomical locations of their biopsy-proven squamous cell carcinomas included palatine tonsil in five and tongue base in three.

Data collection protocols

Data collection and molecular analyses were performed in accordance with the guidelines of the University of Texas McGovern Medical School Committee for the Protection of Human Subjects Institutional Review Board (IRB).

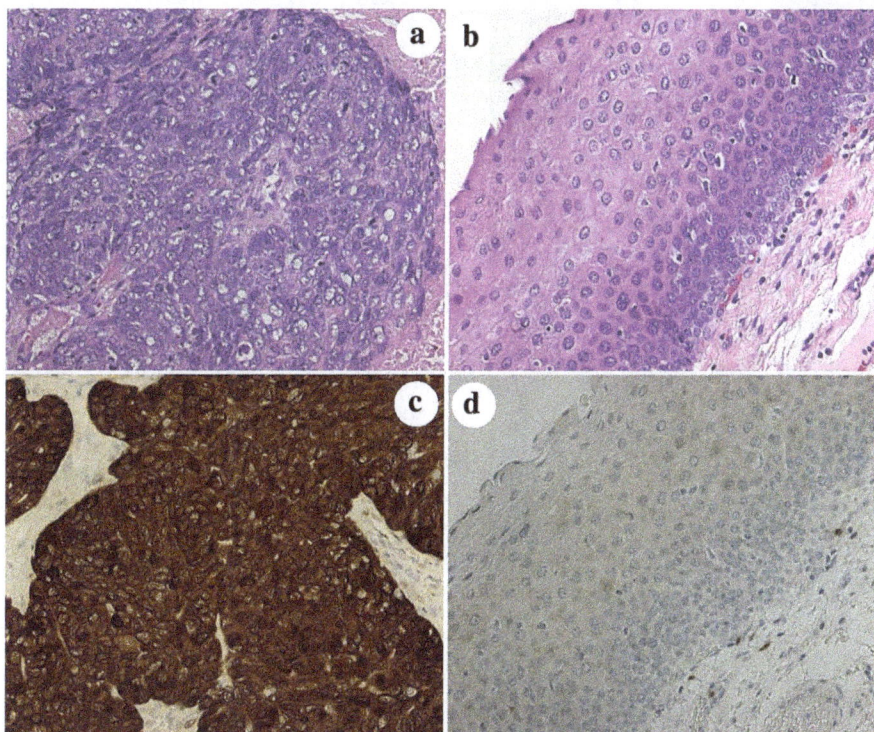

Fig. 1 Patient 8 biopsy specimen with non-keratinizing oropharyngeal carcinoma compared with concurrent non-neoplastic mucosa. H&E and p16INK4a stained sections of non-keratininzing squamous cell carcinoma versus non-neoplastic squamous epithelium (Frames **a** and **c** and **b** and **d**, respectively; note strong DAB brown chromogenic signal for p16INK4a in oropharyngeal carcinoma [Frame **c**] versus absence of expression in non-neoplastic squamous mucosa [Frame **d**]; original magnification ×200 Frames **a**-**d**)

Table 1 Summary of median scores for percentages of Ki-67, p16INK4a, and EZH2, for mitotic indices and for E6/E7 mRNA by individual patient with oropharyngeal carcinoma

Patient	1	2	3	4	5	6	7	8	Median
Ki-67 (MKI67)	80	85	90	60	70	70	60	60	70
Mitotic Index	105	44	36	40	16	55	31	96	42
p16 INK4a (CDKN2A)	100	100	100	100	100	100	100	100	100
EZH2	90	90	90	90	90	90	80	80	90
E6/E7 mRNA	100	100	100	100	50	75	100	100	100

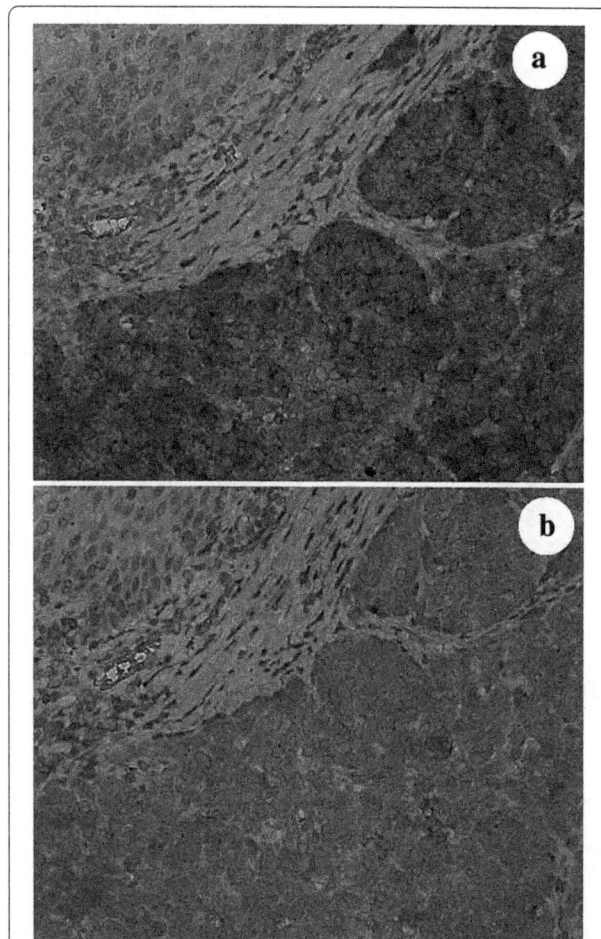

Fig. 2 Patient 8 biopsy specimen with non-keratinizing oropharyngeal carcinoma compared with adjacent non-neoplastic mucosa. Red *RNAscope*® 2.5 HD in-situ hybridization (ISH) assay for HPV-HR18 E6/E7 mRNA performed on the non-keratinizing squamous cell carcinoma revealed strong red chromogenic cytoplasmic expression (4+ semi-quantitative score, see Table 2) in the tumor (lower right and middle, Frame **a**) and no expression in the adjacent non-neoplastic (upper left, Frame **a**). Contrast with the dapβ negative control in Frame **b**. (original magnification ×200 for Frames a and **b**)

Molecular analyses

Molecular analyses included in-situ hybridization for the expression of HPV-HR18 E6/E7 mRNA using the *RNAscope*® technology from Advanced Cell Diagnostics (https://acdbio.com/). Morphoproteomic analysis and biomedical analytics were also performed as part of the molecular analysis in our CLIA and CAP certified Consultative Proteomics Laboratory in order to define the biology of the patients' tumors, to provide correlative expressions, and to ascertain targeted therapeutic options designed to reduce the progression or recurrence of the HPV-associated oropharyngeal carcinomas.

In-situ hybridization

RNAscope® 2.5HD Red Assay was performed to evaluate expression in all 8 tissue specimens. The test assayed 18 high-risk HPV serotypes: HPV-HR18 HPV 16, 18, 26, 31, 33, 35, 39, 45, 51, 52, 53, 56, 58, 59, 66, 68, 73 and 82, E6/E7 mRNA. Hs-PPIB was used as a positive control marker for sample quality control (QC) and to evaluate RNA quality in all the tissue samples. Bacterial gene dapB was used as a negative control. Standard pretreatment assay conditions were determined to be optimal for the samples in the study set. All the samples in the study passed QC with strong PPIB expression and no/negligible dapB background. A semi-quantitative scoring system of 0-4 was utilized.

Morphoproteomics

Morphoproteomic analysis applies bright field microscopy and immunohistochemistry directed against various protein analytes to define the biology of a neoplastic process. The analysis uncovers etiopathogenetic occurrences that might be responsible for the process development and the propensity for it to recur [5, 6]. Immunohistochemical probes were applied against the following protein analytes in unstained sections of the patients' oropharyngeal carcinomas: Ki-67 (G1, S, G2 and M phases of the cell cycle; DakoCytomation, Carpinteria, California, lot #20001030); and enhancer of zeste homolog 2 (EZH2; Cell Signaling Technology, Inc., lot #7). The level of expression of the analytes was graded on a 0 to 3+ scale based on signal intensity indicated by a 3,3′- tetrahydrochloride (DAB) chromogenic (brown) signal, the nuclear estimation of Ki-67 and EZH2 percentages, and mitotic index based on mitotic figures/10 high power fields. The details of the morphoproteomic staining procedure have been previously described [5, 6].

Biomedical analytics

To gain insights into HPV-associated oropharyngeal carcinoma, a standard IPA oropharyngeal pathway network ("ORO") was constructed from key molecules associated with oropharyngeal carcinoma in the Ingenuity Knowledge Base (www.ingenuity.com). Since IPA does not

Table 2 HPV-HR18-E6/E7 mRNA semi-quantitative scoring data by individual patient with oropharnygeal carcinoma

Patient Specimen ID	Hs-PPIB Score (positive control)	dapβ Score (negative control)	QC Pass/Fail	HPV-HR18 E6/E7 mRNA Score
1	4	0	Pass	4
2	4	0	Pass	4
3	4	0	Pass	4
4	4	0	Pass	4
5	3	0	Pass	2
6	3	0	Pass	3
7	4	0	Pass	4
8	4	0	Pass	4

include viral species, E6/E7 and their interactions associated with HPV (hsa05203) ("HPV" network) were extracted from the KEGG pathway database (http://www.genome.jp/kegg/pathway.html) and manually added to the ORO network. A "patient" pathway network was also constructed from the median patient scores and linked to ORO-HPV. From these graphs and additional data mining of the National Library of Medicine's MEDLINE database, a single ORO-HPV network model was constructed using IPA Pathway Designer to represent the key modulation and adaptive responses in the signal transduction processes. Therapies were then linked to the ORO-HPV network model to assess potential benefits.

Results

The IHC workup had established the expression of p16INK4a protein in all cases (Fig. 1, Table 1).

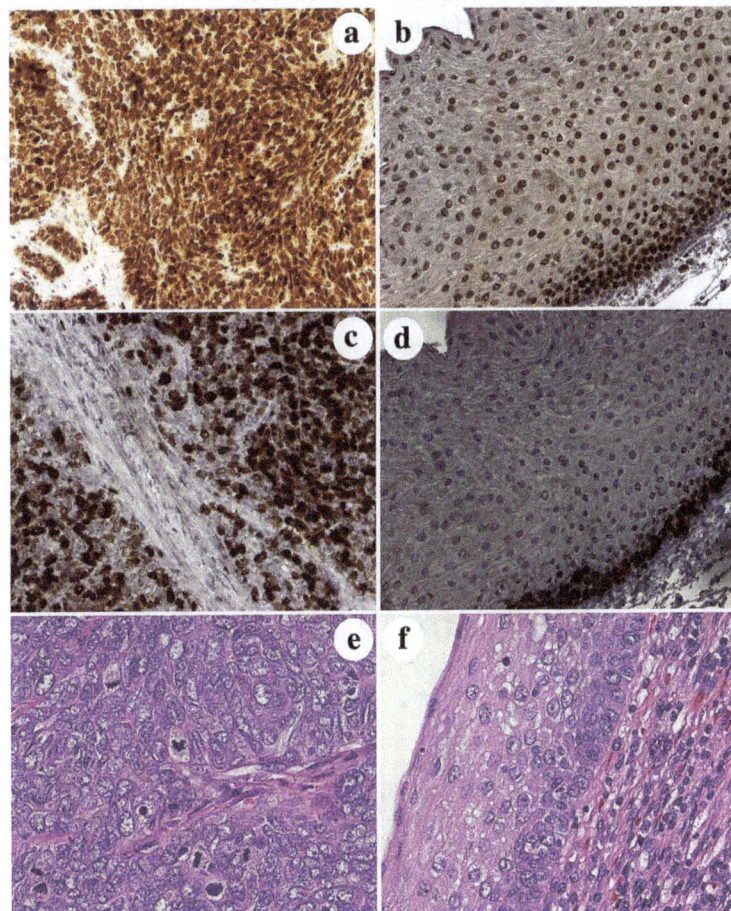

Fig. 3 Patient 8 biopsy specimen with non-keratinizing oropharyngeal carcinoma compared with concurrent non-neoplastic mucosa. Enhancer of zeste homolog 2 (EZH2) and Ki-67 (G1, S, G2 and M phases of the cell cycle) show strong (3+ on a scale of 0-3+) nuclear expression in a majority of the non-keratinizing squamous cell carcinoma (NKSCC) versus similar expression primarily limited to the basal and suprabasal cells of the non-neoplastic squamous mucosa (Frames **a** and **c** versus **b** and **d**, respectively). Mitotic progression in the corresponding H&E coincides with the EZH2 and Ki-67 expression with multiple mitotic figures evident in the NKSCC (Frame **e**) with no mitotic figures in the adjacent non-neoplastic squamous mucosa (Frame **f**). (DAB brown chromogenic signal for frames **a-d**; original magnifications ×200 for frames **a-d** and ×400 for Frames **e** and **f**)

In-situ hybridization

HPV-HR18 E6/E7 was detected at high levels across most samples (score 4) with the exception of patient specimens 5 and 6 that scored at 2 and 3, respectively (see Table 2 and Fig. 2).

Morphoproteomics

Nuclear expressions of EZH2 (enhancer of zeste homolog 2) and Ki-67 (G1, S, G2 and M phases of the cell cycle) and mitotic indices (mitotic figures/10 high power fields) by visual estimation on each case revealed a median of 90% and 70% for EZH2 and Ki-67, respectively and a range of 16 to 105 for the mitotic indices (Table 1 and Fig. 3, frames a and b, c and d, and e and f, respectively for EZH2, Ki-67 expression, and mitotic progression).

Biomedical analytics

In order to provide a visual comparison, biomedical analytics generated a normalized score by patient of the comparative analytes for Ki67, mitotic index, p16INK4a, EZH2 and E6/E7 mRNA. This is illustrated in the bar chart (Fig. 4).

ORO-HPV network model

There were extensive crossover interactions between the HPV pathway and the ORO pathway. Three molecules of interest - EZH2, MKI67 (Ki67) and CDKN2A (p16 INK4a) were present – and affected – in the combined pathway network (not shown.) This combined ORO-HPV network model contained 1086 molecular interactions, or links, in the 3 linked pathways of ORO, HPV, and median patient. Of the 1086 links, 513 bridged between the ORO network and the HPV network. For the patient, the level of CDKN2A affected more molecules associated with HPV than with ORO. In return, more molecules from HPV than ORO affected the patient network, with TP53 and

RB1 being the major influencers. 174 molecules from ORO affected HPV and patients; whereas 224 molecules from HPV affected ORO and patient.

Therapeutic interactions

The complex ORO-HPV network model was edited to focus on the key molecules: E6/E7 mRNA, EZH2, Ki-67 (MK167) plus related interactions from the National Library of Medicine's MEDLINE Database. The potential efficacy of sulforaphane and the metformin and curcumin therapies – the latter in part through the upregulation of microRNAs – were graphically demonstrated (Fig. 5). EZH2 was identified as a possible therapeutic target. It can be seen from the networks that EZH2 (Fig. 5, *upper left*) is a key network point that is activated by E6/E7. Mir-26A can be seen in the upper right hand corner of Fig. 5; it needs to be upregulated to decrease EZH2.

Discussion

This report provides morphoproteomic and mRNA evidence of the association of p16INK4a-HPVinfection with the *E6* and *E7* oncogenes in oropharyngeal carcinoma. The E6 oncoprotein has been shown to bind with and promote the degradation of wild type p53 by activating the ubiquitin ligase E6AP [1, 7], and thereby, potentially to facilitate cell cycle progression [1, 8, 9]. Similarly, the E7 oncoprotein via the upregulation of EZH2 should promote cell cycle progression [1, 4]. Morphoproteomics and biomedical analytics provide correlates in our cases in the form of Ki-67 (G1, S, G2 and M phases) with mitotic progression. The seemingly paradoxical but ineffective increase in p16INK4a, a cyclin-dependent kinase inhibitor [10], coincides with E7 expression in our cases of oropharyngeal carcinoma [1]. In addition to its association with cell cycle progression in our study, enhancer

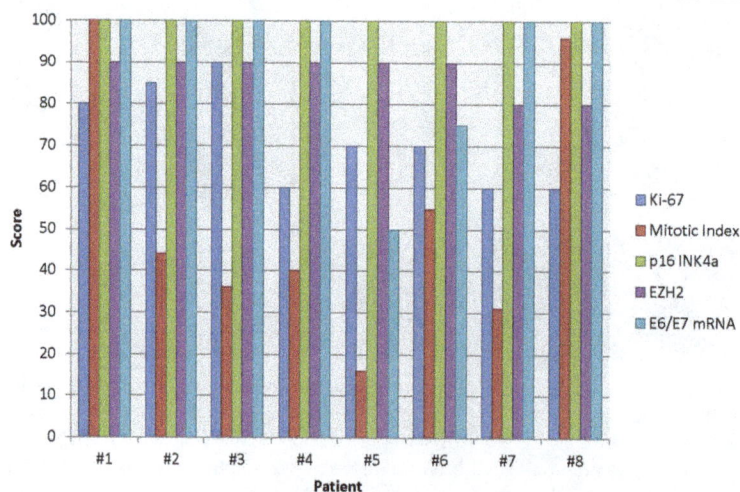

Fig. 4 Bar chart of normalized (median) score by patient of the comparative analytes for Ki67, mitotic index, p16INK4a,EZH2 and E6/E7 mRNA. Comparison of normalized scores. Note that patient #5 has the lowest E6/E7 score (assessed as moderate, 2+), and also the lowest mitotic index (see Tables 1 and 2)

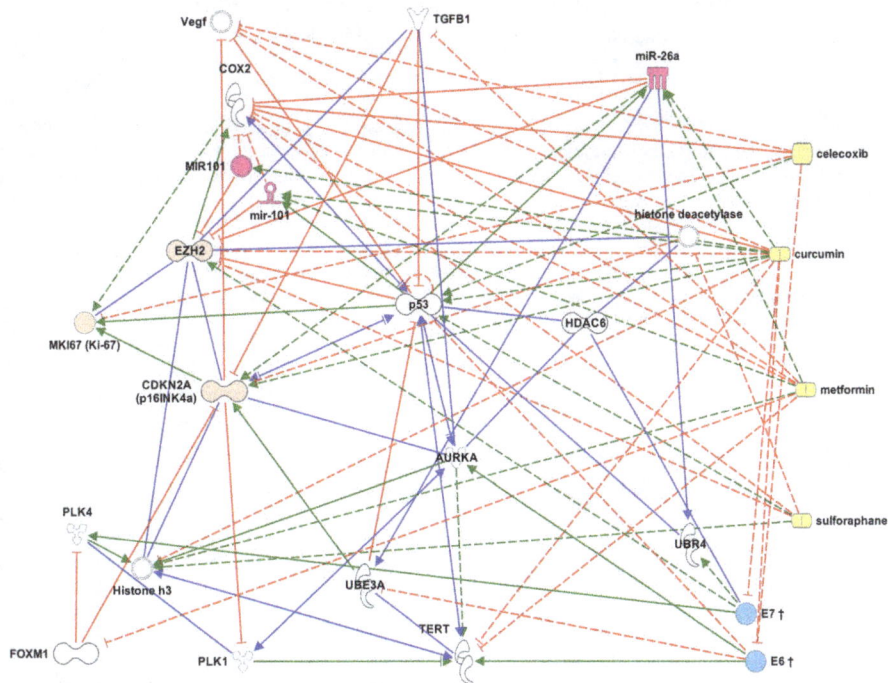

Fig. 5 Potential therapies for ORO-HPV combined pathway. Celecoxib, curcumin, metformin, sulforaphane (*right, yellow*). Scored molecules: CDKN2A, EZH2, MKI67 (*left, light orange*). E6, E7 (*lower right, blue, viral* †). microRNAs: miR-26a, MIR101, miR-101 (*top, pink*)

of Zeste homolog 2 (EZH2) – a histone methyltransferase – is potentially tumorigenic by virtue of the fact that it methylates and inactivates tumor suppressor genes and contributes to a state of proliferation and dedifferentiation in tumors and in facilitating their migratory potential [11–16]. This could account, in part, for the non-keratinizing/poorly keratinizing component of HPV-associated squamous cell carcinomas. The recent manuscript by Idris et al. [17] showed that inhibition of EZH2 has anti-tumorigenic effects on oropharyngeal squamous cell carcinoma (OPSCC) cells in culture that is more pronounced in HPV-positive cell lines. This preclinical evidence plus the results of our study support the applicability of our approach for human patients.

Biomedical analytics confirmed the correlations and the interactive biology of E6/E7 mRNA-associated oropharyngeal carcinoma with the morphoproteomic findings in our study and illustrated the potential targeted therapies of metformin, curcumin, celecoxib and sulforaphane.

Rationale for the application of these agents against HPV-associated oropharyngeal carcinoma are provided as follows: pharmacogenomic upregulation of microRNAs, miR-26a and miR-101, by metformin and a curcumin analog in preclinical studies correspondingly decreased the expression of EZH2 [18, 19] and metformin delays cell cycle progression [20]; curcumin has anti-tumoral activity against HPV-associated cells by selectively inhibiting the expression of viral oncogenes *E6* and *E7* [21, 22];

celecoxib in HPV-18-infected cervical cancer cells has been shown to restore p53 by suppressing viral oncoprotein E6 expression by down-modulating COX-2 and retrieving p53 from COX-2 association [23]; and sulforaphane suppresses EZH2 expression in skin cancer cells via a proteasome-dependent mechanism [24]. Lindsay et al. recently underscored the opportunities for novel therapeutic targets, such as EZH2, in OPC [25]. Although our pilot study was limited by a small patient population, the results are encouraging. We are in the process of developing a specific clinical protocol for patients with a confirmatory biopsy of HPV -oropharyngeal carcinoma (p16INK4a+/EZH2+) with high Ki-67 expression and mitotic progression. The protocol would incorporate the listed therapeutic agents in a combinatorial fashion and be applied following a confirmatory biopsy of HPV-oropharyngeal carcinoma (p16INK4a+/EZH2+ with high Ki-67 expression and mitotic progression) prior to the implementation of standard tumor board-recommended therapy for the individual patient.

Conclusions

Our study showed that p16INK4a-HPV infection is associated with the *E6* and *E7* oncogenes and with the expression of EZH2, Ki-67, and mitotic progression in oropharyngeal carcinoma. This biology lends itself to targeted therapeutic options using metformin, curcumin, celecoxib and sulforaphane as therapeutic strategies to prevent progression or recurrence of disease.

Abbreviations

CAP: College of American Pathologists; CLIA: Clinical Laboratory Improvement Amendments; DAB: 3,3'-Diaminobenzidine; EZH2: Enhancer of zeste homolog 2; H&E: Hematoxylin and eosin stain; HPV: Human papillomavirus; IHC: Immunohistochemistry; IPA: Ingenuity Pathway Analysis; IRB: Institutional Review Board; KEGG: Kyoto encyclopedia of genes and genomes; Ki-67/MKI67: Proliferation marker protein Ki-67; mRNA: messenger ribonucleic acid; p16INK4a/CDKN2A: Cyclin-dependent kinase inhibitor 2A; QC: Quality control; RB1: Retinoblastoma-associated protein; RNA: Ribonucleic acid.

Acknowledgements

The authors thank Pamela Johnston, HT (ASCP) for technical assistance, Bheravi Patel for secretarial support and help with the graphics, and scientists Marie Lauigan and Paul Terinate at Advanced Cell Diagnostics, Newark, CA.

Funding

Funding for this study was obtained from the Morphoproteomics Initiative, University of Texas McGovern Medical School at Houston.

Authors' contributions

RB, MM, RK and SN were involved in all aspects of experimental design, data collection, data analysis and were the main contributors of manuscript preparation. JB was primarily involved in technical aspects of slide analyses. All authors read and approved the final manuscript.

Authors' information

RB is a Professor of Pathology who invented the term "morphoproteomics" in 2003 to help define the biology of disease processes. MM is a Bioinformatics Scientist who invented the term "biomedical analytics" and has developed its applications. RK is Chief of the Division of Head and Neck Surgical Oncology at UTHealth.

Competing interests

The authors declare they have no competing interests.

Author details

[1]Department of Pathology and Laboratory Medicine, at UT Health McGovern Medical School, Houston, TX, USA. [2]Department of Otorhinolaryngology, Head and Neck Surgery at UT Health McGovern Medical School, Houston, TX, USA.

References

1. Spence T, Bruce J, Yip KW, Liu FF. HPV associated head and neck cancer. Cancers (Basel). 2016 Aug 5;8(8):pii:E75. doi:https://doi.org/10.3390/cancers8080075.

2. Ang KK, Harris J, Wheeler R, Weber R, Rosenthal DL, Nguyen-Tan PF, Westra WH, Chung CH, Jordan RC, Lu C, Kim H, Axelrod R, Silverman CC, et al. Human papillomavirus and survival of patients with oropharyngeal cancer. N Engl J Med. 2010;363:24–35.

3. Chang JW, Gwak SY, Shim GA, Liu L, Lim YC, Kim JM, Jung MG, Koo BS. EZH2 is associated with poor prognosis in head-and-neck squamous cell carcinoma via regulating the epithelial-to-mesenchymal transition and chemosensitivity. Oral Oncol. 2016;52:66–74.

4. Holland D, Hoppe-Seyler K, Schuller B, Lohrey C, Maroldt J, Durst M, Hoppe-Seyler F. Activation of the enhancer of zeste homologue 2 gene by the human papillomavirus E7 oncoprotein. Cancer Res. 2008;68(23):9964–72.

5. Brown RE. Morphoproteomics: exposing protein circuitries in tumors to identify potential therapeutic targets in cancer patients. Expert Rev Proteomics. 2005;2(3):337–48.

6. Brown RE. Morphogenomics and morphoproteomics: a role for anatomic pathology in personalized medicine. Arch Pathol Lab Med. 2009;133(4):568–79.

7. Scheffner M, Werness BA, Huibregtse JM, Levine AJ, Howley PM. The E6 oncoprotein encoded by human papillomavirus types 16 and 18 promotes the degradation of p53. Cell. 1990 Dec 21;63(6):1129–36.

8. Feng W, Xiao J, Zhang Z, Rosen DG, Brown RE, Liu J, Duan X. Senescence and apoptosis in carcinogenesis of cervical squamous carcinoma. Mod Pathol. 2007 Sep;20(9):961–6.

9. Feng W, Duan X, Liu J, Xiao J, Brown RE. Morphoproteomic evidence of constitutively activated and overexpressed mTOR pathway in cervical squamous carcinoma and high grade squamous intraepithelial lesions. Int J Clin Exp Pathol. 2009;2(3):249–60.

10. Komata T, Kanzawa T, Takeuchi H, Germano IM, Schreiber M, Kondo Y, Kondo S. Antitumour effect of cyclin-dependent kinase inhibitors(p16 (INK4A), p18(INK4C), p19(INK4D), p21(WAF1/CIP1) and p27(KIP1)) on malignant glioma cells. Br J Cancer. 2003;88(8):1277–80.

11. Yamaguchi H, Hung MC. Regulation and role of EZH2 in cancer. Cancer Res Treat. 2014;46:209–22.

12. Sher F, Boddeke E, Copray S. Ezh2 expression in astrocytes induces their dedifferentiation toward neural stem cells. Cell Reprogram. 2011;13:1–6.

13. Eskander RN, Ji T, Huynh B, Wardeh R, Randall LM, Hoang B. Inhibition of enhancer of zeste homolog 2 (EZH2) expression is associated with decreased tumor cell proliferation, migration, and invasion in endometrial cancer cell lines. Int J Gynecol Cancer. 2013;23:997–1005.

14. Behrens C, Solis LM, Lin H, Yuan P, Tang X, Kadara H, Riquelme E, Galindo H, Moran CA, Kalhor N, Swisher SG, Simon GR, Stewart DJ, et al. EZH2 protein expression associates with the early pathogenesis, tumor progression, and prognosis of non-small cell lung carcinoma. Clin Cancer Res. 2013;19:6556–65.

15. Smits M, Nilsson J, Mir SE, van der Stoop PM, Hulleman E, Niers JM, de Witt Hamer PC, Marquez VE, Cloos J, Krichevsky AM, Noske DP, Tannous BA, Würdinger T. miR-101 is down-regulated in glioblastoma resulting in EZH2-induced proliferation, migration, and angiogenesis. Oncotarget. 2010;1:710–20.

16. Lu J, He ML, Wang L, Chen Y, Liu X, Dong Q, Chen YC, Peng Y, Yao KT, Kung HF, Li XP. MiR-26a inhibits cell growth and tumorigenesis of nasopharyngeal carcinoma through repression of EZH2. Cancer Res. 2011;71:225.

17. Idris S, Lindsay C, Kostiuk M, Andrews C, Côté DW, O'Connell DA, Harris J, Seikaly H, Biron VL. Investigation of EZH2 pathways for novel epigenetic treatment strategies in oropharyngeal cancer. J Otolaryngol Head Neck Surg. 2016;45(1):54.

18. Bao B, Wang Z, Ali S, Ahmad A, Azmi AS, Sarkar SH, Banerjee S, Kong D, Li Y, Thakur S, Sarkar FH. Metformin inhibits cell proliferation, migration and invasion by attenuating CSC function mediated by deregulating miRNAs in pancreatic cancer cells. Cancer Prev Res (Phila). 2012;5:355–64.

19. Bao B, Ali S, Banerjee S, Wang Z, Logna F, Azmi AS, Kong D, Ahmad A, Li Y, Padhye S, Sarkar FH. Curcumin analogue CDF inhibits pancreatic tumor growth by switching on suppressor microRNAs and attenuating EZH2 expression. Cancer Res. 2012;72(1):335–45.

20. Cai X, Hu X, Tan X, Cheng W, Wang Q, Chen X, Guan Y, Chen C, Jing X. Metformin induced AMPK activation, G0/G1 phase cell cycle arrest and the inhibition of growth of esophageal Squamous cell carcinomas in vitro and in vivo. PLoS One. 2015;10(7):e0133349.

21. Divya CS, Pillai MR. Antitumor action of curcumin in human papillomavirus associated cells involves downregulation of viral oncogenes, prevention of NFkB and AP-1 translocation, and modulation of apoptosis. Mol Carcinog. 2006;45:320–32.

22. Chakraborty S, Das K, Saha S, Mazumdar M, Manna A, Chakraborty S, Mukherjee S, Khan P, Adhikary A, Mohanty S, Chattopadhyay S, Biswas SC, Sa G, et al. Nuclear matrix protein SMAR1 represses c-Fos-mediated HPV18 E6 transcription through alteration of chromatin histone deacetylation. J Biol Chem. 2014;289(42):29074–85.

23. Saha B, Adhikary A, Ray P, Saha S, Chakraborty S, Mohanty S, Das K, Mukherjee S, Mazumdar M, Lahiri L, Hossain DM, Sa G, Das T. Restoration of tumor suppressor p53 by differentially regulating pro- and anti-p53 networks in HPV-18-infected cervical cancer cells. Oncogene. 2012;31:173–86.

24. Balasubramanian S, Chew YC, Eckert RL. Sulforaphane suppresses polycomb group protein level via a proteasome-dependent mechanism in skin cancer cells. Mol Pharmacol. 2011;80:870–8.

25. Lindsay C, Seikaly H, Biron V. Epigenetics of oropharyngeal squamous cell carcinoma: opportunities for novel chemotherapeutic targets. J Otolaryngol Head Neck Surg. 2017;46(1):9.

14

Cochlear implant electrode sealing techniques and related intracochlear pressure changes

Ingo Todt[*], Julica Utca, Dania Karimi, Arne Ernst and Philipp Mittmann

Abstract

Background: The inserted cochlear implanted electrode is covered at the site of the round window or cochleostomy to prevent infections and leakage. In a surgically hearing preservational concept, low intracochlear pressure changes are of high importance. The aim of this study was to observe intracochlear pressure changes due to different sealing techniques in a cochlear model.

Methods: Cochlear implant electrode insertions were performed in an artifical cochlear model and the intracochlear pressure changes were recorded in parallel with a micro-pressure sensor positioned in the apical region of the cochlea model to follow the maximum amplitude of intracochlear pressure. Four different sealing conditions were compared: 1) overlay, 2) overlay with fascia pushed in, 3) donut-like fascia ring, 4) donut-like fascia ring pushed in.

Results: We found statistically significant differences in the occurrence of maximum amplitude of intracochlear pressure peak changes related to sealing procedure comparing the different techniques. While the lowest amplitude changes could be observed for the overlay technique (0.14 mmHg $\pm$ 0.06) the highest values could be observed for the donut-like pushed in technique (1.79 mmHg $\pm$ 0.69).

Conclusion: Sealing the electrode inserted cochlea can lead to significant intracochlear pressure changes. Pushing in of the sealing tissue cannot be recommended.

Keywords: Cochlea implant, Round window, Sealing, Intracochlear pressure

Background

Cochlear implantation (CI) is a globally accepted treatment for children and adults with severe-to-profound hearing loss. In recent years, the indications for cochlear implantation have been widened to patients with substantial residual hearing. To avoid complications such as perilymphatic leakage, the loss of residual hearing, vertigo and ascending infections,tight sealing of the cochleostomy or the round window membrane is an important goal for CI surgeons. On the other hand, it has been shown that intracochlear pressure (ICP) changes occur during the implantationprocedure; these are relevant factors in terms of hearing preservation shown clinically and underlined experimentally. ICP changes in a model have been described which correlate to the insertion speed [1] of a cochlear implant electrode insertion. Different forms of opening an artificial round window have been shown to cause significant differences in ICP changes [2, 3], as well as the size of the round window opening and the hydrophilised state of the cochlear implant electrode [4] and post-insertional cable movements [5]. Clinically it has been shown that speed of insertion [6], underwater insertion [7] and the size of the round window opening and moisturisation of the electrode [8] are important factors for hearing preservation.

The aim of the present studywas to investigate the effect of different methods of electrode sealing on the ICP in a model cochlea.

* Correspondence: todt@gmx.net
Department of Otolaryngology, Head and Neck Surgery, Unfallkrankenhaus
Berlin, Warenerstr.7, 12683 Berlin, Germany

Methods

Model and sealing techniques

Pressure sensor

The ICP was measured using a micro-optical pressure sensor 0,8 mm FOP (FISO, Canada). Basically, the tip of the pressure sensor is a hollow glass tube sealed on one end by a plastic thin film diaphragm coated with a reflective surface of evaporated gold. The optical fiber is located in the glass tube with a small distance (50–100 μm) to the diaphragm tip. The optical fiber is attached to a LED light source and to a photodiode sensor. Light from the LED source reaches the sensor tip of the optical fiber, fans out as it exits the fiber and is reflected by the gold-covered flexible diaphragm. The reflected light is sensed by the photodiode. Small amounts of pressure induced distance displacements of the diaphragm, which modulate the intensity of reflected light. The sensor is connected with a module, which is again linked to a computer. Evolution software was used to record the ICP. The time sensitivity of the sensor was 300 measurements per second. Low pass filter was set to 500Hz.

Model

The model was a full-scale model of the cochlea, distributed by Advanced Bionics and MedEl for surgical training with a volume of 87 mm^3 (Fig. 1), which is slightly above the physiological range [9]. The sensor was positioned through a drilled hole in the apical region of the cochlea. The sensor was fixed in its position with fibrin glue and placed within the channel in such a way that the tip was not in contact with the edge of the channel or the ground. Afterwards, the cochlea was microscopically controlled to exclude any enclosed air bubbles. The

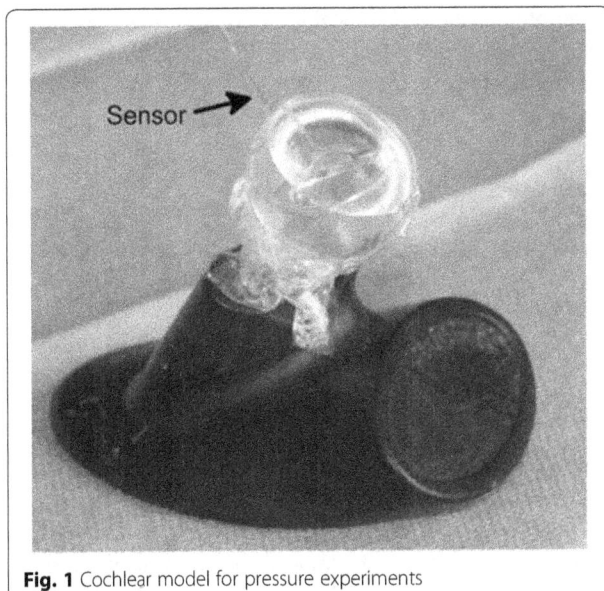

Fig. 1 Cochlear model for pressure experiments

experiments were in series with a sensor in an unchanged position to exclude sensor position-related bias and to allow inter-experimental comparability. All procedures were performed with a High Focus midscalar electrode (Advanced Bionics, Stäfa, Swiss).

Analysis

Statistically, the maximum amplitude of pressure change was calculatedand statistically analysed by an independent t-test (SPSS 10.00). This study was approved by the institutional review board (*IRB-ukb-HNO-2015/10*)

Experiments

1) Overlay sealing:
   The artifical RW opening beside the inserted electrode was covered by a strip of fat. All experiments were performed five times.
2) Overlay sealing with push in:
   The artifical RW opening beside the inserted electrode was covered by a strip of fat. The fat was pushed between the RW edge and electrode. All experiments were performed five times.
3) Donut-like sealing:
   A perforated piece of fat was created, in whichan electrode was inserted. This donut-like seal was inserted into the artifical RW until it was closed. All experiments were performed five times.
4) Donut-like seal pushed in:
   A perforated piece of fat was created, in whichan electrode was inserted. The electrode was inserted and the donut-like seal was pushed down the electrode until the RW was closed. All experiments were performed five times.

Results

A one-way ANOVA was conducted to determine whether the mean maximum ICP (mmHg) was different between the variable sealing techniques. Data are presented as mean ± standard deviation. The mean maximum ICP increased from overlay (1) (0.14 ± 0.06), to donut like (3) (0.44 ± 0.27), to overlay pushed in (2) (0.56 ± 0.3) to donut like push in (1.79 ± 0.69) in that order (Fig. 2).

The differences between these techniques were statistically significant (F(3, 16) = 16.615, $p < 0.001$). The data were normally distributed for each group, asassessed by a Shapiro-Wilks test ($p < 0.05$). Homogeneity of variances was violated, as assessed by Levene's Test of Homogeneity of Variance ($p = 0.003$). Games-Howell post hoc analysis revealed that the difference from donut-like push in (4) to overlay (1) (1.65, 95% CI (0.4 to 2.9)) was statistically significant ($p = 0.019$), as well as from donut- like push in (4) to overlay push in (2) (1.23,

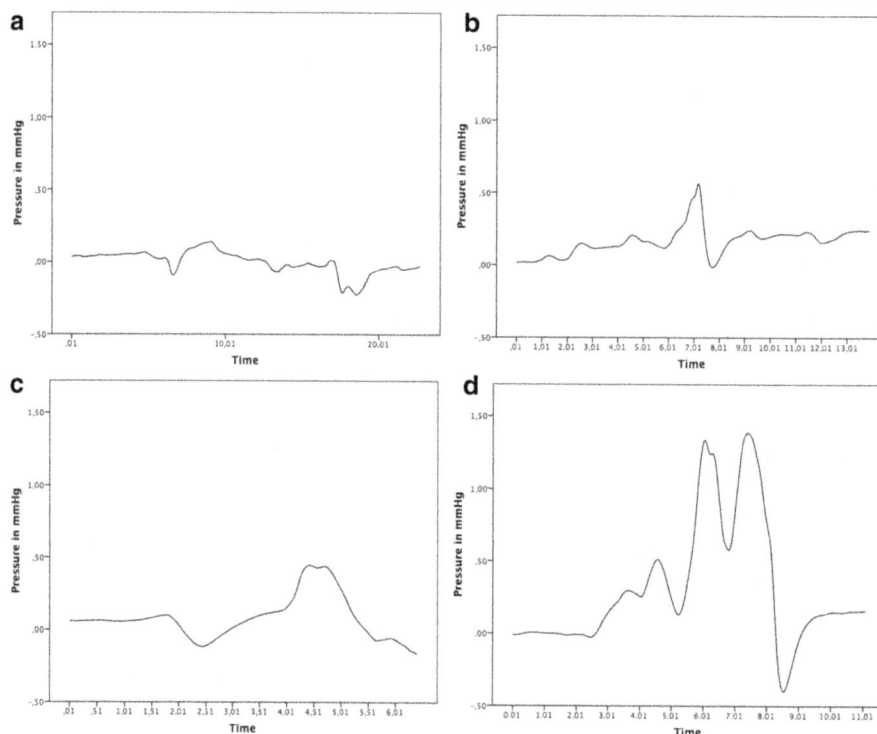

Fig. 2 a Exemplaric pressure change related to an overlay sealing. **b** Exemplaric pressure change related to an overlay push in sealing. **c** Exemplaric pressure change related to a donut-like sealing. **d** Exemplaric pressure change related to a donut-like push in sealing

95% CI (0.04 to 2.43), $p = 0.045$) and from donut-like push in (4) to donut-like (3) (1.36, 95% CI (0.16 to 2.56), $p = 0.031$) (Fig. 3).

Discussion

The sealing of the cochlear implant electrode is so far mostly observed under the aspect of tightness of the seal and a possible interaction of the sealing tissue to induce local fibrosis [10–12]. Our observation focussed on a possible role of the procedure as cause for potentially pathophysiological ICP changes.

Pathophysiologically relevant acoustic levels are assumed to lead to high static ICP change or fast pressure changes with a high angular speed [13, 14]. Experimentally different aspects of the pre-, intra- and postinsertional procedures have been shown to to significantly affect ICP like round window opening [2–4], moisturizing the electrode [4], stabilization of the insertional hand [15], speed of insertion [1], electrode design [16, 17] and postinsertional cable movement [5]. Recent clinical studies underline ICP as an important factor [7, 8].

The packing of a cochlear implant electrode to seal the cochlea led anecdotally to a decrease of the intraoperative EcochG threshold and has an effect on basal ECAP thresholds [18].

This observation led to the question of a possible impact of the sealing procedure on the ICP, which possibly contributes to a decrease of residual hearing.

An impact of the sealing handling of the electrode on the ICP is likely since the seal separates the fluid filled cochlea from the aerated middle ear. By that, every handling is transmitted into the cochlea.

Our observations showed that as long as it is manually attempted to close the local leak, by covering it, pressure remains at a low level (Fig. 2). By trying to further increase the tightness of the seal by a push in or by optimising the circumferential covering, the pressure increases significantly (Fig. 3). The circumferential covering has the effect that movements of the electrode are transmitted into the cochlea like a cylinder stroke in a machine by inducing a sucking and pushing of fluid.

The pressure increase in terms of absolute volume is comparable to a sound pressure equivalent of 130 dB.

The transfer of the observation to the in vivo situation is limited in terms of two main points. The visibility and area to manipulate in vivo is worse related to the limited space through the posterior tympanotomy. This makes a tight circumferential sealing more difficult, as in the experimental situation. Secondly, manipulation around the electrode to reach a tight seal is less likely to be reachable in the in vivo situation, and the amount of handling in terms of touching and moving the electrode should

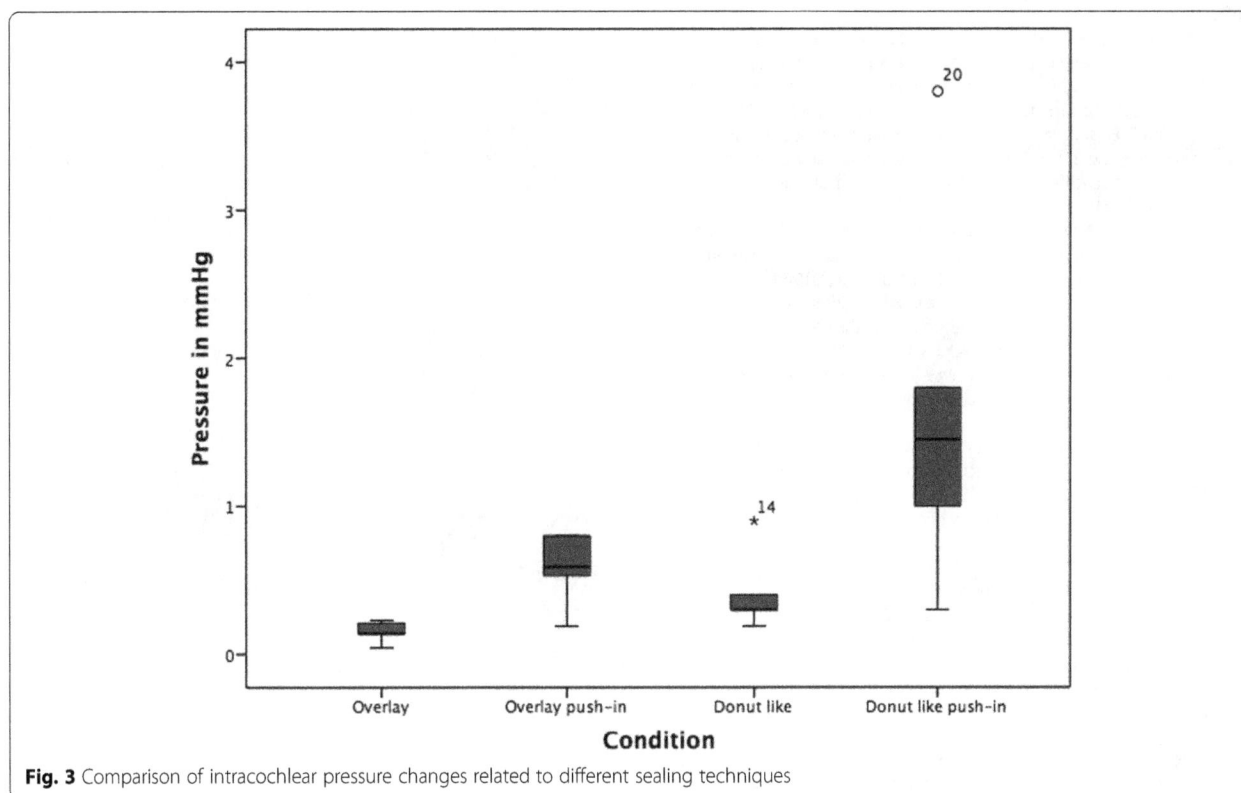

Fig. 3 Comparison of intracochlear pressure changes related to different sealing techniques

be more extensive in vivo. Another point is the used HighFocus MS electrode. It differs from other electrodes by its basal diameter. It can be assumed that in smaller electrodes (e.g., Cochlear slim straight) and larger electrodes (e.g., Medel Flex series) the handling is different and therefore the occurence of ICP is different, too.

Based on our findings, pushing in of a seal should be avoided. A significant difference between a pure overlay of the donut-like technique could not be observed in terms of the generation of pressure. Surgically, not only the aspect of pressure generation and transmission into the cochlea has to be considered. In particular, perilymphatic leakage can be assumed to play a role in hearing preservation. Weakness of the study is the performance of the experiments in a cochlea model. Therefore natural pressure equilibration pathways (e.g., aqueductus cochleae, round window) are not considered in the pressure pattern.

Further studies focussing on the short- and long-term behaviour of seals seems to be of central importance to help to understand the role of the sealing in a hearing preservation concept.

Conclusion

Sealing the inserted cochlea can lead to significant intracochlear pressure changes. Pushing in of the sealing tissue cannot be recommended.

Abbreviations
CI: Cochlear implant; EcochG: Electrocochleography; ICP: Intracochlear pressure; RW: Round window

Acknowledgements
None.

Funding
This study was supported by Advanced Bionics, Stäfa, Switzerland.

Authors' contributions
IT idea, writer. JU helping in manuscript writing, prepering figures. DK collecting data, prepering figures. AE helping in manucript writing. PM analysing data, statistics. All authors read and approved the final manuscript.

Authors' information
IT-head of implant divison. JU-resident. DK-junior resident. AE-head of department. PM-resident

Competing interests
The authors declare that they have no competing interets.

References

1. Todt I, Mittmann P, Ernst A. Intracochlear fluid pressure changes related to the insertional speed of a CI electrode. Biomed Res Int. 2014;2014:507241.

2. Mittmann P, Ernst A, Todt I. Intracochlear pressure changes due to round window opening: a model experiment. Sci World J. 2014;2014:341075.

3. Mittmann P, Ernst A, Mittmann M, Todt I. Optimisation of the round window opening in cochlear implant surgery in wet and dry conditions: impact on intracochlear pressure changes. Eur Arch Otorhinolaryngol. 2016; 273(11):3609–13.

4. Todt I, Ernst A, Mittmann P. Effects of round window opening size and moisturised electrodes on intracochlear pressure related to the insertion of a cochlear implant electrode. Audiol Neurotol Extra. 2016;6:1–8.

5. Todt I, Karimi D, Luger J, Ernst A, Mittmann P. Postinsertional cable movements of cochlear implant electrodes and their effects on intracochlear pressure. Biomed Res Int. 2016;2016:3937196.

6. Rajan GP, Kontorinis G, Kuthubutheen J. The effects of insertion speed on inner ear function during cochlear implantation: a comparison study. Audiol Neurootol. 2013;18(1):17–22.

7. Anagiotos A, Beutner D, Gostian AO, Schwarz D, Luers JC, Hüttenbrink KB. Insertion of cochlear implant electrode array using the underwater technique for preserving residual hearing. Otol Neurotol. 2016;37(4):339–44.

8. Todt I, Mittmann P, Ernst A. Hearing preservation with a midscalar electrode comparison of a regular and steroid/pressure optimised surgical approach in patients with residual hearing. Otol Neurotol. 2016;37(9):e349–52.

9. Kirk EC, Gosselin-Ildari AD. Cochlear labyrinth volume and hearing abilities in primates. Anat Rec (Hoboken). 2009;292:765–76.

10. Robey AB, et al. Effect of cochleostomy size on perilymph fistula control. Laryngoscope. 2010;120(2):373–6.

11. Burghard A, et al. Insertion site and sealing technique affect residual hearing and tissue formation after cochlear implantation. Hear Res. 2014; 312:21–7.

12. Somdas MA, et al. Quantitative evaluation of new bone and fibrous tissue in the cochlea following cochlear implantation in the human. Audiol Neurootol. 2007;12(5):277–84.

13. Böhmer A. Hydrostatic pressure in the inner ear fluid compartments and its effects on inner ear function. Acta Otolaryngol Suppl. 1993;507:3–24.

14. Dancer A, Franke R. Intracochlear sound pressure measurements in guinea pigs. Hear Res. 1980;2(3–4):191–205.

15. Todt I, Ernst A, Mittmann P. Effects of different insertion techniques of a cochlear implant electrode on the intracochlear pressure. Audiol Neurootol. 2016;21(1):30–7.

16. Todt I, Mittmann M, Ernst A, Mittmann P. Comparison of the effects of four different cochlear implant electrodes on intra-cochlear pressure in a model. Acta Otolaryngol. 2017;137(3):235–41.

17. Mittmann P, Mittmann M, Ernst A, Todt I. Intracochlear pressure changes due to 2 electrode Types: An Artificial Model Experiment. Otolaryngol Head Neck Surg. 2017;156(4):712-16.

18. Gordin A, Papsin B, Gordon K. Packing of the cochleostomy site affects auditory nerve response thresholds in precurved off-stylet cochlear implants. Otol Neurotol. 2010;31(2):204–9.

15

Does hyperthyroidism worsen prognosis of thyroid carcinoma? A retrospective analysis on 2820 consecutive thyroidectomies

Fabio Medas[1][*] ⓘ, Ernico Erdas[1], Gian Luigi Canu[1], Alessandro Longheu[1], Giuseppe Pisano[1], Massimiliano Tuveri[2] and Pietro Giorgio Calò[1]

Abstract

Background: Hyperthyroidism is associated with high incidence of thyroid carcinoma; furthermore, tumors arisen in hyperthyroid tissue show an aggressive behavior. Thyroid Stimulating Hormone (TSH) and Thyroid-stimulating antibodies, present in Graves's disease, seem to play a key role in carcinogenesis and tumoral growth.

Methods: We retrospectively reviewed our series of patients who underwent thyroidectomy for thyroid carcinoma. We compared pathological features and surgical outcomes of hyperthyroid versus euthyroid patients.

Results: From 2007 to 2015, 909 thyroidectomies were performed at our institution for thyroid cancer: 87 patients were hyperthyroid and 822 euthyroid. We observed, in hyperthyroid patients, a higher rate of transient hypoparathyroidism (28.1% vs 13.2%; $p < 0.01$) and of node metastases (12.6% vs 6.1%; $p = 0.03$); also local recurrence rate was higher (5.7% vs 2.5%) even if not statistically significant ($p = 0.17$). Five-year disease free survival rate was significant lower in the same group (89.1% vs 96.6%; $p = 0.03$).

Conclusion: Thyroid cancers in hyperthyroid patients have an aggressive behavior, with high incidence of local invasion and a worse prognosis than euthyroid patients. All hyperthyroid patients should undergo a careful evaluation with ultrasound and scintigraphy; in case of suspicious nodules, an aggressive approach, including thyroidectomy and lymphectomy, is justified. In patients with toxic adenoma, thyroid cancer is uncommon, thus a loboisthmectomy can be safely performed.

Keywords: Hyperthyroidism, Thyroid carcinoma, Graves' disease, Thyroidectomy

Background

In the past hyperthyroidism was considered a protective factor for thyroid carcinoma [1]. Nevertheless, since the Fifties some studies [2, 3] reported a high incidence of thyroid carcinoma in patients affected from Graves' disease. From the '90s several authors [4–7] have suggested that not only thyroid carcinoma is frequently associated with hyperthyroidism, especially with Graves' disease, but it also has an aggressive behavior. In this scenario, TSH seems to play a key role: it is known as the most important factor stimulating normal thyroid tissue growth, but it has been reported that it can also stimulate neoplastic thyroid tissue, that contains functional TSH receptors. Filetti and Mazzaferri [4, 8] have observed that thyroid-stimulating antibodies, that are similar to TSH and are present in Graves' disease, may promote tumor growth by activating TSH receptors.

The aim of this retrospective study is to evaluate pathological features and clinical behavior of thyroid carcinoma arising in hyperthyroid patients, and to assess whether there are relevant differences compared with euthyroid patients.

* Correspondence: fabiomedas@gmail.com
[1]Department of Surgical Sciences, University of Cagliari, Cittadella Universitaria, SS554, Bivio Sestu, 09042 Monserrato (CA), Italy
Full list of author information is available at the end of the article

Methods

Study design

After ethical approval by local ethics committee (Independent Ethic Committee, University of Cagliari), we conducted a retrospective study on patients who had undergone thyroidectomy in our Department of General and Endocrine Surgery (University of Cagliari) between January 2007 and December 2015 with pathological diagnosis of thyroid carcinoma. Based on metabolic status, patients were divided into two groups: hyperthyroid patients, including Graves's disease, Toxic Adenoma and Toxic Multinodular Goiter were included in Group A, while euthyroid patients were included in Group B.

All the patients included in group A had received diagnosis of hyperthyroidism, defined as low serum TSH level (< 0.4 mIU/L) with high or normal (subclinic hyperthyroidism) free T4 and free T3 serum levels.

Patients demographics, preoperative data, pathological findings, postoperative complications (including recurrent nerve injury and hypoparathyroidism) and locoregional or distant recurrence were recorded.

Preoperative assessment

All the patients included in the study underwent preoperative physical examination, dosage of serum thyroid hormones including TSH, Tg and anti-Tg antibody and high-resolution ultrasonography of the neck. At the time of surgery, all patients had normal FT3 and FT4 serum levels, including those in group A due to assumption of antithyroid drugs.

In case of suspicious nodules, fine needle aspiration cytology (FNAC) was performed. Preoperative fibrolaryngoscopy was routinely performed to assess vocal folds mobility. In hyperthyroid patients a thyroid scintigraphy was routinely performed.

Surgery. Surgical procedure consisted in extracapsular total thyroidectomy; recurrent laryngeal nerves were routinely exposed until their insertion in larynx, and any attempt to preserve parathyroid glands was performed. In patients with preoperative or intraoperative suspicion of lymph node metastases, central node dissection or radical lateral neck dissection was performed to achieve curative treatment. A subfascial drainage was routinely used.

Postoperative management

Serum calcium level was assayed on first and second postoperative day to promptly detect hypocalcemia: in this case, diagnosis of hypoparathyroidism was confirmed in case of PTH < 10 pg/ml (normal range = 10-65 pg/ml). Drainage was usually removed in second postoperative day. In case of suspected recurrent nerve injury, a fibrolaryngoscopy was performed to assess vocal cord mobility.

Pathological examination

Thyroid cancer was classified according to TNM classification of AJCC (7th edition, 2010). Locally invasive carcinoma was defined as T3 or T4 based on TNM staging.

Follow up

Suppressive L-Thyroxine therapy was routinely administrated. Serum Tg and Tg-antibody levels were assayed every 6 months together with neck ultrasound (US). Diagnosis of recurrent disease was confirmed with US-guided FNC of lymph nodes and Tg washing of FNC aspirates. Patients considered disease-free underwent Tg detection after rhTSH stimulation and neck US.

Hypoparathyroidism and nerve palsy were defined permanent if persisting for more than 12 months after surgery.

Statistical analysis

Chi-squared test was used for categorical data and T-Test for continuous variables. Results were considered statistically significant if p value was ≤0.05. Continuous data are reported as the mean value ± standard error of the mean. Calculations were performed with MedCalc ® 12.7.0.0.

Results

Between January 2007 and December 2015, 2820 patients underwent thyroidectomy at our department: 423 were hyperthyroid and 2398 euthyroid. The incidence of thyroid carcinoma was 20.6% in hyperthyroid patients ($n = 87$) and 34.3% in euthyroid ($n = 822$). In total, 909 patients with diagnosis of thyroid carcinoma were included in the present study. The patients were divided into two groups in accordance with criteria mentioned above: 87 patients were included in group A and 822 in group B.

Table 1 Demographic data and surgical procedure

	Group A ($n = 87$)	Group B (n = 822)	p value
Male	23 (26.4%)	161 (19.6%)	0.17
Female	64 (73.6%)	661 (80.4%)	
Age (years)	51.5 ± 14.2	51.4 ± 15.4	0.81
Surgical procedure			
TT	72 (82.8%)	669 (81.4%)	0.67
TT + CLND	7 (8.0%)	96 (11.7%)	
TT + LND	3 (3.4%)	23 (2.8%)	
Loboisthmectomy	5 (5.7%)	34 (4.1%)	
Operative time (minutes)	107.7 ± 33.4	99.3 ± 28.8	0.61

TT Total thyroidectomy, *CLND* central lymph node dissection, *LND* lateral neck dissection

Demographic data and surgical treatment (Table 1)

Group A: Preoperative diagnosis was Graves' disease in 45 (51.7%) patients, Toxic Multinodular Goiter in 37 (42.5%) and Toxic Adenoma in 5 (5.7%). There were 23 (26.4%) males and 64 (73.6%) females with a mean age of 51.5 ± 14.2 years. Surgical procedure consisted in total thyroidectomy (TT) in 72 (82.8%) cases, associated to central lymph node dissection (CLND) in 7 (8%) patients and lateral neck dissection in 3 (3.4%); a loboisthmectomy was performed in 5 (5.7%) cases. Mean operative time was 107.7 ± 33.4 min.

Group B: There were 161 (19.6%) males and 661 (80.4%) females with a men age of 51.5 ± 15.4 years. The patients underwent to total thyroidectomy (TT) in 669 (81.4%) cases, associated to CLND in 96 (11.7%) patients and lateral neck dissection in 23 (2.8%). A loboisthmectomy was performed in 34 (4.1%) cases. Mean operative time was 99.3 ± 28.8 min.

Surgical outcomes and follow up (Table 2)

Group A. Mean postoperative stay was 2.2 ± 0.8 days; transient hypoparathyroidism was observed in 29 (28.1%) patients and persistent in 4 (4.5%); recurrent nerve injury occurred in 2 (2.2%) cases. Mean follow up was 59.3 ± 29.2 months. Local recurrence was observed in 5 (5.7%) patients with a 5-year disease free survival rate of 89.1%.

Group B: Mean postoperative stay was 2.3 ± 1.2 days. Transient hypoparathyroidism was reported in 109 (13.2%) patients and permanent in 31 (3.7%). Transient recurrent nerve injury was observed in 14 (1.7%) cases. Local recurrence occurred in 21 (2.5%) patients with a 5-year disease free survival rate of 96.6%.

Pathologic data (Table 3)

Group A. Mean tumor size was 2.31 ± 0.9 cm. Papillary thyroid carcinoma was reported in 59 (67.8%) patients, follicular variant of papillary carcinoma in 17 (19.5%), tall cell carcinoma in 3 (3.4%), follicular carcinoma in 5

Table 2 Surgical outcomes and follow up

	Group A (n = 87)	Group B (n = 822)	p value
Postoperative stay (days)	2.2 ± 0.8	2.3 ± 1.2	0.81
Follow-up (months)	59.3 ± 29.24	62.1 ± 19.8	0.77
Transient hypoparathyroidism	29 (28.1%)	109 (13.2%)	<0.01
Permanent hypoparathyroidism	4 (4.5%)	31 (3.7%)	0.93
Recurrent nerve injury	2 (2.2%)	14 (1.7%)	0.97
Local recurrence	5 (5.7%)	21 (2.5%)	0.17
5-year disease free survival rate	89.1%[a]	96.6%[a]	0.03

[a] On 46 patients (Group A) and 621 patients (group B) with at least 5 years of followup

Table 3 Pathologic data

	Group A (n = 87)	Group B (n = 822)	p value
Tumor size (mm)	2.31 ± 0.9	2.35 ± 1.15	0.74
Locally invasive carcinoma	15 (17.2%)	194 (23.6%)	0.22
Multicentric carcinoma	25 (28.7%)	200 (24.3%)	0.43
Node metastasis	11 (12.6%)	50 (6.1%)	0.03
Histopathologic diagnosis			
PTC	59 (67.8%)	464 (56.4%)	0.19
Follicular variant of PTC	17 (19.5%)	190 (23.1%)	
Tall cell carcinoma	3 (3.4%)	23 (2.8%)	
Follicular carcinoma	5 (5.7%)	110 (13.4%)	
Hurtle cell carcinoma	3 (3.4%)	35 (4.3%)	

PTC Papillary thyroid carcinoma

(5.7%) and Hurtle cell carcinoma in 3 (3.4%). A locally invasive carcinoma was found in 15 (17.2%) cases and a multicentric neoplasia in 25 (28.7%). Node metastases were observed in 11 (12.6%) patients.

Group B. Mean tumor size was 2.35 ± 1.15 cm. Papillary thyroid carcinoma was reported in 464 (56.4%) patients, follicular variant of papillary carcinoma in 190 (23.1%), tall cell carcinoma in 23 (2.8%), follicular carcinoma in 110 (13.4%) and Hurtle cell carcinoma in 35 (4.3%). A locally invasive carcinoma was reported in 194 (23.6%) patients and a multicentric tumor in 200 (24.3%). Node metastases were observed in 50 (6.1%) patients.

Comparison between the groups

Demographic data, surgical procedure and operative time were similar between the groups. Incidence of transient postoperative hypoparathyroidism was higher in Group A (p < 0.01), whereas permanent was similar. Pathologic features were similar between the groups, except the incidence of node metastases that was higher in Group A (12.6% vs 6.1%; p = 0.03). Local recurrence was more than twice in group A as much in group B, but not statistically significant (5.7% vs 2.5%; p 0.17). Five-year disease free survival rate was significant lower in Group A (89.1% vs 96.6%; p = 0.03).

Discussion

Before 1950 few cases of association between hyperthyroidism and carcinoma were reported, so that some authors suggested that hyperthyroidism could be a cancer-protective factor [1, 9]. Nevertheless, in the last decades several studies [4–7] have reported that not only thyroid carcinoma occurs with high frequency in hyperthyroid patients, but it also has a more aggressive behavior than usual. Filetti [8] noted that TSH stimulates growth of both normal and cancer cells, and that there are similarities between TSH and thyroid-stimulating anti-bodies in Graves' disease. In fact both activate adenylate cyclase and phospholipase C cascade, with mitogenic and antiapoptotic effects, causing normal thyroid tissue to become hyperplastic and hyperfunctional; further-more, thyroid cancer cells contain functional TSH recep-tors. These evidences support the hypothesis that thyroid-stimulating antibodies and TSH play a key role in carcinoma's pathogenesis.

The prevalence of thyroid carcinoma in hyperthyroid patients varies widely in literature, ranging from 0.5 to over 20% [2, 3, 9–22]. The reason of this wide difference is probably related to patients' selection for surgery, type of surgery and geographical variation of incidence of thyroid carcinoma; in addition, the incidence is higher in retrospective studies that only include patients who underwent thyroidectomy, and lower in studies that in-clude also patients who did not underwent surgery.

Anyway, most of the authors report a higher incidence of thyroid carcinoma in hyperthyroid than euthyroid pa-tients. Sokal [2] found a 20-fold increase of thyroid car-cinoma incidence in patients with hyperthyroidism. Yeh [23], in a large population-based cohort study, analyzed data of 1 million of patients from Taiwan's National Health Insurance database and reported an increased risk of head and neck cancer in patients with hyperthy-roidism, especially for thyroid carcinoma.

We observed in our study a high incidence of carcin-oma in hyperthyroid patients (20.6%) but lower than eu-thyroid patients (34.3%). About this finding, it's important to note that ours is a iodine-deficiency region, thus subclinic hypothyroidism, resulting in chronic in-creased serum TSH levels, may explain the high inci-dence of thyroid carcinoma in euthyroid patients.

Many authors [7, 9, 14] have reported a high frequency of aggressive subtypes of thyroid carcinoma in hyperthy-roidism, being larger, more often multicentric, locally in-vasive or metastatic.

Belfiore [14, 15] described a higher incidence of thy-roid carcinoma in Grave's disease than in toxic adenoma. In addition, he found that tumor with aggressive behav-ior were more frequent in Graves' disease, of intermedi-ate frequency in euthyroid patients and uncommon in toxic adenoma patients. These findings support the hy-pothesis that TSH and thyroid-stimulating antibodies play a key role in tumor genesis and in promoting growth and metastatic spread of thyroid cancer. In fact tumors with an aggressive behavior are less frequent in patients with low or suppressed sereum TSH levels, and, by the other side, more frequent in those with chronic stimulation of TSH receptor by thyroid stimulating antibodies.

These observations are consistent with our findings: we observed an aggressive behavior of tumors arisen in hyperthyroid patients, with a higher incidence of node metastases than in euthyroid patients (12.6% vs 6.1%) and with a worse prognosis (5-year disease free survival of 89.1% compared with 96.6% of euthyroid patients). We did not find larger tumors in hyperthyroid patients, but this could be related, as stated earlier, to chronic TSH stimulation in euthyroid patients due to iodine deficiency.

An Italian study [24] with a long follow-up found not only a lower disease free survival but also a higher disease-specific mortality in patients with thyroid cancer and Grave's disease than in euthyroid patients.

Furthermore, it has been reported that patients with Grave's disease and a palpable nodule are at high risk to have a thyroid carcinoma: in these patients the incidence of thyroid carcinoma reaches 50% [12, 14, 15, 17, 25, 26]. For these reasons, a palpable nodule found in the course of Grave's disease should be strongly considered for surgery.

A fine needle aspiration cytology (FNAC) from nod-ules could be taken into account, but diagnosis is often difficult due to cytomorphologic changes as a conse-quence of the disease and of antithyroid drug treatment. In addition, radioiodine treatment produce cellular aty-pia that can lead to erroneous diagnosis of malignancy; therefore FNAC should be performed prior to radioio-dine therapy.

The extent of surgery in hyperthyroid patients with preoperative diagnosis of carcinoma has been matter of debate. Because of the aggressive behavior of the tumor, an aggressive approach, including total thyroidectomy with prophylactic central lymph node dissection, seems justified in these cases, following current trend in thy-roid surgery [27–33]. By the other side, patients with Grave's disease or multinodular toxic goiter in whom no suspicion of carcinoma exists, should be treated with only total thyroidectomy.

Patients with toxic adenoma are usually treated with loboisthmectomy. If pathological examination demon-strates a carcinoma, removal of contralateral lobe is not necessary in case of small (<1 cm), unifocal, low-risk, intrathyroidal nodules and no lymph node metastases. In our series, we found only 5 cases of carcinoma arisen in patients with toxic adenoma; all of them had under-gone loboisthmectomy and diagnosis of carcinoma was incidental. Pathologic diagnosis was in all the cases pap-illary microcarcinoma, thus none of them required a subsequent contralateral lobectomy.

According to literature [34–37], we observed in our series a higher incidence of transient hypoparathyroid-ism in hyperthyroid patients (28.1%) than in euthyroid (13.2%; $p < 0.01$). Common causes of postoperative hypo-calcemia are damage, devascularization or inadvertent removal of parathyroid glands, but another cause that has been postulated for hyperthyroid patients is "hungry bone syndrome", due to postoperative reversal of thyrotoxic osteodystrophy [38]. It's therefore necessary a careful follow-up with serum calcium measurement to promptly detect hypocalcemia, and, where appropriate, adequate calcium supplementation should be administrated to prevent hypocalcemia-related symptoms.

Finally, it should be pointed out that, being aware of the aggressive behavior of thyroid cancer in hyperthyroid patients, a more aggressive surgical approach could have been carried out in hyperthyroid rather than euthyroid patients, resulting, for example, in more extensive lymphectomies with higher incidence of complications and even of detected node metastases; thus, this could represent a bias of this study.

Conclusion

Thyroid cancers arisen in hyperthyroid gland have an aggressive behavior, with high incidence of local invasion and a worse prognosis than euthyroid patients, especially in patients with Graves' disease. A careful evaluation with ultrasound and scintigraphy should be routinely performed in hyperthyroid patients; in case of suspicious nodules, an aggressive approach, including thyroidectomy and lymphectomy, is justified. A FNAC of the nodule could be helpful, even if its results are often inconclusive. Thyroid cancer is uncommon in patients with toxic adenoma, thus these patients can be safely treated with a loboisthmectomy.

Abbreviations
FNAC: Fine Needle Aspiration Cytology; Tg: Thyroglobulin; TSH: Thyroid Stimulating Hormone; US: Ultrasound

Acknowledgements
Not applicable.

Funding
This research did not receive any specific grant from funding agencies in the public, commercial, or not-for-profit sectors.

Authors' contributions
FM: Participated substantially in conception, design, and execution of the study and in the analysis and interpretation of data; also participated substantially in writing, drafting, and editing of the manuscript. EE: Participated substantially in conception, design, and execution of the study and in the collection, analysis and interpretation of data. GLC: Participated substantially in execution of the study and in the analysis and interpretation of data. AL: Participated substantially in conception and execution of the study and in the collection, analysis and interpretation of data. GP: Participated substantially in conception and execution of the study and in the collection and interpretation of data. MT: Participated substantially in conception and design of the study and in the interpretation of data. PGC: Partecipated substantially in conception and execution of the study and in the analysis and interpretation of data; also partecipated substantially in the drafting and editing of the manuscript. All authors read and approved the final manuscript.

Competing interests
The authors declare that they have no competing interests.

Author details
[1]Department of Surgical Sciences, University of Cagliari, Cittadella Universitaria, SS554, Bivio Sestu, 09042 Monserrato (CA), Italy. [2]Istituto Pancreas, Policlinico Borgo Roma, AOUI Verona, Piazzale L.A. Scuro, 10, 37134 Verona, Italy.

References
1. Means JH. The thyroid and its diseases, vol. 482. Philadelphia: JB Lippincott Co; 1937.
2. Sokal JE. Incidence of malignancy in toxic and nontoxic nodular goiter. JAMA. 1954;154:1321–5.
3. Shapiro SJ, Friedman NB, Perzik SL, Catz B. Incidence of thyroid carcinoma in graves' disease. Cancer. 1970;26:1261–70.
4. Mazzaferri EL. Thyroid cancer and graves' disease. J Clin Endocrinol Metab. 1990 Apr;70(4):826–9.
5. De Rosa G, Testa A, Maurizi M, Satta MA, Aimoni C, Artuso A, Silvestri E, Rufini V, Troncone L. Thyroid carcinoma mimicking a toxic adenoma. Eur J Nucl Med. 1990;17(3-4):179–84.
6. Kim WB, Han SM, Kim TY, Nam-Goong IS, Gong G, Lee HK, Hong SJ, Shong YK. Ultrasonographic screening for detection of thyroid cancer in patients with graves' disease. Clin Endocrinol. 2004;60(6):719–25.
7. Pazaitou-Panayiotou K, Michalakis K, Paschke R. Thyroid cancer in patients with hyperthyroidism. Horm Metab Res. 2012;44(4):255–62. https://doi.org/10.1055/s-0031-1299741. Epub 2012 Feb 14
8. Filetti S, Belfiore A, Amir SM, Daniels GH, Ippolito O, Vigneri R, Ingbar SH. The role of thyroid-stimulating antibodies of graves' disease in differentiated thyroid cancer. N Engl J Med. 1988;318(12):753–9.
9. Beahrs OH, Pemberton JJ, Black BM. Nodular goiter and malignant lesions of the thyroid gland. J Clin Endocrinol Metab. 1951;11(10):1157–65.
10. Farbota LM, Calandra DB, Lawrence AM, Paloyan E. Thyroid carcinoma in graves' disease. Surgery. 1985;98:1148–53.
11. Pacini F, Elisei R, Di Coscio GC, Anelli S, Macchia E, Concetti R, Miccoli P, Arganini M, Pinchera A. Thyroid carcinoma in thyrotoxic patients treated by surgery. J Endocrinol Investig. 1988;11(2):107–12.
12. Dobyns JM, Sheline GE, Workman JB, Tompkins EA, McConahey WM, Becker DV. Malignant and benign neoplasms of the thyroid in patients treated for hyperthyroidism: a report of the cooperative Thyrotoxicosis therapy follow-up study. J Clin Endocrinol Metabl. 1974;38:976–98.
13. Ocak S, Akten AO, Tez M. Thyroid cancer in hyperthyroid patients: is it different clinical entity? Endocr Regul. 2014 Apr;48(2):65–8.
14. Belfiore A, Garofalo MR, Giuffrida D, Runello F, Filetti S, Fiumara A, Ippolito O, Vigneri R. Increased aggressiveness of thyroid cancer in patients with graves' disease. J Clin Endocrinol Metab. 1990;70(4):830–5. Review
15. Belfiore A, Russo D, Vigneri R, Filetti S. Graves' disease, thyroid nodules and thyroid cancer. Clin Endocrinol. 2001;55(6):711–8.
16. Vaiana R1, Cappelli C, Perini P, Pinelli D, Camoni G, Farfaglia R, Balzano R, Braga M. Hyperthyroidism and concurrent thyroid cancer. Tumori. 1999; 85(4):247–52.
17. Senyurek Giles Y, Tunca F, Boztepe H, Kapran Y, Terzioglu T, Tezelman S. The risk factors for malignancy in surgically treated patients for graves' disease, toxic multinodular goiter, and toxic adenoma. Surgery. 2008;144(6):1028–36. discussion 1036-7
18. Phitayakorn R, Morales-Garcia D, Wanderer J, Lubitz CC, Gaz RD, Stephen AE, Ehrenfeld JM, Daniels GH, Hodin RA, Parangi S. Surgery for graves' disease: a 25-year perspective. Am J Surg. 2013;206(5):669–73. https://doi.org/10.1016/j.amjsurg.2013.07.005.
19. Weber KJ, Solorzano CC, Lee JK, Gaffud MJ, Prinz RA. Thyroidectomy remains an effective treatment option for graves' disease. Am J Surg. 2006; 191(3):400–5.
20. Calò PG, Tatti A, Farris S, Malloci A, Nicolosi A. Differentiated thyroid carcinoma and hyperthyroidism: a frequent association? Chir Ital. 2005;57(2): 193–7.
21. Edmonds CJ, Tellez M. Hyperthyroidism and thyroid cancer. Clin Endocrinol. 1988;28(2):253–9.
22. Vázquez-Quintana E, Vázquez-Torres DE. Hyperthyroidism and thyroid carcinoma. Am Surg. 2016;82(9):257–8.

23. Yeh NC, Chou CW, Weng SF, Yang CY, Yen FC, Lee SY, Wang JJ, Tien KJ. Hyperthyroidism and thyroid cancer risk: a population-based cohort study. Exp Clin Endocrinol Diabetes. 2013;121(7):402–6.

24. Pellegriti G, Mannarino C, Russo M, Terranova R, Marturano I, Vigneri R, Belfiore A. Increased mortality in patients with differentiated thyroid cancer associated with graves' disease. J Clin Endocrinol Metab. 2013;98(3):1014–21.

25. Stocker DJ, Foster SS, Solomon BL, Shriver CD, Burch HB. Thyroid cancer yield in patients with graves' disease selected for surgery on the basis of cold scintiscan defects. Thyroid. 2002;12(4):305–11.

26. Kraimps JL, Bouin-Pineau MH, Mathonnet M, De Calan L, Ronceray J, Visset J, Marechaud R, Barbier J. Multicentre study of thyroid nodules in patients with graves' disease. Br J Surg. 2000;87(8):1111–3.

27. Calò PG, Conzo G, Raffaelli M, Medas F, Gambardella C, De Crea C, Gordini L, Patrone R, Sessa L, Erdas E, Tartaglia E, Lombardi CP. Total thyroidectomy alone versus ipsilateral versus bilateral prophylactic central neck dissection in clinically node-negative differentiated thyroid carcinoma. A retrospective multicenter study. Eur J Surg Oncol. 2017;43(1):126–32.

28. Agrawal N, Evasovich MR, Kandil E, Noureldine SI, Felger EA, Tufano RP, Kraus DH, Orloff LA, Grogan R, Angelos P, Stack BC Jr, McIver B, Randolph GW. Indications and extent of central neck dissection for papillary thyroid cancer: an American head and neck society consensus statement. Head Neck. 2017;39(7):1269–79.

29. Conzo G, Tartaglia E, Avenia N, Calò PG, de Bellis A, Esposito K, Gambardella C, Iorio S, Pasquali D, Santini L, Sinisi MA, Sinisi AA, Testini M, Polistena A, Bellastella G. Role of prophylactic central compartment lymph node dissection in clinically N0 differentiated thyroid cancer patients: analysis of risk factors and review of modern trends. World J Surg Oncol. 2016;14:149.

30. Calò PG, Pisano G, Medas F, Marcialis J, Gordini L, Erdas E, Nicolosi A. Total thyroidectomy without prophylactic central neck dissection in clinically node-negative papillary thyroid cancer: is it an adequate treatment? World J Surg Oncol. 2014;12:152.

31. Conzo G, Calò PG, Sinisi AA, De Bellis A, Pasquali D, Iorio S, Tartaglia E, Mauriello C, Gambardella C, Cavallo F, Medas F, Polistena A, Santini L, Avenia N. Impact of prophylactic central compartment neck dissection on locoregional recurrence of differentiated thyroid cancer in clinically node-negative patients: a retrospective study of a large clinical series. Surgery. 2014;155(6):998–1005.

32. Conzo G, Avenia N, Ansaldo GL, Calò P, De Palma M, Dobrinja C, Docimo G, Gambardella C, Grasso M, Lombardi CP, Pelizzo MR, Pezzolla A, Pezzullo L, Piccoli M, Rosato L, Siciliano G, Spiezia S, Tartaglia E, Tartaglia F, Testini M, Troncone G, Signoriello G. Surgical treatment of thyroid follicular neoplasms: results of a retrospective analysis of a large clinical series. Endocrine. 2017; 55(2):530–8.

33. Gambardella C, Tartaglia E, Nunziata A, Izzo G, Siciliano G, Cavallo F, Mauriello C, Napolitano S, Thomas G, Testa D, Rossetti G, Sanguinetti A, Avenia N, Conzo G. Clinical significance of prophylactic central compartment neck dissection in the treatment of clinically node-negative papillary thyroid cancer patients. World J Surg Oncol. 2016;14(1):247.

34. Bojic T, Paunovic I, Diklic A, Zivaljevic V, Zoric G, Kalezic N, Sabljak V, Slijepcevic N, Tausanovic K, Djordjevic N, Budjevac D, Djordjevic L, Karanikolic A. Total thyroidectomy as a method of choice in the treatment of graves' disease - analysis of 1432 patients. BMC Surg. 2015;15:39.

35. Miah MS, Mahendran S, Mak C, Leese G, Smith D. Pre-operative serum alkaline phosphatase as a predictive indicator of post-operative hypocalcaemia in patients undergoing total thyroidectomy. J Laryngol Otol. 2015;129(11):1128–32.

36. Tamatea J, Tu'akoi K, Conaglen JV, Elston MS, Meyer-Rochow GY. Thyroid cancer in graves' disease: is surgery the best treatment for graves' disease? ANZ J Surg. 2014;84(4):231–4.

37. Chen Y, Masiakos PT, Gaz RD, Hodin RA, Parangi S, Randolph GW, Sadow PM, Stephen AE. Pediatric thyroidectomy in a high volume thyroid surgery center: risk factors for postoperative hypocalcemia. J Pediatr Surg. 2015; 50(8):1316–9.

38. See AC, Soo KC. Hypocalcaemia following thyroidectomy for thyrotoxicosis. Br J Surg. 1997;84(1):95–7.

16

Identifying high quality medical education websites in Otolaryngology: a guide for medical students and residents

Nathan Yang[1], Sarah Hosseini[1], Marco A. Mascarella[2], Meredith Young[3,4], Nancy Posel[5], Kevin Fung[6] and Lily H. P. Nguyen[2,3*]

Abstract

Background: Learners often utilize online resources to supplement formalized curricula, and to appropriately support learning, these resources should be of high quality. Thus, the objectives of this study are to develop and provide validity evidence supporting an assessment tool designed to assess the quality of educational websites in Otolaryngology- Head & Neck Surgery (ORL-HNS), and identify those that could support effective web-based learning.

Methods: After a literature review, the Modified Education in Otolaryngology Website (MEOW) assessment tool was designed by a panel of experts based on a previously validated website assessment tool. A search strategy using a Google-based search engine was used subsequently to identify websites. Those that were free of charge and in English were included. Websites were coded for whether their content targeted medical students or residents. Using the MEOW assessment tool, two independent raters scored the websites. Inter-rater and intra-rater reliability were evaluated, and scores were compared to recommendations from a content expert.

Results: The MEOW assessment tool included a total of 20 items divided in 8 categories related to authorship, frequency of revision, content accuracy, interactivity, visual presentation, navigability, speed and recommended hyperlinks. A total of 43 out of 334 websites identified by the search met inclusion criteria. The scores generated by our tool appeared to differentiate higher quality websites from lower quality ones: websites that the expert "would recommend" scored 38.4 (out of 56; CI [34.4–42.4]) and "would not recommend" 27.0 (CI [23.2–30.9]). Inter-rater and intra-rater intraclass correlation coefficient were greater than 0.7.

Conclusions: Using the MEOW assessment tool, high quality ORL-HNS educational websites were identified.

Keywords: Medical education, Assessment tool, Online resources

Background

Over the past decade, there has been a proliferation of sources of medical information available in both formal and informal contexts [1, 2]. Formal platforms include scientific journals and peer-reviewed evidence-based resources (e.g., UpToDate), whereas less formal platforms may include medical education websites and lectures or tutorials available on video-sharing websites (e.g., You-Tube). As evidence-based medicine (EBM) increasingly guides decision-making, access to online resources allows trainees to access up-to-date information in a timely manner [3]. Since the introduction of EBM, medical schools have gradually adopted these concepts and taught the principles of EBM to students through various methods including online instructions [3]. At the core of EBM are skills such as recognizing a knowledge gap, searching for literature and appraising the evidence [3]. Searching for pertinent and reliable medical information may thus be of particular difficulty and importance for

* Correspondence: lily.hp.nguyen@gmail.com
Podium Presentation. 69th Annual Meeting of the Canadian Society of Otolaryngology- Head & Neck Surgery. June 6–9, 2015. Winnipeg, MB.
[2]Department of Otolaryngology – Head and Neck Surgery, McGill University, Montreal, QC, Canada
[3]Center for Medical Education, McGill University, Montreal, QC, Canada
Full list of author information is available at the end of the article

medical students and residents, who are simultaneously acquiring medical knowledge and learning appraisal skills.

Despite such potential challenges, learners across the medical education continuum are likely to seek and appraise online resources in order to fit their learning needs and complement their formal curricula. This may particularly be true for specialties such as Otolaryngology-Head and Neck Surgery (ORL-HNS), where learning objectives and content vary significantly among medical schools [4]. Current literature within medical education research has shown that students appreciate online learning for its accessibility, ease of use, freedom of navigation, and high image quality [4, 5]. Although, there are currently multiple definitions for the term "online learning," most authors agree that this term refers to the access of learning experiences via the use of some technology [6]. At the moment, various medical specialties have assessed web-based resources pertaining to their field, with the majority focusing on educational websites for patient teaching. However, few specialties have described educational websites available to complement formal undergraduate medical education or residency training, and a paucity of data exists in the realm of ORL-HNS.

In light of the challenges that medical trainees face when searching for reliable information and the need for complementary resources in ORL-HNS, the objectives of this study are

1. To assess the quality of educational websites in Otolaryngology- Head & Neck Surgery (ORL-HNS) using an assessment tool and identify those that could support effective web-based learning for medical students and residents.
2. To develop and provide validity evidence supporting the Modified Education in Otolaryngology Website (MEOW) assessment tool designed to assess the quality of ORL-HNS education websites.

Methods
In order to identify high quality educational websites in Otolaryngology- Head & Neck Surgery (ORL-HNS), we engaged in a multi-stage development process:

1. Identifying and modifying a medical education website assessment tool
2. Conducting the web search to identify available websites
3. Assessing the quality of identified websites using the assessment tool
4. Providing evidence supporting validity and reliability of the assessment tool

Identifying and modifying a medical education website assessment tool
The first step of this study was to identify a website assessment tool that could objectively identify high-quality educational websites in ORL-HNS. In order to do so, we engaged in a literature search describing medical website assessment tools using PubMed and Google Scholar. Search terms included: "medical websites evaluation tool" and "medical websites quality." Articles highlighting the important elements of a medical education website or describing existing quality assessment tools were reviewed [2, 5–15]. Previously validated assessment tools designed to assess the quality of consumer health information websites such as the DISCERN instrument, the LIDA instrument and Health on the Net Foundation's Health Website Evaluation tool could not be used given their limitations when applied to educational websites designed for medical trainees [13–15]. In the end, the Medical Education Website Quality Evaluation Tool (MEWQET) developed and validated for pathology websites by Alyusuf et al. was deemed to be the tool most aligned with the goal of this study. The MEWQET is in fact designed to assign a score out of 100 points by assessing 43 scoring items within 12 different categories such as authorship, content accuracy and navigability.

After identifying the MEWQET, experts in otolaryngology, medical informatics and medical education were invited to critically appraise the tool and determine its applicability to our study. After reviewing the scoring grid, it was deemed via consensus that the MEWQET could be modified to condense the website assessment process and make it more applicable to ORL-HNS websites, as several items limit its use to non-pathology related websites.

In order to modify the tool, the panel of experts reviewed each of the scoring grid's items. Items that the authors felt were not applicable to ORL-HNS websites were discarded. Similarly, additional items important in the evaluation of medical education websites as demonstrated by the literature review were also added, including summary statements. The panel of experts also reviewed all 12 categories of the original tool. The categories were either renamed, merged or discarded. Items of the modified tool were then re-organized into the new categories.

In regards to the scoring of individual items, scores were either preserved or adapted in order to reflect their relative importance as per the original tool with input from our expert panel. Indeed, items with binary answers were attributed a maximum of 1, 2 or 3 points, and items with three possible answers were given a maximum of 2, 3 or 6 points. In the end, the total maximal score for each category also reflected the relative importance of the category as per the expert panel and the original tool.

The finalized modified version of the tool was called the Modified Education in Otolaryngology Website (MEOW) assessment tool.

Conducting the web search to identify available websites
ORL-HNS education websites were identified using the Startpage (www.startpage.com), a Google-based search engine, to allow for reproducible search results between raters (contrary to other search engines which generate search results based on navigational history and user location). Search results were generated using the following search strategy: ("Otolaryngology" OR "head and neck surgery" OR "ENT") AND ("resources" OR "learn" OR "educational"). The first 50 hits and all hyperlinks within these websites were analyzed. This number was decided in order to obtain the targeted pool of approximately 250 websites to be evaluated, aligned with approaches described in previous work [7]. Website inclusion criteria consisted of websites that were free of charge, in English language, targeted for ORL-HNS education, and targeted to undergraduate medical education (UGME) students/ postgraduate medical education (PGME) in ORL-HNS. Websites consisting of online manuals and textbooks, journal articles, databases or search engines were excluded.

Assessing the quality of identified websites using the assessment tool
Two raters (SH, NY) conducted the initial search to determine which websites to include and appraise in the study. The raters determined via consensus whether the website targeted: a) medical students, b) residents or c) both categories of students. This was done by reviewing the educational objectives set by the Medical Council of Canada, Royal College of Physicians and Surgeons of Canada, American Academy Otolaryngology-Head and Neck Surgery, and Accreditation Council for Graduate Medical Education (ACGME) prior to identifying content area relevant to each learner level [16–19]. Lastly, both raters used the MEOW assessment tool to assess all included websites independently twice, one week apart. Each website was thus scored four times - once by each rater on the first day, and a second time by each rater one week later. Scores were averaged across both raters on both days for all included websites in order to identify the top 3 websites for UGME, PGME and both categories.

Providing evidence supporting construct validity and reliability of the tool
In order to provide evidence supporting construct validity of the MEOW assessment tool, scores were compared to the ratings of a content expert. This expert was Mariana Smith (MS), an outside practicing academic otolaryngologist who completed additional training at McGill University and with previous research experience. She was selected to minimize biases, as she was not involved in the development of any of the websites. Furthermore, she was blinded to the scores generated by the MEOW assessment tool. In order to provide evidence supporting validity, the rating otolaryngologist was first asked to classify 30% of websites included in this study into 1 of 3 categories: 1) Definitely recommend, 2) Maybe recommend and 3) Not recommend. These websites were randomly selected, and classification was made as per the expert's view of the website's educational value for medical students, residents or both. Mean MEOW assessment tool scores of websites found in each category (definitely recommend, maybe recommend, and not recommend) were compared. An analysis of variance (ANOVA) and ninety-five percent confidence intervals were calculated in order to determine statistically significant differences between the mean score of websites falling in each recommendation categories.

Website scores obtained from the MEOW assessment tool were analyzed for intra- and inter-rater reliability. Given that all websites included in this study were assessed by each rater one week apart, intra-rater reliability was measured by the scores given by the same rater to the same website. As for inter-rater reliability, mean scores obtained for each website from each rater were compared. The intraclass correlation coefficient was calculated for both intra- and inter-rater reliabilities using SPSS 20.0. The authors determined that a coefficient of more than 0.7 was the cut-off for good reliability [7].

Results
Tool modification
After eliminating and modifying more than 23 out of the 43 items from the previously existing assessment tool in the field of pathology, a total of 20 items blueprinted to 8 categories were included in our final assessment tool: the Medical Education in Otolaryngology Website (MEOW) assessment tool [7]. These categories included items targeted at assessing: authorship, credibility and disclosure (6 items), frequency of revision (1 item), content quality (4 items), interactivity (1 item), graphic elements (2 items), layout and design (2 items), navigability (2 items) and available hyperlinks to other resources (2 items).

In the end, the total maximal score for each category of items was considered to ensure that the proportion of points attributed to each category reflected the importance of the category as per the Medical Education Website Quality Evaluation Tool (MEWQET) with input from our expert panel. A maximum score of 56 could be attributed to a given website. The finalized version of

Table 1 The Modified Education in Otolaryngology Website (MEOW) assessment tool

Category	Criteria	Weight	Score
1. Authorship, Credibility & Disclosure	1.1 Disclosure of authorship? If yes (pick one)	No = 0	
	A. Authors' name(s), credentials and contact information	A = 3	
	B. Authors' name(s) with credentials	B = 2	
	C. Authors' name(s)	C = 1	
	1.2 If author's credentials are given, author is (if multiple authors, the majority are)		
	A. Otolaryngologist	A = 2	
	B. Other healthcare professional/scientist	B = 1	
	C. Other	C = 0	
	1.3 Disclosure of institution? If yes (pick one)		
	A. Educational, non-profit or government domain	A = 3	
	B. Other	B = 0	
	1.4 Is there an editorial review process?	Yes = 3 No = 0	
	1.5 Is the email of the webmaster provided for feedback?	Yes = 2 No = 0	
	1.6 Are references provided?	Yes = 2 No = 0	
2. Frequency of Revision	2.1 When was the website (including references) last updated?		
	A. <1 year	A = 2	
	B. ≥1 year but <5 years	B = 1	
	C. Other	C = 0	
3. Content Quality	3.1 Breadth. Does the information provided cover aspects pertinent to the field of interest?		
	A = Adequate	A = 6	
	B = Somewhat adequate	B = 3	
	C = Inadequate	C = 0	
	3.2 Depth. Is the information provided adequately detailed for the intended audience?		
	A = Adequate	A = 6	
	B = Somewhat adequate	B = 3	
	C = Inadequate	C = 0	
	3.3 Accuracy. Is the information accurate?		
	A = Accurate	A = 6	
	B = Somewhat accurate	B = 3	
	C = Inaccurate	C = 0	
	3.4 Does the website have summary statements/take-home points?	Yes = 2 No = 0	
4. Interactivity	4.1 Are there any interfaces requiring relevant action on the part of the learner (e.g., quizzes, self assessments, interactive figures)?		
	A. Definitely	A = 6	
	B. Somewhat	B = 3	
	C. No/Does not apply	C = 0	
5. Graphic Elements & Media	5.1 Are graphic/media elements included to provide additional information or to clarify existing content?		
	A. Present and pertinent	A = 2	
	B. Present	B = 1	
	C. Other	C = 0	
	5.2 Are graphic/media elements well integrated in the website?	Yes = 1	

Table 1 The Modified Education in Otolaryngology Website (MEOW) assessment tool *(Continued)*

		No = 0
6. Layout & Design	6.1 Clear/professional display of available information?	Yes = 1 No = 0
	6.2 Is the website user-friendly, having a logical layout and intuitive?	Yes = 2 No = 0
7. Navigability & Speed	7.1 Does the website contain a search engine or table content?	Yes = 2 No = 0
	7.2 Was the website or server accessible in a timely manner?	Yes = 2 No = 0
8. Hyperlinks	8.1 Are there any links to provide relevant additional information?	Yes = 2 No = 0
	8.2 If links are provided, are they active (≥90% of total links)?	Yes = 1 No = 0

the modified tool, the MEOW assessment tool, can be found in Table 1.

Website assessment

A total of 334 websites were identified using the search strategy described above. Of this total, 87% (291/334) were excluded (164 websites not meeting inclusion criteria, 96 website duplicates and 31 inactive links; see Fig. 1). Of the 43 included websites, 22 were considered to be targeting medical student-level educational objectives, 14 targeting resident-level objectives and seven targeting both groups. Using the MEOW assessment tool, the total scores of websites ranged from 20 to 56. The total mean score for all websites was 34.3 ± 7.8. For individual categories of websites, the mean score for websites targeted to medical students, residents and both types of learners were 31.6 ± 7.5, 35.0 ± 5.9 and 41.6 ± 7.1, respectively. The distribution of scores of all websites is demonstrated in Fig. 2. A list of the 3 websites that obtained the highest scores using the modified assessment tool for each type of learner is included in Fig. 3. The highest scoring sites included medical education websites developed by the American Academy of Otolaryngology- Head & Neck Surgery (ORL-HNS), the Canadian Society of ORL-HNS, and two Canadian universities.

Construct validity and reliability assessments

For intra-rater reliability, intra-class correlation coefficients were 0.98 (CI [0.94–0.99]) and 0.94 (CI [0.84–0.98]) for the two raters. Regarding inter-rater reliability, intra-class correlation coefficient was 0.86 (CI [0.76–0.92]). Scores generated by the assessment tool related to the perceptions of quality made by the blinded academic otolaryngologist, with an average evaluation score of 38.4/56 (CI [34.4–42.4]) for "definitely recommend" websites, 36.2/56 (CI [33.2–39.1]) for "maybe recommend" websites and 27.0/56 (CI [23.2–30.9]) for "not recommended" websites. ANOVA analysis revealed that the differences between the means were statistically significant ($F(2, 13) = 4.13$, $p < 0.05$).

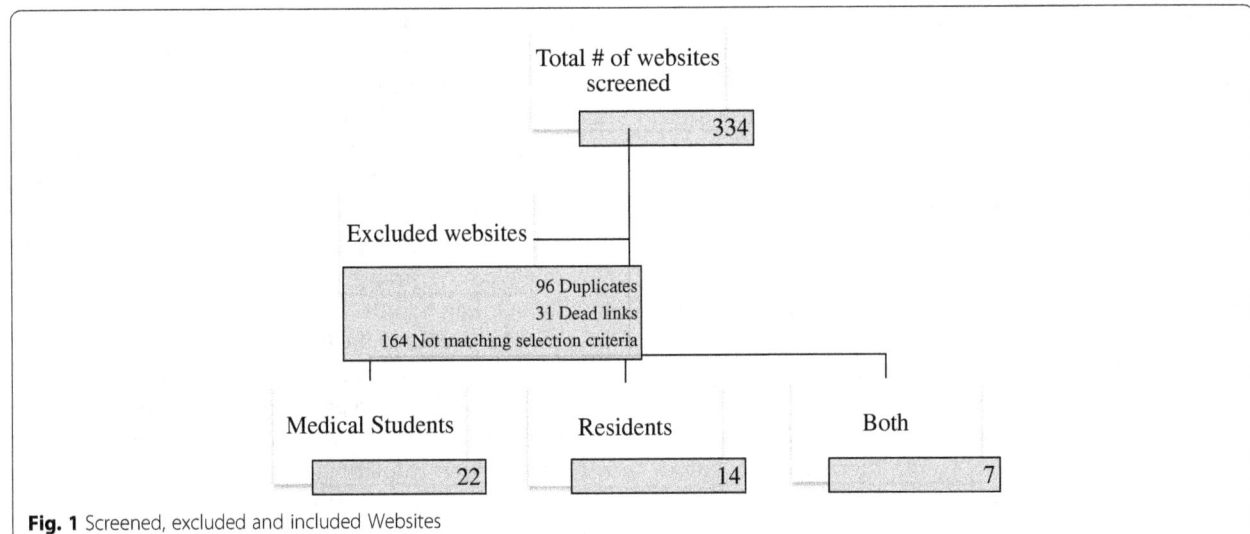

Fig. 1 Screened, excluded and included Websites

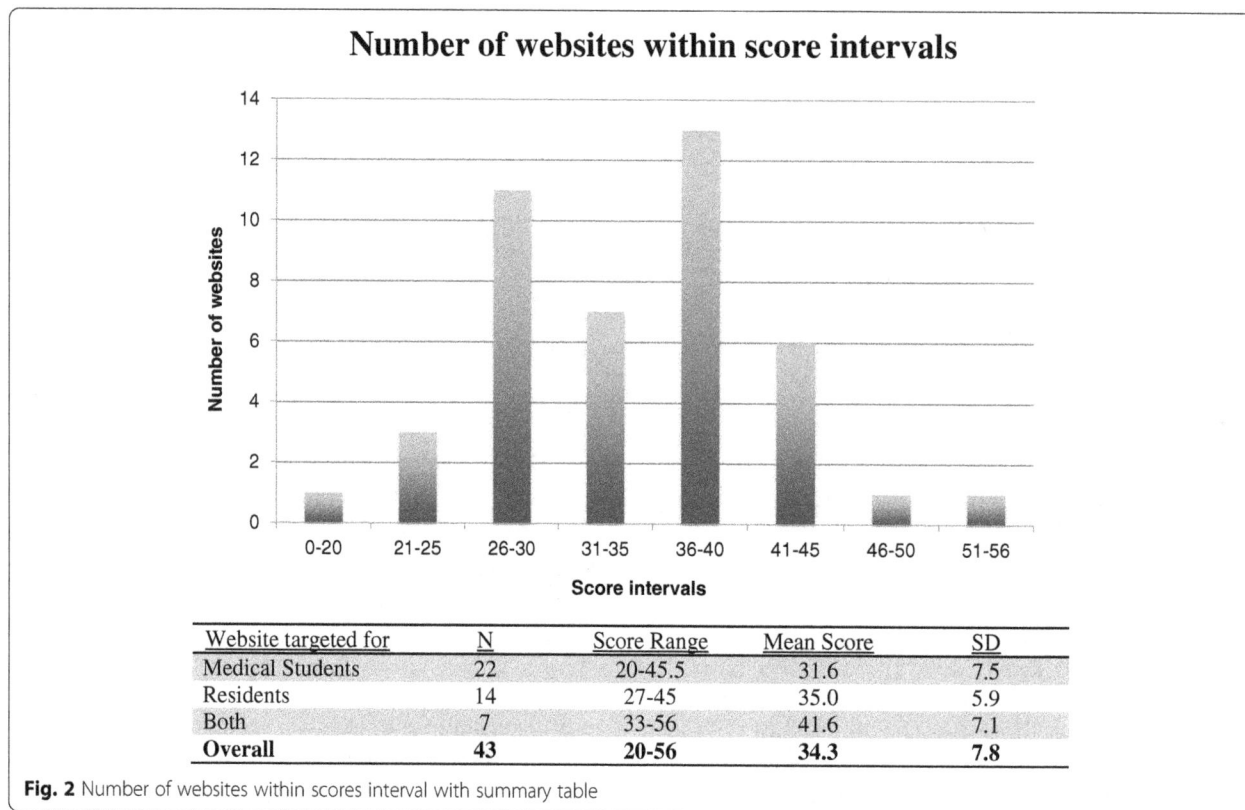

Fig. 2 Number of websites within scores interval with summary table

Website targeted for	N	Score Range	Mean Score	SD
Medical Students	22	20-45.5	31.6	7.5
Residents	14	27-45	35.0	5.9
Both	7	33-56	41.6	7.1
Overall	**43**	**20-56**	**34.3**	**7.8**

Discussion

The goal of this study was to assess and identify high quality online resources in Otolaryngology- Head and Neck Surgery (ORL-HNS) for both medical students and residents. The intent behind providing such a list of websites was to facilitate access to high quality educational content for medical trainees, and provide academic physicians with recommendable resources for their undergraduate and post-graduate programs. Indeed, given that most medical schools only offer brief clinical exposure to the specialty, students may not be inclined to purchase new reference material. Providing access to free, high-quality, readily available online material may thus enhance the learning experience. To our knowledge, no other study has previously identified such resources in the field of ORL-HNS.

Prior to this study, only one assessment tool that allows for grading of medical education websites for health professionals through a scoring system existed [7]. A standardized tool for the assessment of medical education websites arose from the need to assess and compare the quality of a website objectively and systematically rather than intuitively. As medical education websites allows for more independent learning, recognizing reliable sources of information becomes crucial for any medical practitioner. The ability to recognize and utilize high quality learning materials is

a key component in evidence-based medicine and continuing professional development. Although using the Medical Education Website Quality Evaluation Tool (MEWQET) or Modified Education in Otolaryngology Website (MEOW) assessment tool may not be necessary to accomplish such appraisal, both assessment tools highlight the important components of high quality educational websites in all specialties. In fact, these tools could be of potential value to medical educators who seek to design educational websites for various medical specialties.

Our findings suggest that there may be a paucity of online resources specific to ORL-HNS with content that specifically aligns with the learning objectives set forth by national licensure committees for medical students and residents. Indeed, of the 334 websites screened, only 43 met inclusion criteria. We believe that multiple factors are at the basis of the paucity of available material. First, the use of a single search strategy rather than multiple ones, and limiting our search to the first 50 websites and their hyperlinks may have affected the total number of found websites. For instance, the University of Iowa's head and neck website (https://iowaheadneckprotocols.oto.uiowa.edu) is a potentially useful online resource that outlines operative steps in various otolaryngology procedures that was not uncovered by the search strategy. This website was therefore not formally assessed with the MEOW

Both level of training

http://www.entnet.org/content/cool	• American Academy of Otolaryngology- Head & Neck Surgery • Case-Based Learning • MEOW Score= 56/56
http://emedicine.medscape.com/otolaryngology	• Medscape • Text on anatomy, embryology, pathology, surgery, radiology • MEOW Score= 43.5/56
http://www.drtbalu.com/index.html	• DrtBalu's Otolaryngology Online • Text, videos, quizzes, presentations on various medical & surgical topics • MEOW Score= 43/56

Medical Students

http://www.uwoent.ca/node/30**	• Western University • Case-Based Learning, Anatomy • MEOW Score= 45.5/56
http://learnent.ca/	• LearnENT • Physical exam, pertinent additional resource • MEOW Score= 45/56
http://home.comcast.net/~wnor/index.htm	• Anatomy of the Head & Neck • Anatomy and quizz • MEOW Score= 41/56

Residents

http://www.entusa.com/entvideos.htm	• ENTUSA • Surgical Videos, presentations, text on medical & surgical topics • MEOW Score= 45/56
https://www2.aofoundation.org/wps/portal/surgery?showPage=diagnosis&bone=CMF&segment=Overview	• AO Foundation • Surgical indications, approach and management for maxillofacial surgery • MEOW Score= 41.5/56
http://www.utmb.edu/otoref/	• Dr Quinn's online textbook of otolaryngology • Ground Round presentations on various medical topics • MEOW Score= 40/56

Fig. 3 The three top scoring websites for Medical students, Residents and both level of training as evaluated using the MEOW assessment tool. **Alternative website address: http://www.schulich.uwo.ca/otolaryngology/undergraduate/clerkship.html

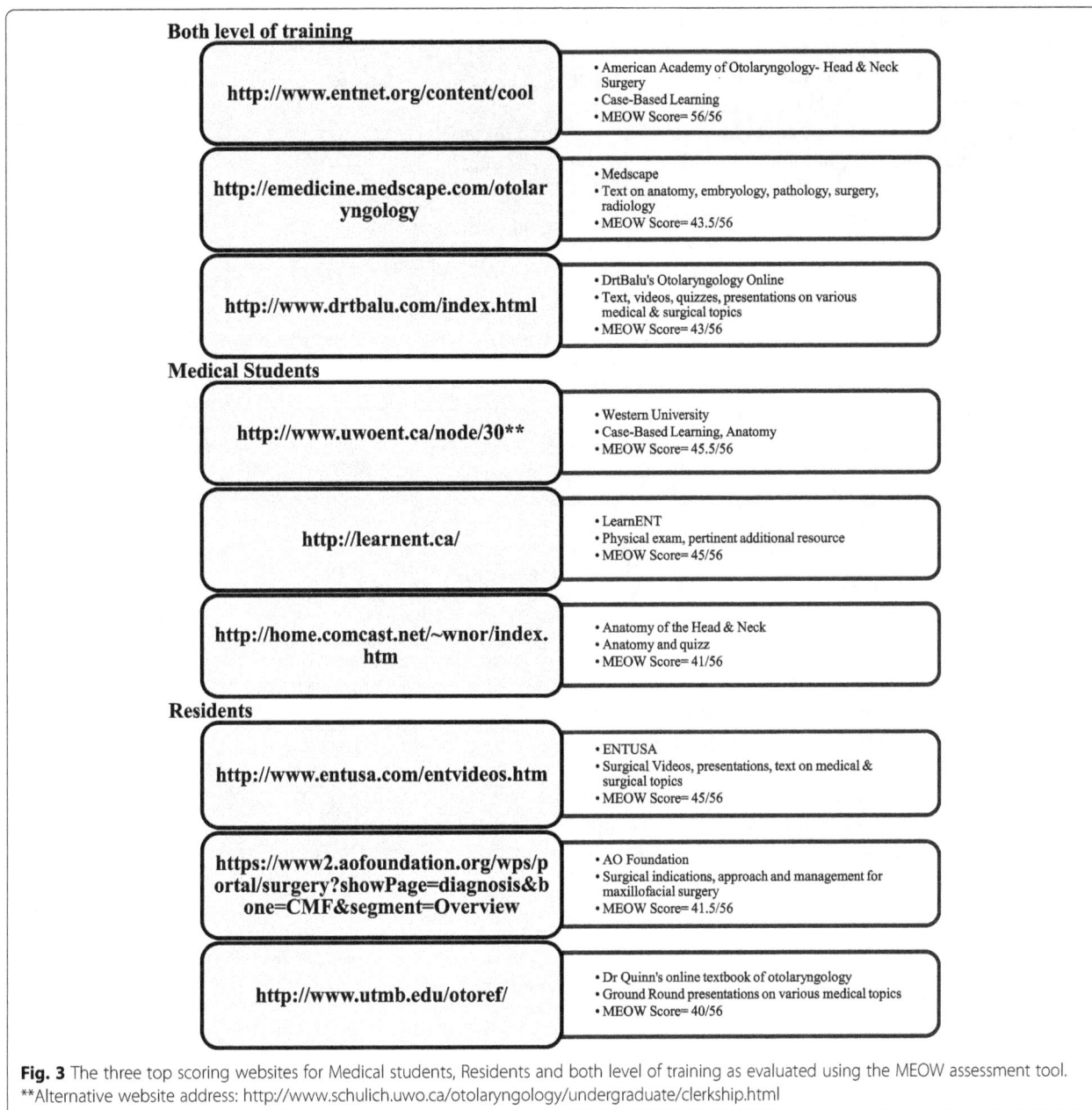

assessment tool (Fig. 3). Other factors limiting the number of available websites may include the need for multiple experts (content, medical education, web development experts) and cost for educational websites development, and the perceived and actual need for educational ORL-HNS websites. Future studies should aim at determining how these websites are being used, whether they are meeting the needs of the users, and whether the number of educational websites in ORL-HNS is comparable to other medical specialties. Such information would help determine whether more educational online resources should be developed for this specialty.

When looking at the quality of available websites, scores generated by the MEOW assessment tool varied widely suggesting a spectrum in website quality. Although higher scoring websites tended to come from known organizations or institutions, one website designed by an independent otolaryngologist with unknown affiliation was highly rated. In fact, although this website did not score well in the authorship, disclosure and credibility category, the content and remainder elements resulted in an overall high score. This suggests that the modified assessment tool speaks to multiple components of quality, and how multiple factors play into the design of good education material. Nevertheless, given that raters could not be blinded to the source of websites in our study, we cannot exclude that websites from well-known organizations were unintentionally scored more favorably. This should perhaps lead us to reconsider the weight of certain authorship elements in the conceptualization of 'credible' resources for online learning.

Our study has several limitations. In addition to the limitations pertaining to our search strategy and potential selection bias due to raters' knowledge of the websites' source, inter-rater reliability may have been affected given that both raters worked collaboratively to include or exclude screened websites. Scores generated by the MEOW tool were significantly different between websites that were rated as "recommend" and "maybe recommend" by an expert ORL-HNS educator from those that were rated as "not recommend." However, although there seems to be a trend, no statistically significant difference was demonstrated between websites' scores in the first two categories. While, this may be due to the relative small sample size, such finding may suggest that the MEOW assessment tool is most useful in differentiating high and average quality websites from lower quality ones.

Conclusions

Online learning resources constitute integral sources of information for today's learners, but are associated with variable quality. The Modified Education in Otolaryngology Website (MEOW) assessment tool has been shown to be a validated instrument that can objectively assess educational websites for medical trainees. With its application, we were able to identify high-quality educational websites pertaining to the field of ORL-HNS that could enhance the learning experience of medical trainees.

Abbreviations
ACGME: Accreditation Council for Graduate Medical Education; EBM: Evidence-based medicine; MEOW: Modified Education in Otolaryngology Website; MEWQET: Medical Education Website Quality Evaluation Tool; ORL-HNS: Otolaryngology- Head & Neck Surgery; PGME: Postgraduate medical education; UGME: Undergraduate medical education

Acknowledgment
We would like to thank Dr Mariana Smith for taking the time to provide her opinion on websites included in our study. Her contribution allowed us to correlate scores from our assessment tool to the opinion of a content expert, and evaluate construct validity. We are sincerely grateful for her help that was generously offered to us.

Funding
This study did not receive funding from any source. No author received financial remuneration from any of the websites evaluated. Authors involved in development of some of the websites were not involved in website assessment.

Authors' contributions
NY, SH, MA, MY, NP, KF and LHPN designed the study. NY, SH and MA designed the pilot assessment tool. MY, NP, KF and LHPN reviewed the pilot assessment tool and finalized it. NY and SH conducted the data extraction. NY, SH, MA, MY, NP, KF and LHPN conducted data analysis. All authors participated in writing and reviewing the manuscript. All authors read and approved the final manuscript.

Competing interests
KF was involved in the development of one of the website. However, the author was not involved in website assessment. The authors do not have any other potential competing interests.

Author details
[1]Faculty of Medicine, McGill University, Montreal, QC, Canada. [2]Department of Otolaryngology – Head and Neck Surgery, McGill University, Montreal, QC, Canada. [3]Center for Medical Education, McGill University, Montreal, QC, Canada. [4]Department of Medicine, McGill University, Montreal, QC, Canada. [5]McGill Molson Medical Informatics, McGill University, Montreal, QC, Canada. [6]Department of Otolaryngology – Head and Neck Surgery, Western University, London, ON, Canada.

References
1. Drenth JPH. Proliferation of authors on research reports in medicine. Sci Eng Ethics. 1996;2(4):469–80.
2. Jain T, Barbieri RL. Website quality assessment: mistaking apples for oranges. Fertil Steril. 2005;83(3):545–7.
3. Maggio LA, Tannery NH, Chen HC, ten Cate O, O'Brien B. Evidence-based medicine training in undergraduate medical education: a review and critique of the literature published 2006–2011. Acad Med. 2013;88(7):1022–8. doi:10.1097/ACM.0b013e3182951959.
4. Fung K. Otolaryngology- head and neck surgery in undergraduate medical education: advances and innovations. Laryngoscope. 2015;125 Suppl 2:S1–14. doi:10.1002/lary.24875. Epub 2014 Aug 14.
5. Potomkova J, Mihal V, Cihalik C. Web-based instruction and its impact on the learning activity of medical students: a review. Biomed Pap Med Fac Univ Palacky Olomouc Czech Repub. 2006;150:357. 35.
6. Moore JL, Dickson-Deane C, Galyen K. e-Learning, online learning and distance learning environments: are they the same? Internet High Educ. 2011;14:129–32.
7. Alyusuf RH, Prasad K, Abdel Satir AM, Abalkhail AA, Arora RK. Development and validation of a tool to evaluate the quality of medical education websites in pathology. J Pathol Inform. 2013;4:29–3539. 120729. eCollection 2013.
8. Moustakis V, Litos C, Dalivigas A, Tsironis L. Website Quality Assessment Criteria. Ninth International Conference on Information Quality. 2004. p. 59–73. http://mitiq.mit.edu/ICIQ/Documents/IQ%20Conference%202004/Papers/WebsiteQualityAssessmentCriteria.pdf. Accessed 19 Oct 2015.
9. Lewiecki EM, Rudolph LA, Kiebzak GM, Chavez JR, Thorpe BM. Assessment of osteoporosis-website quality. Osteoporos Int. 2006;17:741–52.
10. Hasan L, Abuerlrub E. Assessing the quality of web sites. Appl Comput Inform. 2011;9(1):11–29.
11. Posel N, Fleiszer D, Shore BM. 12 tips: guidelines for authoring virtual patient cases. Med Teach. 2009;31(8):701–8. doi:10.1080/01421590902793867.
12. Silberg WM, Lundberg GD, Musacchio RA. Assessing, controlling, and assuring the quality of medical information on the Internet: Caveant lector et viewor- let the reader and viewer beware. JAMA. 1997;277(15):1244–5.
13. Discern online: Quality criteria for consumer health information- Background. 2017. http://www.discern.org.uk/background_to_discern.php. Accessed 14 Apr 2017.
14. Minervation: Evidence based healthcare consultancy- Is the LIDA website assessment tool valid. 2012. http://www.minervation.com/does-lida-work. Accessed 14 Apr 2017.
15. Health on the Net Foundation- Health website evaluation tool. 2010. http://www.hon.ch/HONcode/Pro/HealthEvaluationTool.html. Accessed 14 Apr 2017.

16. Objectives for the Qualifying Examination. 2015. http://apps.mcc.ca/ Objectives_Online/objectives.pl?lang=english&loc=help#Version. Accessed 14 Apr 2017.

17. Objectives of Training in the specialty of Otolaryngology- Head and Neck Surgery. 2015. http://www.royalcollege.ca/cs/groups/public/documents/ document/y2vk/mdaw/~edisp/tztest3rcpsced000926~2.html. Accessed 22 May 2017.

18. COCLIA. AAO Member Engagement Portal. 2015. http://portal.entnet.org/ aaohns_Portal/Education/COCLIA/portal/coclia/onlineguide/cocliamain.aspx. Accessed 14 Apr 2017.

19. The Otolaryngology Milestone Project. 2013. http://www.acgme.org/ acgmeweb/Portals/0/PDFs/Milestones/OtolaryngologyMilestones.pdf. Accessed 14 Apr 2017.

17

In-office laryngeal procedures (IOLP) in Canada: current safety practices and procedural care

Yael Bensoussan[1][*] [iD] and Jennifer Anderson[2]

Abstract

Background: The advent of chip tip technology combined with advanced endoscopy has revolutionized the field of laryngology in the past decade. Procedures such as transnasal esophagoscopy, site-specific steroid injections, injection laryngoplasty and laryngeal laser treatment can now be performed in the office setting under local anaesthesia. Although In-Office Laryngeal Procedures (IOLPs) have become standard-of-care in many American and several Canadian centers, there are no guidelines regulating the practice of these procedures. The goal of this report was to evaluate the current method of IOLP delivery in Canada.

Methods: An electronic survey was dispersed to 22 practicing Canadian laryngologists to assess safety and procedural care measures undertaken when performing IOLP. The survey consisted of 37 questions divided into 6 categories; 1) Demographic data 2) Facilities 3) Staff/personnel 4) Patient screening/monitoring 5) Procedure and emergency equipment 6) Reporting of adverse events.

Results: Data was collected for 16/22 laryngologists (72.7% response rate). Only 1 respondent did not perform IOLP. All performed injection augmentation laryngoplasty. Most performed laryngeal biopsies, intramuscular injection and/or electromyography guided injection for the treatment of spasmodic dysphonia and glottic/subglottic steroid injections. Only 4 respondents performed in-office KTP laser. Significant variation was found in procedural processes including intra procedural monitoring, anticoagulation screening, access to emergency equipment and documentation.

Conclusion: Our survey demonstrates that the delivery of IOLP in Canada varies considerably. The construct of IOLP practice guidelines based on the evidence with consistent documentation would promote safe, efficient and quality care for patient with voice disorders.

Keywords: Office-based procedures, Patient safety, Laryngology procedures, Awake procedures, Patient tolerance, Complications

Background

The advent of chip tip technology combined with advanced endoscopy including port access has revolutionized the field of laryngology in the past decade [1–4]. Procedures such as laryngeal biopsies, transnasal esophagoscopy, steroid injection, injection augmentation and laryngeal laser treatment can be performed in the office setting on awake patients with videoendoscopic guidance.

In office laryngology procedures (IOLP) have specific advantages over traditional surgical management for the treatment of laryngeal pathology such as improved access, shorter procedure time and less cost [4–6]. In safety measures, IOLP with local/topical anaesthesia also represent reduced risk by avoiding general anaesthesia and other surgery associated risk inherent to suspension laryngoscopy (injury to dentition, tongue/mucosal, TMJ/jaw). In patients with significant comorbidities or anatomic limitations who are not suitable or are at a high risk of complications to undergo a general anaesthetic with suspension laryngoscopy, IOLP is a viable alternative to treatment which was not available previously.

---
* Correspondence: yael.bensoussan@mail.utoronto.ca
[1]Department of Otolaryngology Head & Neck Surgery, University of Toronto, Toronto, ON, Canada
Full list of author information is available at the end of the article

Disease outcomes, safety, and tolerance of these procedures in awake patients have been explored in the literature [4–7]. Although IOLP have now become 'routine' practice in many American and several Canadian centers, to date, there are no guidelines regulating the practice of these procedures despite potential adverse events and complications.

The purpose of this study was to report the current practices in terms of safety measures and procedural processes for IOLP in the Canadian health system.

Methods

An electronic survey was dispersed to 22 practicing Canadian laryngologists trough an electronic survey platform to assess safety and procedural measures undertaken when performing IOLP. Canadian laryngologists were identified through the membership list of the Canadian Society of Otolaryngology – Head & Neck Surgery (CSOHNS) (self-reported laryngologists) and by contacting Otolaryngology departments of each Canadian university. The list was then reviewed by the senior academic laryngologist (J.A) at our institution and recent graduates were added to the list. Once the list was completed, laryngologists were contacted by email and/or phone and received a link to complete the anonymous survey through the electronic platform. Data was collected in a cross-sectional fashion between November 2016 and June 2017.

The survey consisted of 37 questions divided into 6 categories; 1) demographic data 2) facilities 3) staff/personnel 4) patient screening/monitoring 5) procedure and emergency equipment 6) monitoring and reporting. After the demographic section, participants were asked if they performed IOLP. A negative answer ended the questionnaire, whereas a positive answer opened further questions. The full survey questions are available in the electronic version of this manuscript in Additional file 1.

Results

The survey was completed by 16 of the 22 laryngologists (72.7% response rate) with an equal number or male and female laryngologists. The majority of the respondents were fellowship trained (87.5%). Complete demographics data is summarized in Table 1.

Fifteen out of 16 respondents (93.8%) reported performing IOLP. Only 1 respondent did not perform IOLP despite fellowship training due to concerns raised from their hospital administration about safety for these procedures. As such, the remaining questions of the survey were answered by 15 respondents.

Injection laryngoplasty was the most performed procedure (15/15), followed by laryngeal biopsies (11/15), botulinum toxin A injections for spasmodic dysphonia (11/15) and video endoscopic guided glottic/subglottic

Table 1 Demographic data of participating Canadian Laryngologists

Variable	Respondents N = 16 (%)
Gender	
Male	8 (50.0)
Female	8 (50.0)
Province of practice	
Ontario	7 (43.8)
Alberta	3 (18.8)
Manitoba	2 (12.5)
British Columbia	2 (12.5)
Quebec	1 (6.25)
Nova Scotia	1 (6.25)
Years in practice	
Less than 5 years	5 (31.3)
5 to 10 years	4 (25.0)
10 to 20 years	3 (18.8)
More than 20 years	4 (25.0)
Fellowship training	
Yes	14 (87.5)
No	2 (12.5)

steroid injection (10/15). Four respondents reported performing in office KTP laser in their clinic which were all hospital-based. Other procedures included transnasal esophagoscopy, esophageal dilation, and bronchoscopy as summarized in Fig. 1.

Facilities

All respondents reported performing IOLP in a clinic within a hospital. One third (33.3%) of laryngologists also perform the procedures out-of hospital in a private clinic or office outside the main hospital facility, between 2 to 4 km away from their base hospital.

Staff/personnel

Fifty three percent (8/15) respondents indicated that their assistant/nursing staff had received some form of IOLP related training. Human resources available for assistance to perform IOLP was variable and included registered nurses, otolaryngology trainees, speech language pathologist and physician assistants. On the other hand, 80.0% of respondents indicated their staff/assistants have training for emergency situations such as CPR (cardiopulmonary resuscitation) or ACLS (advanced cardiovascular life support) training.

Patient screening and monitoring

Participants were asked to describe if there was exclusion criteria used to screen patients before IOLP (Table 2.).

Types of procedures performed

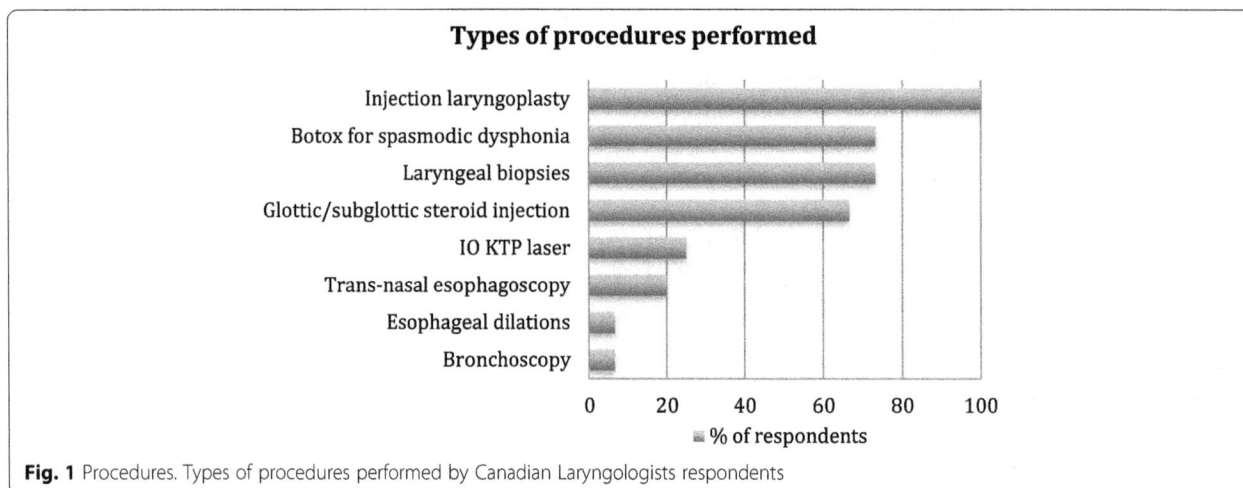

Fig. 1 Procedures. Types of procedures performed by Canadian Laryngologists respondents

Three laryngologists (20.0%) indicated there had no exclusion criteria for these types of procedures.

The survey results demonstrated considerable variability in whether or not patients were instructed to discontinue anticoagulation medication by their laryngologist prior to undergoing IOLP (Table 3). More than 20% of respondents reported performing IOLP for patients on therapeutic levels of warfarin. However, none of these laryngologists were performing laser treatment.

Sixty per cent (9/15) of laryngologists use pre-medication such as an anxiolytic (i.e. lorazepam) for some patients whereas 40.0% indicated that premedication or sedation was never used.

The majority of the laryngologists (86.7%) did not require patients to be NPO before their procedure.

Only 35.7% of laryngologists reported systematically measuring and documenting vital signs as part of their procedure protocol. In terms of patient monitoring, only 1 laryngologist reported taking post-procedure vital signs.

Most centres monitored patients post IOLP for 15–30 min (73.3%), and in some cases, less than 15 min (20.0%) and rarely over 30 min (6.7%).

Most laryngologists always ask patients to be accompanied after a procedure (66.7%). Two of the three laryngologists who reported not requiring that patients be accompanied perform full range of procedures described previously including KTP laser procedures (Table 4).

Procedure and emergency equipment
The majority of laryngologists surveyed use chip tip video endoscopy (93.3%), and 40% also use fiberoptic scopes to perform IOLP. A variety of local anaesthesia techniques were reported. For nasal anaesthesia, half of the respondents use packing whereas the remaining use spray technique. The agents used include lidocaine, or a mix of lidocaine and xylometazoline. For laryngeal anaesthesia, transcutaneous/transtracheal injection of lidocaine and topical lidocaine delivered via a port catheter in the endoscopy were the most commonly used techniques (60.0% and 53.3%). Other methods less often utilized were the use of nebulizer/mist inhaled lidocaine,

Table 2 Exclusion criteria reported

Exclusion criteria	Number of times reported (n = 15)
Intolerance to office scope/ severe gag	6
Significant anxiety	4
Poor Anatomy/obesity	4
Poor lung function/02 requirement	2
Lesion too bulky for KTP	2
Neuromuscular disease	1
Uncontrolled hypertension	1
Allergy to lidocaïne	1
Unable to understand English	1
None	3

Table 3 Antiplatelet/anticoagulation management

	Would Continue N = 15 (%)	Would Stop[a] N = 15 (%)	Would perform IOLP if patient cannot stop
ASA 81 mg	11 (73.3)	4 (26.7)	15 (100.0)
NSAIDs	12 (80.0)	3 (20.0)	13 (86.7)
Clopidogrel	5 (33.2)	10 (66.7)	7 (46.7)
New agents (i.e. dabigatran)	8 (53.5)	7 (46.7)	5 (33.3)
Warfarin	3 (20.0)[b]	12 (80.0) [c]	4 (26.7)[d]

[a] Stop from 3 to 7 days prior to procedure
[b] 1 respondent specified if INR less than 3.5
[c] With or without bridging
[d] 1; only for injection laryngosplasty, 1; only if INR over 2.5 (hold or modify)

Table 4 Procedural care questions

Procedural care	Respondents n = 15 (%)
Do you use sedation/pre-medication?	
Yes, for anxious patients	9 (60.0)
No, Never	6 (40.0)
Do you ask your patient to be NPO before the procedure?	
Yes	2 (13.3)
No	13 (86.7)
How long are patients monitored post-procedure?	
Less than 15 min	3 (20.0)
15–30 min	11 (73.3)
More than 30 min	1 (6.7)
Do you ask patients to be accompanied post procedure?	
Yes	10 (66.7)
No	3 (20.0)
Depending on procedure	1 (6.7)
Only if pre-medicated	1 (6.7)

endotracheal lidocaine spray, laryngojet and superior laryngeal nerve block.

In terms of emergency equipment, 80.0% of respondents have access to a crash cart and defibrillator, 73.3% have access to material to treat an allergic reaction, and 66.7% have access to material to treat a laryngospasm in the case of severe complication (Fig. 2). Out of the 3 respondents who said not having a crash cart in their facility, 1 reported he had access to one 500 m away from the clinic facility.

Monitoring and reporting of adverse events

In an open-ended question about adverse events and complications encountered by laryngologists, only minor complications were reported such as patient anxiety, intolerance, intractable gag, coughing, vomiting, vasovagal episodes, discomfort and pain. One laryngologist

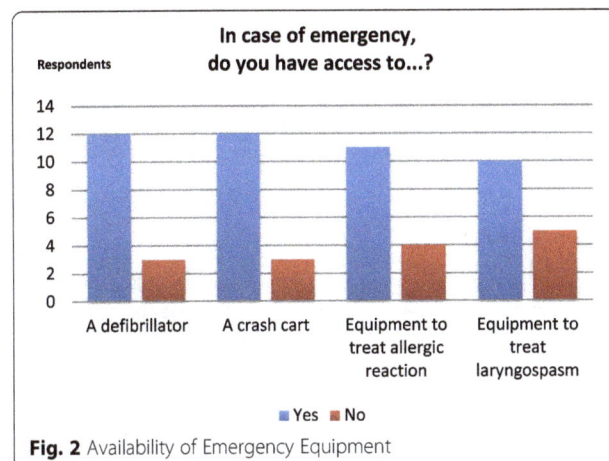

Fig. 2 Availability of Emergency Equipment

reported a minor laryngospasm adverse event, spontaneously resolving after termination of the procedure and patient monitoring.

Eleven out of 15 physicians (73.3%) document of the dosage of topical and/or injected local anaesthesia used during the procedure. All surveyed laryngologists dictate and/or write procedure notes in the medical chart. In addition, two respondents also have a nursing note added to the chart. One laryngologist keeps a separate binder for injectables where dosages and materials are documented. One respondent used a standardized laser flow sheet and safety checklist for all laser procedures.

In terms of reporting of adverse events, all respondents indicated that the patients' electronic or paper medical record was used for documentation. One respondent also uses a separate adverse event hospital log for standardized reporting.

Discussion

The purpose of this national survey was to describe the procedural practices used to conduct IOLP in Canada. This initiative was motivated by the fact that there are presently no guidelines on procedure and safety measures for IOLP.

Operating room procedures are regulated by detailed protocols including surgical timeout and debriefing, instruments counts, nursing and anaesthesia monitoring, and laser safety protocol as well as standardized documentation [8–11]. Although patients are not undergoing general anaesthesia, in-office laryngology procedures have potential significant risks.

Any use of sedation or local anaesthesia poses a potential risk of allergic reaction or toxicity [12]. Moreover, the specific risks of airway manipulation of the awake, nonintubated patients are particularly of concern in our specialty. Although largely minor complications such as vasovagal episodes, minor airway bleeding, discomfort, pain, patient intolerance are reported in the literature, some authors have encountered laryngospasm, airway bleeding, and lidocaine toxicity during these procedures [2, 3, 6, 7, 13]. More recent reports from several authors describe non-negligible hemodynamic effects during IOLP including severe tachycardia and hypertension [14–16].

Our survey results suggest that although most laryngology practices are equipped in case of adverse events, a significant percentage of respondents (20.0–33.3%) reported no access to medical resources in order to treat laryngospasm or allergic reactions. In case of an emergency situation when in a hospital setting, any serious adverse event can be supported through usual emergency procedure I.E. code blue. However, immediately accessible emergency resources such suction (bleeding, secretions), arrest cart (standardized medical treatment) and defibrillator are reasonable for patient safety.

In an office setting outside the hospital, access to these resources may be limited or unavailable. One third of the responding laryngologists reported practicing in such a setting.

When looking at the literature from other specialties performing office- based procedure, several associations of surgeons have published guidelines to regulate these practices and ensure patient safety. The American Academy of Dermatology recently published explicit guidelines for the use of local anaesthesia in office-based dermatological surgery (2016) [17]. These guidelines detail evidence on types of agents, methods of delivery, and potential complication. Among other recommendations, they suggest calculation and documentation of local anaesthetic use for each patient to prevent adverse toxicity events. The Society of American Gastrointestinal Endoscopic Surgeons (SAGES) has also issued guidelines regulating endoscopy practices [18]. The published document includes recommendations in terms of facilities and physical environment, training of staff, patient selection and NPO status, patient monitoring, equipment, medication requirements and documentation.

Although there are no published guidelines in laryngology, several authors have recommended some measures to promote patient safety. Madden et al. suggested a cardiovascular pre-screening tool to prevent avoidable complications for high risk patients [19]. The protocol consists of measuring vital signs at the pre-operative appointment to screen patients and refer to the appropriate physician before exposing patients to avoidable risks. Yung et al. also suggested the monitoring of vitals during these procedures after reporting significant changes in BP and HR [14]. The results of the present survey suggests that less than 40% of Canadian laryngologists measure vital signs prior to or after IOLP. There is no current data that describes American laryngologists practices in terms of vital signs monitoring during these procedures.

The analysis of the survey responses also demonstrates that similar to other surgical specialties, office based procedures are increasingly being performed in laryngology in Canada. Brown et al., from Halifax, had already described the trend in 2012 by reporting the results of a survey detailing the composition of practice and technology used by Canadian laryngologists [20]. At that time, the authors identified 11 laryngologists in Canada. According to our data, the self-reported laryngologists in practice have doubled in the last 5 years ($n = 22$) with one third of out respondents in practice less than 5 years. The variety and complexity of procedures performed on awake patient have also increased with now at least 4 laryngologists performing in-office KTP laser in Canada.

There may be some influence on delivery of novel procedures due to resource restrictions and physician remuneration based on provincial fee schedules. For example,

in eastern Canada and a few academic centres in Ontario, physicians are on a full salary and are not limited by the lack of a specific procedure code in offering these novel treatment options. However, in western Canada (British Columbia and Alberta) there is no specific fee code for in office laser treatment. Laryngeal augmentation and botox injection however have has a code in the schedule in most provinces. In Ontario and Quebec, a specific business case was submitted to the provincial health organization which approved in office laser laryngeal procedures. It is important to take into consideration safety requirements may vary between institutions as well. The survey did not have specific questions regarding differences in institutional restrictions or provincial remuneration.

Another limitation of this study is the relative risks of the various types of IOLP. For example. A 30 min endoscopic laser treatment for extensive RRP likely does not have the same degree of risk as a unilateral injection for spasmodic dysphonia (usually less than 5 min) which may therefore influence exclusion criteria or the need for cessation of anticoagulants prior to procedures. However, all the IOLP listed in our survey require manipulation of the upper airway in an awake patient and safety measure such as access to emergency equipment, training of assistants, and standardized reporting of adverse events are recommended.

Conclusion

IOLPs are increasingly practiced in the laryngology field in the Canada. Our survey demonstrates that practices in terms of safety and procedural care remain variable. Practice enhancement strategies should focus on providing more structured guidelines to regulate IOLP and promote patient safety.

Acknowledgements
We want to thank the Canadian Society of Otolaryngology who helped identify Canadian laryngologists.

Funding
Not applicable.

Authors' contributions
JA, senior author, participated in the elaboration of the survey questions, identified Canadian laryngologists, supervised the study and revised the manuscript. YB participated in the elaboration of the survey questions, collected and analyzed the data. Both authors read and approved the final manuscript.

Competing interests
All the authors mentioned above have no conflict of interests to disclose.

Author details
[1]Department of Otolaryngology Head & Neck Surgery, University of Toronto, Toronto, ON, Canada. [2]Department of Otolaryngology-Head and Neck Surgery, University of Toronto, St-Michael's Hospital, 30 Bond Street, Toronto, ON M5B 1W8, Canada.

References
1. Rosen CA, et al. Advances in office-based diagnosis and treatment in laryngology. Laryngoscope. 2009;119(Suppl 2):S185–212.
2. Shah M, Johns M. Office-based laryngeal procedures. Otolaryngol Clin N Am. 2013;46:75–84.
3. Naidu H, Noordzij JP, Samim A, Jalisi S, Grillone GA. Comparison of efficacy, safety, and cost-effectiveness of in-office cup forcep biopsies versus operating room biopsies for laryngopharyngeal tumors. J. Voice Off. J. Voice Found. 2012;26:604–6.
4. Lippert D, et al. In-office biopsy of upper airway lesions: safety, tolerance, and effect on time to treatment. Laryngoscope. 2015;125:919–23.
5. Pitman MJ, Lebowitz-Cooper A, Iacob C, Tan M. Effect of the 532nm pulsed KTP laser in the treatment of Reinke's edema. Laryngoscope. 2012;122:2786–92.
6. Andrade Filho PA, Carrau RL, Buckmire RA. Safety and cost-effectiveness of intra-office flexible videolaryngoscopy with transoral vocal fold injection in dysphagic patients. Am J Otolaryngol. 2006;27:319–22.
7. Koss SL, Baxter P, Panossian H, Woo P, Pitman MJ. Serial in-office laser treatment of vocal fold leukoplakia: disease control and voice outcomes. Laryngoscope. 2017;127:1644–51.
8. WHO | WHO surgical safety checklist and implementation manual. WHO. Available at: http://www.who.int/patientsafety/safesurgery/ss_checklist/en/. Accessed 1 Nov 2017.
9. Norton E. Implementing the universal protocol hospital-wide. AORN J. 2007;85:1187–97.
10. Dillon KA. Time out: an analysis. AORN J. 2008;88:437–42.
11. Baxter DA. Laser safety in the operating room. Insight Am Soc Ophthalmic Regist Nurses. 2006;31:13–4.
12. Eggleston ST, Lush LW. Understanding allergic reactions to local anesthetics. Ann Pharmacother. 1996;30:851–7.
13. Del Signore AG, Shah RN, Gupta N, Altman KW, Woo P. Complications and failures of office-based endoscopic Angiolytic laser surgery treatment. J Voice Off J Voice Found. 2016;30:744–50.
14. Yung KC, Courey MS. The effect of office-based flexible endoscopic surgery on hemodynamic stability. Laryngoscope. 2010;120:2231–6.
15. Tierney WS, Chota RL, Benninger MS, Nowacki AS, Bryson PC. Hemodynamic parameters during Laryngoscopic procedures in the office and in the operating room. Otolaryngol–Head Neck Surg Off J Am Acad Otolaryngol-Head Neck Surg. 2016;155:466–72.
16. Morrison MP, et al. Hemodynamic changes during otolaryngological office-based flexible endoscopic procedures. Ann Otol Rhinol Laryngol. 2012;121:714–8.
17. Kouba DJ, et al. Guidelines for the use of local anesthesia in office-based dermatologic surgery. J Am Acad Dermatol. 2016;74:1201–19.
18. Heneghan S, Myers J, Fanelli R, Richardson W, Society of American Gastrointestinal Endoscopic Surgeons. Society of American Gastrointestinal Endoscopic Surgeons (SAGES) guidelines for office endoscopic services. Surg. Endosc. 2009;23:1125–9.
19. Madden LL, et al. A cardiovascular prescreening protocol for unmonitored in-office laryngology procedures. Laryngoscope. 2017;127:1845–9.
20. McNeil ML, Brown TFE. Laryngology in Canada: results of a national survey. J Otolaryngol - Head Neck Surg J Oto-Rhino-Laryngol Chir Cervico-Faciale. 2012;41:65–70.

18

The molecular mechanisms of increased radiosensitivity of HPV-positive oropharyngeal squamous cell carcinoma (OPSCC): an extensive review

Changxing Liu[1], Daljit Mann[2], Uttam K. Sinha[1] and Niels C. Kokot[1*]

Abstract

Head and neck carcinomas (HNCs) collectively are the sixth most common cancer with an annual incidence of about 400,000 cases in the US. The most well-established risk factors for HNCs are tobacco and alcohol abuse. With the increasing public awareness, the incidence of HNCs is decreasing. But there is an increasing incidence of oropharyngeal squamous cell carcinoma (OPSCC) has been observed during the last decade. This phenomena is associated with persistent infection with high-risk HPV. HPV associated OPSCC patients tend to be younger males of high socioeconomic status. The increasing incidence causes a significant loss to social resources, given that it's reported that HPV associated OPSCC represents about 60% of OPSCC cases. There is a growing amount of data supporting the hypothesis that HPV-associated OPSCC has a better survival rate due to a higher sensitivity to chemotherapy and radiotherapy as compared to HPV-unrelated OPSCC. Although the HPV positivity is associated with increased radio-sensitivity, the underlying mechanisms are not yet fully understood. This review summarizes the current knowledge on the effects of HPV infection and its carcinogenesis on the radiosensitivity of OPSCC, from the molecular to histologic level, providing a comprehensive insight of this special tumor entity.

Keywords: HPV-positive oropharyngeal squamous cell carcinoma, Radiosensitivity, HPV, P53

Background

Head and neck carcinomas (HNCs) collectively are the sixth most common cancer with an annual incidence of ~ 400,000 cases [1], and represent about 3.5% of all malignant tumors in western societies [2, 3] and other parts of the world. Nearly 90% of these cancers are head and neck squamous cell carcinomas (HNSCCs). The most well-established risk factors for HNSCC are tobacco and alcohol abuse [4]. HPV involvement in head and neck carcinogenesis was initially reported 30 years ago [5]; however, it was just recently recognized as an emerging risk factor for oropharyngeal squamous cell carcinoma (OPSCC) [6].

OPSCC arises in the oropharynx, the middle region of the throat that includes the soft palate, the base of the tongue, the tonsils, and the lateral and posterior walls of the throat. According to the American Cancer Society's most recent estimates for 2016, in the United States, about 48,330 people are estimated to get oral cavity or oropharyngeal cancers, and an estimated 9570 people will die of these cancers. An increasing incidence of OPSCC has been observed during the last decade [7–10]. This rise in incidence is mostly occurring in individuals aged 40–55 years, without environmental risk factors, and is associated with persistent infection with high-risk HPV [11]. HPV-positive OPSCC patients tend to be younger than HPV(–) patients [12]. Tonsil and oropharyngeal cancers increased in male predominance over the last 30 years, despite a decline in smoking, which may be linked to the decreasing proportion of HPV-negative cancers; while changes in sexual activity may be reflected in increasing proportion of HPV-positive cancers [11]. Recently, HPV

* Correspondence: Niels.Kokot@med.usc.edu
[1]USC Tina and Rick Caruso Department of Otolaryngology-Head and Neck Surgery, Keck Medicine of USC, University of Southern California, Los Angeles, CA 90033, USA
Full list of author information is available at the end of the article

associated OPSCC represents about 60% of OPSCC cases compared to 40% in the previous decade.

There is a growing amount of data supporting the hypothesis that HPV-related tumors have a better survival rate due to a higher sensitivity to chemotherapy and radiotherapy as compared to HPV-unrelated HNSCC [12]. This significant difference in etiology and outcomes has been recognized by the AJCC, and new staging guidelines have been released to reflect the data [13]. DNA damage in HPV-related and HPV-unrelated HNSCC cell lines occurs by different mechanisms, which illustrate the reasons for the increased sensitivity of HPV-related OPSCC [14]. HPV positivity is associated with increased radio-sensitivity in probably multiple, not yet understood pathways [15–20]. This review summarizes the current literature on the effects of radiation therapy on OPSCC cell lines and how HPV infection alters these mechanisms to create a higher sensitivity to treatment.

Radiation in OPSCC treatment

Radiation has a significant role in the management of head and neck squamous cell carcinomas (HNSCCs). Strategies to use radiation for the treatment of HNSCC have improved significantly during the past two decades, primarily through the use of IMRT techniques and through the addition of chemoradiotherapy. Radiation delivered postoperatively in the adjuvant setting significantly improves eradication of locoregional disease, and organ-sparing approaches for pharyngeal and laryngeal cancers that rely on chemoradiation as the primary treatment modality yields high rates of disease control [21]. The goal of radiation as a cancer treatment is to preferentially kill cancer cells over normal cells. This is achieved by both direct and indirect damage at different cellular levels of radiated tissue. Radiotherapy can injure nuclear DNA, nuclear membrane, organelles, and the cell membrane.

Nuclear DNA is the major target of radiation, and the two principal mechanisms of radiation induced damage are direct ionization damage to DNA, and indirect damage by free radicals formed in the microenvironment of the DNA by water radiolysis. The indirect damage from free radicals plays a larger role in inducing DNA damage, so it is important to recognize that oxygen is required to trigger the injury. This is one of the reasons that intra-tumor hypoxia can induce radioresistance [22].

Recent findings from the Radiation Therapy Oncology Group (RTOG) 0129 trial demonstrated that patients with oropharyngeal squamous cell carcinoma (OPSCC) that is positive for human papillomavirus (HPV) had significantly improved overall survival and progression-free survival, whereas HPV-negative OPSCCs treated with primary radiation therapy and cisplatin had significantly reduced locoregional control and overall survival [15].

These findings have opened the window for personalized medicine based on the molecular signature of the tumor. In fact, 2 RTOG trials were conceived based on this concept, and those trials were designed to evaluate the role of treatment de-intensification in HPV-positive OPSCCs (RTOG 1016) and the role of treatment intensification in HPV-negative OPSCCs (RTOG 1221). Thus, HPV positivity or expression of the p16 protein, a surrogate marker for HPV infection in OPSCC, appears to be a prognostic biomarker and is a potential predictive biomarker in HNSCC.

Radiobiology of cancer treatment

Cancer cells have different radiosensitivities during the various cell cycle phases. For instance, during the M phase, all chromosomes are condensed and located in the middle of nucleus to form a larger target. All the DNA repair mechanisms are shut down, cells can lose large fragments of DNA, and any injury will be fixed in place. This contributes to cells having the highest sensitivity to radiation during the M-phase of the cell cycle. In contrast, during the S phase, DNA repair mechanisms are activated, and chromosomes are loosely arranged in the nucleus allowing cells in the S phase to be the most resistant to radiation [23] (Fig. 1).

There are several classes of DNA damage that can occur with radiotherapy, which include base pair injury, base pair deletion, cross linkage, single strand break or double strand break. When DNA is damaged by radiation, the first response for the cell is to arrest the cell cycle, then check and repair DNA injuries [22]. The result may lead to either repair of the insult or some type of cell death. Minimal damage can be repaired and the

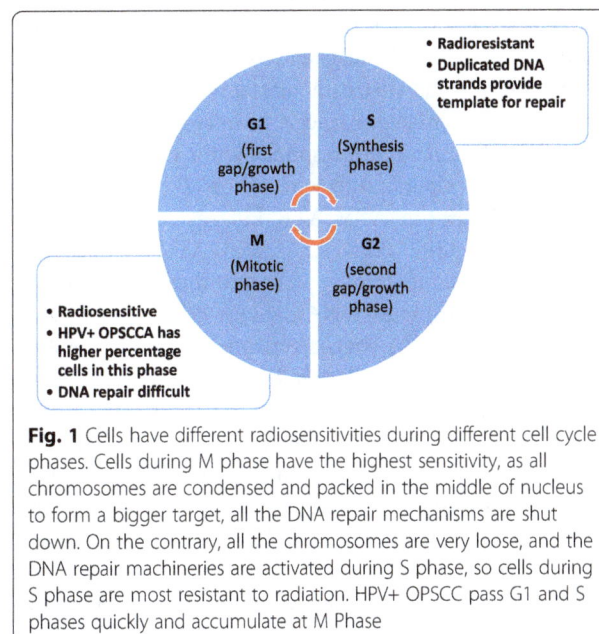

Fig. 1 Cells have different radiosensitivities during different cell cycle phases. Cells during M phase have the highest sensitivity, as all chromosomes are condensed and packed in the middle of nucleus to form a bigger target, all the DNA repair mechanisms are shut down. On the contrary, all the chromosomes are very loose, and the DNA repair machineries are activated during S phase, so cells during S phase are most resistant to radiation. HPV+ OPSCC pass G1 and S phases quickly and accumulate at M Phase

cancer cell will resume proliferation and duplication. Cancer cells have several different mechanisms to repair the damage caused by radiation, and the mechanism that is used depends on the class of induced damage. However, if the damage is severe and unable to be repaired, apoptosis or other cell death pathways will be initiated. Double strand DNA breaks most commonly lead to cell death as all other types of injury are more likely to be repaired [22].

DNA double strand breaks (DSBs) are repaired primarily by two mechanisms: non-homologous end-joining (NHEJ) and homologous recombination (HR) [24]. The mechanism of repair is dependent on the type and time of injury. NHEJ is utilized for simple and primary DSBs, and HR for clustered and secondary DSBs that occur post-radiation. The cell cycle phase at the time of injury is an important factor as well. For example, damage induced during G1 phase tend to be repaired with NHEJ, and during the S and G2 cell cycle phases are more likely to be repaired by HR. If the DNA damage is unable to be repaired, the cell pathways will induce cell apoptosis, senescence, or mitotic catastrophe. The final cell pathway depends on the functional status of cell cycle checkpoints and p53 [25].

Role of p53 and Rb protein in cell cycle regulation
Normal cells have 3 checkpoints during a cell cycle: G1, G2 and M (spindle assembly) checkpoints. These checkpoints confirm that cells are ready to continue proliferation without error. G1 checkpoint controls the passage of G1 into S phase. It mainly verifies that the size of the cell and the environment are correct and favorable to continue. The G2 &M checkpoints mainly prevent the cell from entering mitosis (M phase) if the genome is damaged, which is almost exclusively internally controlled [26].

P53 is a transcription factor known to be an important regulator in DNA damage and repair. Phosphorylation of p53 permits downstream interaction with additional transcriptional cofactors, and is ultimately important for activation of target genes responsible for cell cycle arrest, DNA repair, apoptosis and senescence [27]. P53 is a substrate for both the ATM/ATR kinases, as well as for CHK1/CHK2 [28]. Both ATM and ATR belong to a structurally unique family of serine-threonine kinases. P53 induction by acute DNA damage begins when DNA double-strand breaks trigger activation of ATM or ATR kinases [29]. Phosphorylation of p53 occurs at several sites. As a consequence, activation enhances p53 stability and activity, and regulates the transcriptional activation of a number of downstream target genes, such as p21, GADD45, 14–3-3, Bax, and Mdm2 [29]. This process acts as a major regulator in cell cycle arrest, apoptosis, senescence, DNA repair, metabolism, and even invasion and metastasis. This role has led to p53 to also be known as the molecular node in the radiation response [28].

Another important protein family in cell cycle regulation is the Rb protein family, which plays a pivotal role in negative control of the cell cycle by acting as a major G1 checkpoint controller, blocking S-phase entry and cell growth. The Rb protein family includes three members which repress gene transcription required for transition from G1 to S phase, by directly binding to the transactivation domain of transcription factor E2F. When cells are activated, Rb protein will be phosphorylated and releases E2F. In turn, E2F-dependent genes will be transcribed and accelerate cell passage from G1 checkpoint into S phase. When DNA is damaged from radiation therapy, p53 will be phosphorylated and stabilized by ATM or ATR. It will then inhibit Rb protein from releasing E2F via p21 protein. This results in arrest of cell cycle at the G1 checkpoint [30].

P53 induced apoptosis/senescence
When the damage is too severe and the repair fails, the cell processes will be switched towards cell death. P53 can induce cell apoptosis through an extrinsic or intrinsic pathway. However, radiation therapy primarily acts via the intrinsic pathway. In the intrinsic pathway, eventual accumulation of cytoplasmic P53 induces pro-apoptotic genes Bax, PUMA, and Noxa [31]. Bax will insert into the mitochondrial membrane, creating a permeable outer mitochondrial membrane. This leads to the release cytochrome c and triggers cell death through the caspase cascade. In the extrinsic apoptotic pathway, p53 will induce expression of apoptosis receptors CD95/Fas, KILLER/DR5, and the CS95/Fas Ligand. Activation of these receptors leads to downstream induction of the caspase cascade as well, ultimately leading to apoptosis and cell death [31].

Cells with greater expression of p53 are generally more prone to respond to radiation therapy and are considered to be more radiosensitive. Radiation induced apoptosis regulated by p53 is the main mechanism of cell death in cells of myeloid and lymphoid origin [27]. Radiation-induced intrinsic apoptosis occurs within a few hours following radiation exposure in the interphase before mitosis. However, if cells have already passed the interphase stage and are in M phase, other cell death mechanisms will be activated, including senescence and mitotic catastrophe [27].

Senescence is a state of permanent cell cycle arrest which can be induced by radiation, and is another mechanism to prevent cancer cell growth. When DNA damage is irreparable, a chronic DNA damage response signal is produced to create cell cycle arrest. This state of arrest prevents damaged DNA from being propagated to daughter cells. Senescence caused by radiation is induced by p53 and p21. Senescent cells do not divide but may remain metabolically active. As a result, they may still possess the ability to secrete both tumor suppressing and tumor promoting factors which could lead to an inflammatory response to the tumor, or stimulate cancer cell growth [27, 28] (Fig. 2).

Mitotic catastrophe

Mitotic catastrophe is an event in which cell death happens during mitosis or as a consequence of aberrant mitosis. There are two predominant proposed mechanisms for the induction of mitotic catastrophe. The first mechanism is from a combination of radiation induced DNA damage and dysfunction cell cycle checkpoints. Checkpoint inactivation generally occurs when tumor cells have mutated or inactivated p53. This would allow a cell with damaged DNA to progress passed the G2/M checkpoint. Since p53 is also important in DNA repair, mitotic catastrophe will be the more likely fate of tumor cells in this phase [32]. The second proposed mechanism is by hyperamplification of centrosomes. This will lead abnormal chromosome segregation and create cells with multiple nuclei, and or several micronuclei. Centrosome hyperamplification is also more prevalent in cells without functional p53, and results in mitotic catastrophe. These cells can survive for several days after initial radiation, but undergo cell death either by delayed necrosis, delayed apoptosis, or induced senescence. Mitotic catastrophe is considered to be the major cell death mechanism by which solid tumors respond to clinical radiotherapy [33].

HPV in OPSCC radiotherapy

Human papillomavirus (HPV) is a small, non-enveloped DNA with a circular, double-stranded viral genome. Nearly all our knowledge of the mechanisms by which HPV causes cellular proliferation and neoplasia are from research of HPV in cervical cancer. This research can be extrapolated to HPV associated OPSCC, as the most common high-risk HPV genotypes in head in neck cancers is also HPV genotypes 16 and 18 [34]. Besides the obvious difference in anatomic location, there may be some difference in the natural history of HPV infection in cervical cells when compared to oropharyngeal cells, and in the manifestation of HPV associated neoplasia in the two tissues. From studies in women with cervical HPV infection, only 5–10 per 100,000 progresses to malignant cervical disease. On the other hand, preventative screening for oropharyngeal infection is not currently the standard of practice and therefore studies to compare cervical infection rates to head and neck infection rates are not available. However, the fundamental molecular mechanisms by which HPV encoded proteins circumvent cell-cycle control are likely to be the same, irrespective of tissue localization [35]. It is also important to understand that p16 overexpression is used as a surrogate marker to identify actively infected HPV cells, and has been incorporated into the new 8th edition AJCC staging guidelines [34, 13]. Immunohistochemistry assays are cost effective and widely available in most laboratories and therefore serves as an excellent surrogate marker [34]. However, more accurate testing for specific high risk genotypes should be considered to further classify responsiveness to therapy in future studies.

The infection and proliferation of HPV is unique. New HPV virions are only produced once the initially infected cell has undergone mitosis and one of the daughter cells has differentiated. HPV does not encode proteins directly responsible for replication of its own DNA. Instead, it uses the host cell replication machinery. HPV encoded proteins disrupt multiple cellular signaling pathways to

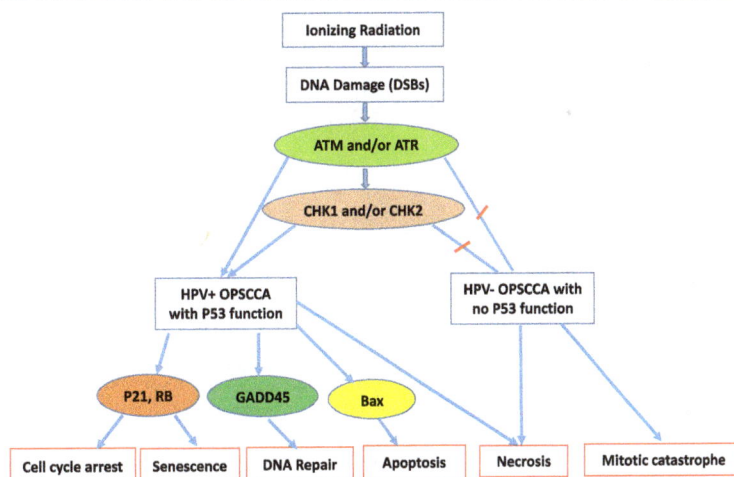

Fig. 2 P53 is the most important regulator in DNA damage. P53 is a substrate for both the ATM and ATR kinases, as well as for CHK1 and CHK2. Phosphorylation of p53 allows its interaction with transcriptional cofactors, transcribes and activates its target genes for extensive cell responses, such as cell cycle arrest, DNA repair, apoptosis and senescence. When DNA damage is difficult to be repaired, it will induce cell apoptosis, senescence, or mitotic catastrophe. The final death pathway depends on the function of checkpoints and the status of p53

maintain infected cells in a proliferative state that facilitates viral persistence and replication [34]. The primary viral proteins responsible for disruption of the host cell-cycle, and most significant in oncogenesis, are the E6 and E7 oncoproteins.

E6/E7 Oncoproteins

Expression of both viral E6 and E7 oncogenes is consistently maintained in infected cells to inhibit the functions of p53 and Rb tumor suppressor pathways. E6 oncogene expression will lead to ubiquitination and subsequent degradation of p53 protein. This allows for dysregulation of both G1/S and G2/M cell cycle checkpoints leading to genomic instability. E6 oncoprotein also has the ability to activate cellular telomerase through transcriptional upregulation of the catalytic subunit of human telomerase. This allows the infected cell to maintain telomere length, which is an important step in cellular immortalization and transformation [36].

HPV E7 oncoproteins have a complementary effect to E6 oncoproteins by binding and inactivating the Rb protein family. This results in overactivation of E2F transcription factor with upregulation of cell cycle genes, and transition of cell from G1 to S phase and an increase in DNA synthesis and cell proliferation. Inactivation of Rb proteins also results in increased levels of p16, an inhibitor of cdk4/cyclin D, by a feedback control mechanism. Therefore, high levels of p16 expression serves as a specific diagnostic biomarker for tumor infected with HPV [36] (Fig. 3).

Pathologic and genetic profile differences

There are also some differences in pathological characteristics when comparing HPV-positive tumors to HPV-negative tumors. It has been shown that HPV-positive OPSCC normally shows no surface dysplasia or keratinization, has lobular growth with infiltrating lymphocytes, and often demonstrates baseloid variation. On the other hand, HPV negative OPSCC, histologically shows keratinizing tumor cells with abundant pink cytoplasm composed in discrete nests [35] (Fig. 4).

Gene profiling of HPV positive and HPV negative oropharyngeal cancer has shown that HPV-positive cancers have a significantly different genetic expression profile. Differences were particularly common among genes involved in DNA regulation and repair (CDKN2A, LIG1, MCM6, E2F, CDT1, PARP2, SMC4, CDC7, etc.), cell cycle (MLLT6, PTTG1, CUL4A, LIG1, SASS6, etc.), and chemotherapy/radiotherapy-sensitivity (CCND1, TYMS, STMN1, RBBP4) [37].

Epigenetic modifications mainly effect tumorigenesis by DNA methylation, histone modification and miRNA expression. These mechanisms and their role in OPSCC is thoroughly summarized in a recent review by Lindsay et al. [38]. Briefly, HPV- positive OPSCC has been shown to have increased areas of DNA methylation when compared to HPV-negative tumors which are associated with genome wide hypomethylation. One proposed mechanism of this difference is from DNA methyltransferase (DNMT) dysregulation as there is increased expression of the protein in HPV positive tumors, likely from the viral oncoproteins E6 and E7 discussed above. The authors also discuss the histone methyltransferase EZH2 as a possible HPV-positive tumor marker that may have a role in regulating cell proliferation. EZH2 is another downstream product of the E7 oncoprotein and is therefore closely associated with HPV positive malignancies. There is still

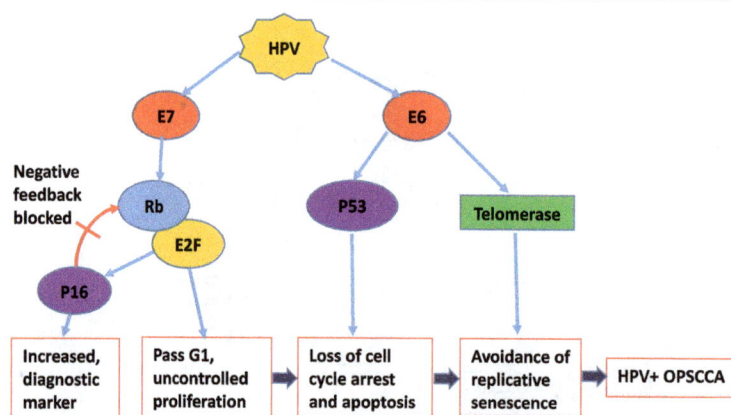

Fig. 3 E6 and E7 are the main oncoproteins. They are encoded by HPV and disrupt or usurp multiple cellular signaling pathways to maintain infected cells in a proliferative state that facilitates viral persistence and replication. HPV E7 oncoprotein inactivates the Rb protein family, resulting in over-activation of E2F transcription factor with increased transition of cell from G1 to S phase and cell proliferation. Inactivation of Rb proteins also results in increased levels of p16, a marker for HPV infection diagnosis. E6 degrades p53 protein, deregulating cycle checkpoints, and activates telomerase through the transcriptional upregulation of an important subunit of human telomerase, maintaining the telomere length. E7 and E6 have complementary effects

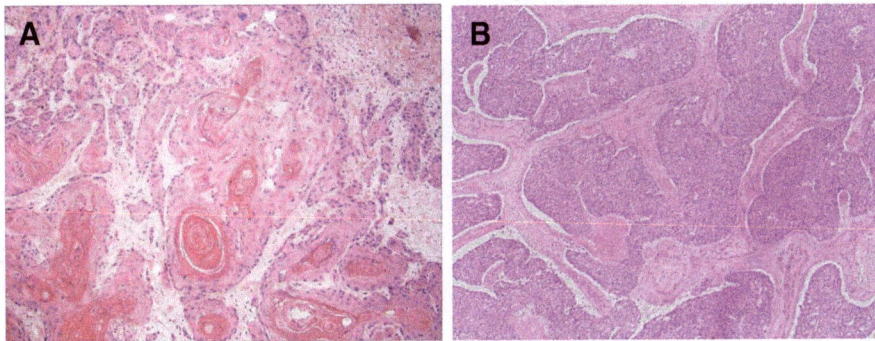

Fig. 4 Histological characteristics of HPV-positive and HPV-negative OPSCC. HPV-positive OPSCC normally shows no surface dysplasia or keratinization, it has lobular growth with infiltrating lymphocytes, and often demonstrates baseloid variation. Photo (**a**) is HPV– OPSCC, keratinizing tumor cells with abundant pink cytoplasm in discrete nests. Photo (**b**) shows HPV+ OPSCC, nonkeratinizing hyperchromatic tumor cells with ill-defined borders, abundant mitoses and areas of necrosis

further research required on the topic of micro and non-coding RNA and its epigenetic effects on OPSCC [38]. There are a few chemotherapy agents under study that target these epigenetic differences, however there are no trials summarized for OPSCC specifically and they show poor activity against solid tumors. Although there may be epigenetic difference between HPV- positive and HPV- negative OPSCC, further research is required to determine outcomes of targeted radiation therapy and if the differing response can be partially attributed to the epigenetic profiles.

HPV-positive OPSCC response to radiation

HPV-positive cancer cells have different gene profiles. Studies show that there are no significant differences in the average number of mutated genes, however, the gene expression levels are significantly different (347 differentially expressed genes) in HPV-positive vs HPV-negative cancers [39]. Differences were particularly common among genes involved in DNA regulation and repair, cell cycle regulation, and chemotherapy/radiotherapy-sensitivity. These differences allow for increased sensitivity to radiation in HPV-positive cells [39]. This leads us to the main mechanisms that lead to an improved response to radiation therapy: Altered DNA repair, reduced hypoxic regions, and increased cellular immune response.

In HPV-positive oropharyngeal cancer cells, p53 is still wild type and has normal functions. Although the concentration is low due to degeneration induced by E6 oncoprotein, it remains detectable and can be induced with radiation. When radiation breaks down double stranded DNA, p53 will be activated as discussed above. In HPV-negative OPSCC, p53 is mutated and cell cycle arrest will not occur. However, in HPV-positive tumors, there remains a basal level of functioning p53. This will activate cell cycle arrest and induce quick cell apoptosis if the DSBs are severe [40]. Increased p53 levels should

also allow for a better response to radiation therapy in HPV-positive cells [41]. However, in one study which looked at radiation effects on 5 cell lines of HPV positive tumors, there was minimal evidence of apoptosis at the dosage of radiation studied, and instead found a substantial number of cells arrested in G2 phase associated with DNA DSB [42]. The authors concluded that the increased sensitivity was therefore more likely to be from the inability to repair DSB caused by the radiation. Future studies will need to address these differing opinions when a greater number of cell lines are available to study.

As previously discussed, P16 is over-expressed in HPV-positive OPSCC, which will impair DNA repair system by precluding Rad51 from access to the DNA damage site [43]. This causes a shift in the repair mechanism from homologous to non-homologous, and will lead to more errors. Misrepair of damaged DNA may lead to increased cell apoptosis if functioning p53 is available.

Another reason for the increased sensitivity to radiation is the consistently activated E2F from HPV E7 oncoprotein degradation of Rb protein family. This will promote cell cycle advancement from G1 to S phase, and as a result, all HPV-positive cells will accumulate at G2/M phases. In this phase, cells are more sensitive to radiation as the chromosomes are more densely packed, and DNA repair function is weak [41, 42].

Oxygen is important for radiotherapy and the formation of free radicals. Most solid tumors have hypoxic centers, and cancer cells are resistant to radiation because oxygen is not available to from free radicals in the microenvironment of the DNA to cause damage. Also, oxygen is important in fixating injury induced by radiation. Under hypoxic conditions, DNA damage is reduced (mainly by –SH-containing compounds), which leads to cell survival. Hypoxia-inducible factor 1α (HIF1α) is stabilized under hypoxic conditions, which leads to the upregulation of genes involved in cell survival [44]. HPV-positive OPSCCs are less hypoxic than negative ones, and the lack of hypoxia inside HPV-positive tumors could contribute to the improved radiosensitivity [40, 45]. This theory is supported by a retrospective analysis of the DAHANCA 5 trials performed by Lassen et al., which concludes that hypoxic radioresistance may not be relevant in HPV associated tumors since there is no benefit from hypoxic radiosensitization [45].

HPV-positive tumors have stronger T cells tumor infiltration and the higher radiosensitivity of HPV-positive OPSCC might be partially due to a more effective immune response following radiation. Tumor cell injury and inflammation induced by radiation lead to the release of tumor antigens and HPV viral antigens, which can trigger a stronger immune response [33, 44, 46, 47]. These findings have been confirmed in studies of immune-incompetent mice with HPV positive tumors that show improved outcomes with transplant of wild type immune cells and improved outcomes in mice given an E6/E7 oncogene vaccination prior to treatment [48].

Conclusions

Over the past few decades, the number of oropharyngeal cancers linked to HPV has risen dramatically. HPV DNA is now found in about 2 out of 3 oropharyngeal cancers and in a much smaller fraction of oral cavity cancers. HPV-positive OPSCC tends to respond favorably to radiotherapy when compared to HPV-negative OPSCC. DNA damage in HPV-related and HPV-unrelated HNSCC cell lines occurs by different mechanisms. Low level wild type p53 is the key molecule for the enhanced radiosensitivity of HPV-positive OPSCC. The enhanced responsiveness of HPV-positive OPSCC to radiotherapy may also be due to a higher cellular radiosensitivity secondary to cell cycle dysregulation and impaired DNA DSB repair, and other factors including immune response and fewer hypoxic regions. However, all pathways are still not completely understood and require further research.

Abbreviations
DSB: Double strand breaks; HNCs: Head and neck cancers; HNSCC: Head and neck squamous cell carcinomas; HPV: Human papilloma virus; OPSCC: Oropharyngeal squamous cell carcinoma

Authors' contributions
CL composed the manuscript, DM contributed to drafting and revising the manuscript, US and NK provided critical revisions to the manuscript. All authors read and approved the final manuscript.

Competing interests
The authors declare that they have no competing interests.

Author details
[1]USC Tina and Rick Caruso Department of Otolaryngology-Head and Neck Surgery, Keck Medicine of USC, University of Southern California, Los Angeles, CA 90033, USA. [2]Keck School of Medicine, University of Southern California, Los Angeles, CA 90033, USA.

References
1. Duray A, Descamps G, Decaestecker C, et al. Human papillomavirus DNA strongly correlates with a poorer prognosis in oral cavity carcinoma. Laryngoscope. 2012;122(7):1558–65.
2. Ferlay J, Parkin DM, Steliarova-Foucher E. Estimates of cancer incidence and mortality in Europe in 2008. Eur J Cancer. 2010;46(4):765–81.
3. Siegel R, Naishadham D, Jemal A. Cancer statistics, 2012. CA Cancer J Clin. 2012;62:10–29.
4. Osei-Sarfo K, Tang XH, Urvalek AM, Scognamiglio T, Gudas LJ. The molecular features of tongue epithelium treated with the carcinogen 4-nitroquinoline-1-oxide and alcohol as a model for HNSCC. Carcinogenesis. 2013;34(11):2673–81.
5. Syrjänen K, Väyrynen M, Castrén O. Morphological and immunohistochemical evidence of human papilloma virus involvement in the dysplastic lesions of the uterine cervix. Int J Gynecol Obstet. 1983;21(4):261–9.
6. IARC working group on the evaluation of carcinogenic risks to humans. Biological agents. Volume 100 B. A review of human carcinogens. IARC Monogr Eval Carcinog Risks Hum. 2012;100(Pt B):1–441.
7. Hong AM, Grulich AE, Jones D, et al. Squamous cell carcinoma of the oropharynx in Australian males induced by human papillomavirus vaccine targets. Vaccine. 2010;28(19):3269–72.
8. Näsman A, Attner P, Hammarstedt L, et al. Incidence of human papillomavirus (HPV) positive tonsillar carcinoma in Stockholm, Sweden: an epidemic of viral-induced carcinoma? Int J Cancer. 2009;125(2):362–6.
9. Syrjänen S. HPV infections and tonsillar carcinoma. J Clin Pathol. 2004; 57(5):449–55.
10. Article O. HPV and other risk factors of oral cavity / oropharyngeal cancer in the Czech Republic. Control. 2005:181–5.
11. Chaturvedi AK, Engels EA, Pfeiffer RM, et al. Human papillomavirus and rising oropharyngeal cancer incidence in the United States. J Clin Oncol. 2011;29(32):4294–301.
12. Lajer CB, Von Buchwald C. The role of human papillomavirus in head and neck cancer. APMIS. 2010;118(6–7):510–9.
13. Lydiatt WM, Patel SG, O'Sullivan B, et al. Head and neck cancers—major changes in the American joint committee on cancer eighth edition cancer staging manual. CA Cancer J Clin. 2017;67(2):122–37.
14. Arenz A, Ziemann F, Mayer C, et al. Increased radiosensitivity of HPV-positive head and neck cancer cell lines due to cell cycle dysregulation and induction of apoptosis. Strahlenther Onkol. 2014;190(9):839–46.
15. Ang KKP, Harris J, Wheeler R, et al. Human papillomavirus and survival of patients with oropharyngeal cancer. N Engl J Med. 2011;363(1):24–35.
16. Fakhry C, Psyrri A, Chaturvedhi A. HPV and head and neck cancers: state-of-the-science. Oral Oncol. 2014;50(5):353–5.
17. Gillison ML, D'Souza G, Westra W, et al. Distinct risk factor profiles for human papillomavirus type 16-positive and human papillomavirus type 16-negative head and neck cancers. J Natl Cancer Inst. 2008;100(6):407–20.
18. Kumar B, Cordell K, Lee J. Response to therapy and outcomes in oropharyngeal cancer are associated with biomarkers including human papillomavirus, epidermal growth factor receptor, gender and smoking. Int J Radiat Oncol Biol Phys. 2007;69(2 Suppl):S109–11.
19. Weinberger PM, Yu Z, Haffty BG, et al. Molecular classification identifies a subset of human papillomavirus- associated oropharyngeal cancers with favorable prognosis. J Clin Oncol. 2006;24(5):736–47.
20. Posner MR, Lorch JH, Goloubeva O, et al. Survival and human papillomavirus in oropharynx cancer in TAX 324: a subset analysis from an international phase III trial. Ann Oncol. 2011;22(5):1071–7.
21. Wang X, Hu C, Eisbruch A. Organ-sparing radiation therapy for head and neck cancer. J Surg Oncol. 2008;97(8):697–700.
22. Minafra L, Bravatà V. Cell and molecular response to IORT treatment. Transl Cancer Res. 2014;3(1):32–47.
23. Mishra K, Dayal R, Singh A, Pandey A. Reactive oxygen species as mediator of tumor radiosensitivity. J Cancer Res Ther. 2014;10(4):811.
24. Kim BM, Hong Y, Lee S, et al. Therapeutic implications for overcoming radiation resistance in cancer therapy. Int J Mol Sci. 2015; 16(11):26880–913.

The molecular mechanisms of increased radiosensitivity of HPV-positive oropharyngeal squamous cell...

125

25. Lauber K, Ernst A, Orth M, Herrmann M, Belka C. Dying cell clearance and its impact on the outcome of tumor radiotherapy. Front Oncol. 2012;2:116.

26. Hein AL, Ouellete MM, Yan Y. Radiation-induced signaling pathways that promote cancer cell survival (review). Int J Oncol. 2014;45(5):1813–9.

27. Eriksson D, Stigbrand T. Radiation-induced cell death mechanisms. Tumor Biol. 2010;31(4):363–72.

28. Bieging KT, Mello SS, Attardi LD. Unravelling mechanisms of p53-mediated tumour suppression. Nat Rev Cancer. 2014;14(5):359–70.

29. Abraham RT. Cell cycle checkpoint signaling therough the ATM an ATR kinases. Genes Dev. 2001;15:2177–96.

30. Fouse Shaun D, Nagarajan RPCJ. Genome-scale DNA methylation analysis. Biochemistry. 2010;9(6):400–14.

31. Haupt S, Berger M, Goldberg Z, Haupt Y. Apoptosis - the p53 network. J Cell Sci. 2003;116(Pt 20):4077–85.

32. Caruso RA, Branca G, Fedele F, et al. Mechanisms of coagulative necrosis in malignant epithelial tumors. Oncol Lett. 2014;8(4):1397–402.

33. Golden EB, Pellicciotta I, Demaria S, Barcellos-Hoff MH, Formenti SC. The convergence of radiation and immunogenic cell death signaling pathways. Front Oncol. 2012;2(August):88.

34. Mirghani H, Amen F, Moreau F, et al. Human papilloma virus testing in oropharyngeal squamous cell carcinoma: what the clinician should know. Oral Oncol. 2014;50(1):1–9.

35. Daniel LM, Michael DP. And M. Sharon S. Virology and molecular pathogenesis of human papillomavirus (HPV)-associated oropharyngeal squamous cell carcinoma. Biochem J. 2012;443(2):339–53.

36. Bol V, Gregoire V. Biological basis for increased sensitivity to radiation therapy in HPV-positive head and neck cancers. Biomed Res Int. 2014;

37. Lohavanichbutr P, Houck J. Genomewide gene expression profiles of HPV-positive and HPV-negative oropharyngeal cancer: potential implications for treatment choices. Arch Otolaryngol Head Neck Surg. 2009;135(2):180–8.

38. Lindsay C, Seikaly H, Biron VL. Epigenetics of oropharyngeal squamous cell carcinoma: opportunities for novel chemotherapeutic targets. J Otolaryngol Head Neck Surg. 2017;46(1):9.

39. Zhang P, Mirani N, Baisre A, Fernandes H. Molecular heterogeneity of head and neck squamous cell carcinoma defined by next-generation sequencing. Am J Pathol. 2014;184(5):1323–30.

40. Kimple RJ, Smith MA, Blitzer GC, et al. Enhanced radiation sensitivity in HPV-positive head and neck cancer. Cancer Res. 2013;73(15):4791–800.

41. Ziemann F, Arenz A, Preising S, et al. Increased sensitivity of HPV-positive head and neck cancer cell lines to x-irradiation ± cisplatin due to decreased expression of E6 and E7 oncoproteins and enhanced apoptosis. Am J Cancer Res. 2015;5(3):1017–31.

42. Rieckmann T, Tribius S, Grob TJ, et al. HNSCC cell lines positive for HPV and p16 possess higher cellular radiosensitivity due to an impaired DSB repair capacity. Radiother Oncol. 2018;107(2):242–6.

43. Dok R, Kalev P, Van Limbergen EJ, et al. P16INK4a impairs homologous recombination-mediated DNA repair in human papillomavirus-positive head and neck tumors. Cancer Res. 2014;74(6):1739–51.

44. Barker HE, Paget JTE, Khan A, Harrington KJ. The tumour microenvironment after radiotherapy: mechanisms of resistance and recurrence. Nat Rev Cancer. 2015;15(7):409–25.

45. Lassen P, Eriksen JG, Hamilton-Dutoit S, et al. HPV-associated p16-expression and response to hypoxic modification of radiotherapy in head and neck cancer. Radiother Oncol. 2018;94(1):30–5.

46. Cid-Arregui A. Therapeutic vaccines against human papillomavirus and cervical cancer. Open Virol J. 2009;3:67–83.

47. Mirghani H, Amen F, Tao Y, Deutsch E, Levy A. Increased radiosensitivity of HPV-positive head and neck cancers: molecular basis and therapeutic perspectives. Cancer Treat Rev. 2015;41:844–52.

48. Spanos WC, Nowicki P, Lee DW, et al. Immune response during therapy with cisplatin or radiation for human papillomavirus–related head and neck cancer. Arch Otolaryngol Head Neck Surg. 2009;135(11):1137–46.

19

Correlation between gonial angle and dynamic tongue collapse in children with snoring/sleep disordered breathing – an exploratory pilot study

S. Anderson[3,4,5], N. Alsufyani[1,2,3], A. Isaac[3,4,5], M. Gazzaz[3,4,5] and H. El-Hakim[3,4,5*] (iD)

Abstract

Background: Drug induced sleep endoscopy (DISE) is hoped to identify reasons of failure of adenotonsillectomy (AT) in treating pediatric sleep disordered breathing (SDB). Maxillomandibular disproportion has been studied as another association which may explain alternative pathogenesis of SDB. We aimed to explore the relation between the size of the gonial angle and inclination of the epiglottis measured from cone beam CT (CBCT) and tongue base collapse based on DISE in children with SDB.

Method: A retrospective chart review was conducted at a tertiary pediatric center. Children (6-17 years old) assessed at a multi-disciplinary Upper Airway Clinic, diagnosed with SDB and maxillo-mandibular disproportion (MMD), and who underwent DISE were eligible. Variables obtained from the electronic medical records of the clinic and prospective database included demographics, comorbidities, surgeries performed, investigations, DISE findings and CBCT findings. The gonial angle of subjects with and without tongue base collapse (TBC) on SNP were compared.

Results: In total 29 patients (13 male, 8 female) age 6-17 (median= 9) were eligible for the study from January 2009 – July 2016. We included 11 subjects, and 10 comparators. The mean gonial angle of the TBC group was 139.3°± 7.6°, while that of the comparison group was 129.4°±3.5 (mean difference -9.937, 95% CI of -15.454 to - 4.421, P = 0.001, power of test 0.95). Additionally, the mean inclination of the epiglottis had a mild positive correlation (r=0.32, $p<0.05$) with the gonial angle, in the whole cohort.

Conclusions: This pilot study suggests that TBC may be mediated by a wider gonial angle in children with SDB patients. The posterior tilt of the epiglottis on CBCT may be a surrogate sign of TBC.

Keywords: Pediatric sleep disordered breathing, Maxillo-mandibular disproportion, Gonial angle, Adeno-tonsillectomy, Drug induced sleep endoscopy, Pharyngeal collapse

Background
The American Academy of Otolaryngology – Head and Neck Surgery defines Pediatric sleep disordered breathing (SDB) as difficulty in breathing during sleep, which can range from habitual snoring to obstructive sleep

* Correspondence: hamdy.elhakim@albertahealthservices.ca
Presented on the podium at the Annual meeting of the Canadian Society of Otolaryngology Head & Neck Surgery, Saskatoon, Sask, June 2017.
[3]University of Alberta, Edmonton, AB, Canada
[4]Division of Pediatric Surgery, Department of Surgery, Stollery Children's Hospital, Edmonton, AB, Canada
Full list of author information is available at the end of the article

apnea [1]. Current evidence suggests a strong association with multiple negative outcomes which include cardiovascular, metabolic, behavioral and learning consequences, as well as increased rate of nocturnal enuresis [1–6]. The risk factors for SDB include male sex, obesity, African American ethnicity, asthma, and allergies [7]. Given the high prevalence of 4–11% [8, 9], and the negative associations, scrutiny of the pathogenesis of risk factors and effectiveness of treatment offered is of great importance. Current guidelines consider adenotonsillectomy (AT) as the first line surgical solution for pediatric SDB [10]. However, as much as 20 to 40% of patients treated for SDB with AT fail to improve, resulting in a noteworthy volume who need further treatment [11, 12].

Although prevalence estimates and the negative outcomes of pediatric SDB are well described within the literature, there is a paucity of data regarding predictive factors for failure of AT [13]. Previously identified independent risk factors of failure include age, obesity, chronic rhinitis, deviated nasal septum and tonsil size. We expect other patient related variables which are yet to be accounted for, or researched, to play a role. In the late 1800's Tomes was one of the first to described an association with upper airway obstruction and morphological facial changes due to adenoid hypertrophy which he termed "adenoid facies" [14]. Since then research has supported this finding with changes in the nasal passage and gonial angle as a result of upper airway obstruction [15, 16]. The gonial angle is that formed by the mandibular plane and ramus, Fig. 1. A large gonial angle would indicate backwards (clockwise) rotation of the mandible causing the tongue/tongue base to be situated inferiorly-posteriorly and potentially cause pharyngeal airway obstruction. Furthermore, it can cause the development of anterior open bite thus promoting or enabling mouth breathing. Whereas retrognathia indicates a small jaw regardless of its angle relative to the horizontal plane. They are separate entities, possibly can occur together or independently.

On the other hand, there are two patterns of pharyngeal compromise that may occur in SDB, namely pharyngeal obstruction or collapse, and can be identified on drug induced sleep endoscopy (DISE) or imaging [17, 18]. The pharynx may exhibit collapse upon inspiration in concentrically, lateral wall to lateral wall, or at the tongue base level [17]. The significance and associations related to each type of collapse has neither been studied nor determined to date. But the proponents of DISE argue that its findings may provide an insight into the mechanisms of airway dysfunction for which there may be solutions other than traditional procedures. Therefore, we sought to conduct an exploratory study to find a phenotypic marker (gonial angle) associated with SDB in which base of tongue collapse is found upon DISE.

Methods

Study design

A retrospective chart review was conducted at the Stollery Children's Hospital, Edmonton, Alberta, Canada in order to explore the relationship between the gonial angle and pharyngeal collapse at the base of tongue in children with SDB. This study received IRB ethics approval (Pro00067134). Eligible children were those assessed at the multidisciplinary Upper Airway Clinic for a combination of persistent symptoms of SDB and maxillo-mandibular disproportion (MMD) from January 2009 till July 2016. Disciplines involved in this clinic are Pediatric Orthodontics, Pulmonary medicine, and Otolaryngology- Head and Neck Surgery.

The inclusion criteria comprised ages 6–17 years old, Pediatric Sleep Questionnaire (PSQ) score over 33 [19], features of MMD requiring radiologic assessment by cone beam computerized tomography (CBCT), and having undergone DISE (and being eligible for operative treatment). All patients were scanned with the same CBCT machine in the seated-natural head position, asked to rest their tongues at the anterior teeth, and the total scan time was 4.8 s. The study group were those who exhibited tongue base collapse (TBC) on DISE, whereas the comparison group did not. We excluded children who had a history of maxillo-facial trauma or surgery, congenital craniofacial abnormalities or syndromes, and those who had incomplete data (including those with an incomplete view of the epiglottis or mandible on CBCT).

Variables were collected from electronic medical records, the electronic repository of CBCT, surgical database of the otolaryngologist and video documentation of the performed DISE. These included demographics, diagnoses, procedures performed, McGill score for overnight sleep oximetry [20], gonial angle measurement, inclination of the epiglottis on CBCT, type of pharyngeal collapse on DISE, and surgery performed.

DISE was conducted using a uniform technique and reported in a structured format that was previously

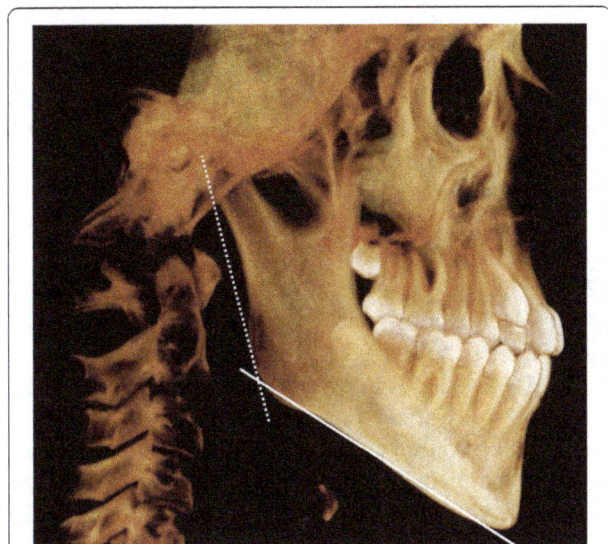

Fig. 1 Lateral 3D image reconstructed from CBCT showing the gonial angle; formed by the mandibular plane (solid line) and ramus plane (dotted line)

validated. The patients were kept spontaneously breathing throughout the assessment in the operating room, using Remifentanyl 2–2.5 mcg/ml and infusion rates of Propofol varying from 200 to 350 mcg/kg/min titrated for response to stimulation [18]. DISE was always conducted under the same anesthetic where the surgery planned will take place.

Measures

A certified maxillo-facial radiologist conducted two one-on-one training sessions for a senior medical student on preforming the CBCT measurements. The medical student measured the angle of the mandible (gonial angle) and inclination of the epiglottis. Prior to performing the actual measurements, an intra and inter-rater assessment on a sample ($n = 10$) of patients, not included in this pilot, demonstrated 0.95 agreement (Cohen's kappa) between the student and the expert.

Prior to any measurement, the CBCT volume was adjusted such that the Frankfort plane (eye-ear plane) and interorbital line were parallel to the horizontal plane, and any right-left rotations were corrected. The gonial angle, as conventionally described, was that between the intersection of the ramus and the mandibular lines (Fig. 1) [21]. The inclination of the epiglottis was measured as the angle at the intersection between the horizontal plane and a line drawn through long axis of the epiglottis (Fig. 2). The latter was chosen based on an observation by the multidisciplinary group of a possible association between large gonial angle and posterior tilt of the epiglottis, which may affect airflow into the laryngeal inlet.

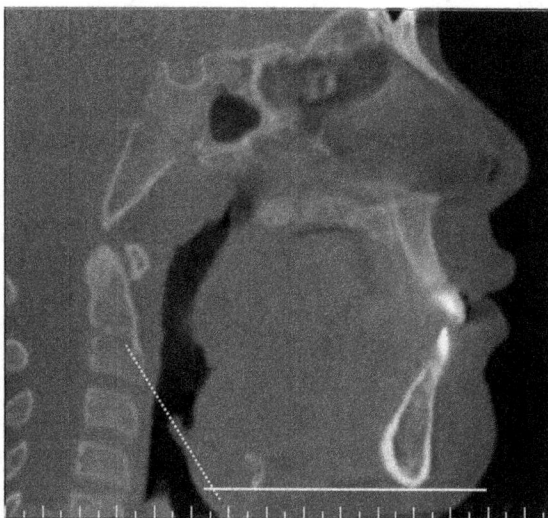

Fig. 2 Sagittal CBCT image showing the inclination of epiglottis; the angle formed by the long axis of epiglottis (dotted line) relative to the horizontal plane (solid line)

The assessor of the gonial angle and the epiglottic inclination was unaware of the type of collapse in the pharynx. The subjects were recruited from a database which was intended for use in another project.

Outcome measures

The primary outcome measure was the difference between means of gonial angles of study and comparison groups. The secondary outcome measure was the correlation between epiglottic inclination and gonial angle.

Statistical analysis

Basic descriptive statistics were conducted to obtain the mean and standard deviation of the angle of mandible and the inclination of the epiglottis. An independent sample T-test was used to assess the statistical variance between the study and comparison gonial angles. Pearson r correlation analysis and r^2 statistics were conducted between the angle of mandible and inclination of the epiglottis. All analyses were conducted and completed using SPSS 23.

Results

In total 29 eligible patients, 18 male and 11 female ages 6–12 (median = 9) were identified (Fig. 1). Eighteen of whom met the inclusion criteria as study group, and 11 as the comparator group (Table 1) and Fig. 3. Seven patients out of the study group and one out of the comparator group were excluded, Fig. 2. As a result, we included 11 (seven males) valid subjects and 10 (six were males) valid comparators. In the comparison group, four patients exhibited lateral and six circumferential pharyngeal collapse upon SNP.

The median age for the study group was 9 years (range = 6–12) and 7 (range 6–13). for the comparison group. Comorbidities and types of surgeries are summarized in Table 1. AT was the most common surgery performed followed by adenoidectomy. There was no difference between the parameters of the sleep oximetry between the two groups (Table 2).

The mean gonial angle of the study group were 139.3° ± 7.6° (95% CI 134.8–143.8), as opposed to 129.4° ± 3.5° (95% CI 127.2–131.6) in the comparison group which were significantly different ($p < 0.01$). The mean difference is − 9.937 (95% CI of − 15.454 to − 4.421, $P = 0.001$). The effect size is 1.675 and is large. Since the study group values were not normally distributed, Mann Whitney test was also run and the difference between the medians was still significant. However, the mean difference between the epiglottic inclination in the study (123.0° ± 4.6°) and the comparison groups (121.45° ± 6.94°) was 1.932 (95% CI -3.389 to 7.252, $P = 0.457$), which was not significant, but the test was short of the recommended power of 0.8 (0.05).

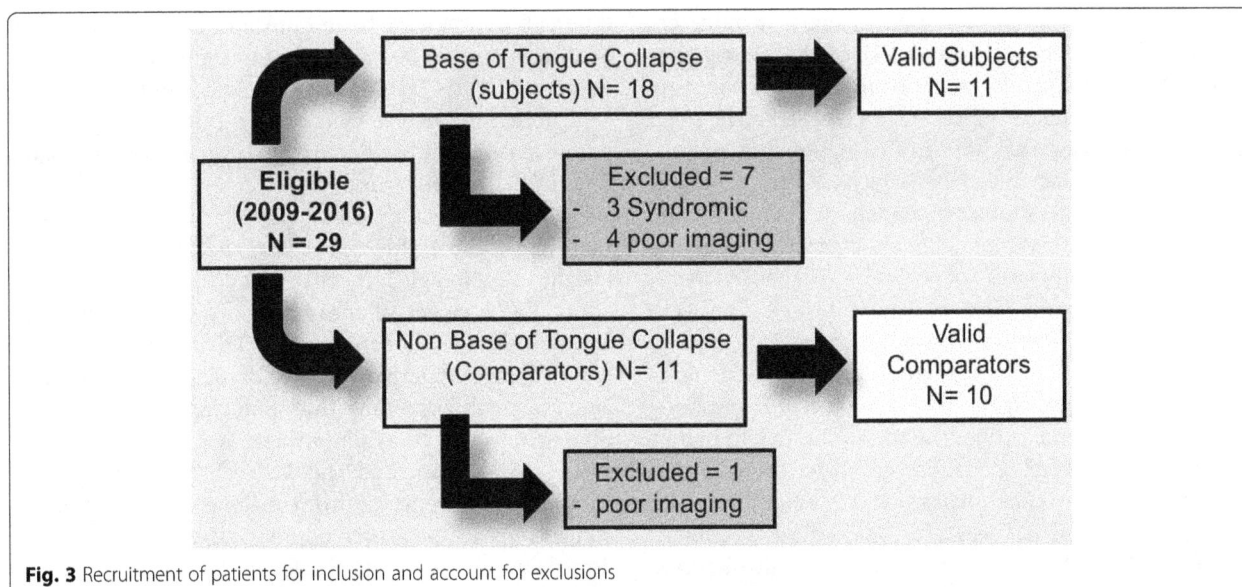

Fig. 3 Recruitment of patients for inclusion and account for exclusions

Analysis of our secondary outcome showed that within the whole cohort, inclination of the epiglottis had a mild positive correlation ($r = 0.32$, $p < 0.05$) between gonial angle and inclination of the epiglottis.

Discussion

Current recommended first line surgical treatment for SDB is AT [10]. However, given the significant proportion of patients who fail to receive benefit from such treatment, evidence providing insight into predictors of the pathophysiology of patients SDB could reduce unnecessary and ineffective surgical procedures. Gonial angle, was chosen based on the clinical observation of the interdisciplinary airway team during the six years' experience in the clinical and radiographic assessment of children with MMD and Snoring/Sleep Disordered Breathing.

Our exploratory study demonstrated that the children with SDB and MMD who exhibited TBC has a larger mean gonial angle (139.3° ± =7.6°), than their counterparts who exhibit different types of collapse (129.4° ± 3.5°), and more than the reported mean values of gonial angle for this age group in the literature (133.96° ± =7.6°) [21]. A mild positive correlation ($r = 0.32$, $p < 0.05$) was also found between the size of the gonial angle and the inclination or posterior tilt of the epiglottis. This suggests that downward growth of the mandible might be associated with that particular type of pharyngeal tongue collapse.

This is the first study to investigate how dynamic endoscopic findings during chemically induced sleep can relate to static 3D imaging (CBCT) in children with SDB. There is a surging interest into the role of imaging in assessing SDB in children and specifically in orthodontic and maxillofacial literature [18]. In the adult literature, a systematic review was conducted to assess the most important anatomical characteristics of the upper airway related to the pathogenesis of obstructive sleep

Table 1 Comparison between means of gonial angle of the study and comparison group. 95CI: 95% confidence interval

Parameter	Subjects (n of 11)	Comparison (n of 10)
Male: female	7:4	6:4
Age in years (median & range)	9 (6–12)	7 (5–12)
Comorbidities		
Chronic rhinitis	4	5
Obesity	0	1
Asthma	1	2
Surgeries performed		
Adenotonsillectomy	6	5
Tonsillectomy	1	2
Adenoidectomy	4	3

Table 2 Sleep oximetry parameters

Parameter	Subjects	Comparison
McGill Oximetry Score		
1	3 (27%)	0 (0%)
2	5 (46%)	7 (70%)
3	3 (27%)	3 (30%)
4	0 (0%)	0 (0%)
Mean Desaturation Index ± SD	6.4 ± 4.6	7.2 ± 5.5
Mean SaO2 Saturation ± SD	96.1 ± 2.2	95.7 ± 3.1
Mean SaO2 Nadir ± SD	86.2 ± 5.4	83.8 ± 6.5

apnea by analyzing the three-dimensional parameters (using different imaging modalities) of the airway column. The minimum cross-sectional area was the only one that was reduced consistently in obstructive sleep apnea (OSA) patients. The majority of the studies were of fair quality and quite heterogenous precluding a meta-analysis [22]. Another systematic review, this time in the pediatric literature [23], indicated that multiple cepahlometric measures of children diagnosed with MMD are statistically different between those who were asymptomatic and those with primary snoring and/or SDB. However, given the modest differences demonstrated, the clinical significance was deemed questionable. Alsufyani et al. [18] in a review of the literature indicated that several modalities had been used to perform three-dimensional analysis and measurements of the airway of SDB patients before and after treatment, including magnetic resonance imaging, multi-detector computed tomography and CBCT. The group commented that aside from the well known inherent advantages and disadvantages of each modality (expense, radiation exposure, physics inadequacies) the authors highlighted the challenges remaining with respect to image acquisition, three-dimensional reconstruction and analysis. Thus far nearly all the work concentrates on static measures (be them two dimensional of volume related) and how they relate to cross sectional polysomnographic parameters and their changes after various treatment lines.

Some of this work is in support of our observation. For example, Finkelstein et al. [24], in 2000 studied a group of children with nasal obstruction and counterparts without, all of whom did not have tonsillar enlargement and were otherwise healthy. They explored the relation between cephalometric measures and the severity of their symptoms (5 grade severity ranging from none to nasal obstruction with universally observed snoring and obstructive symptoms during sleep – but no objective or validated sleep parameters). An increased gonial angle was associated with increased symptoms which was statistically significant, and interestingly within the values which we reported and more than those reported for normative values, although including wider age group than ours. In another clinical study by Iwasaki and coinvestigator [25], after treating 28 subjects with rapid maxillary expansion, a significant increase in pharyngeal airway volume was demonstrated which they related to improvement in tongue position.

However, the study that may lend support to our work was done by Watanabe and colleagues [26]. In a study of the impact of body habitus and craniofacial parameters on pharyngeal closing pressures, SDB adult patients were found to have receded mandibles, with longer faces and downward mandibular growth. The angle reflecting the development of the mandible was significantly

different between SDB and normal patients (mean of 36.0° range of 34.0°– 41.5° versus a mean of 30.5° and range of 27.0°–33.0°, $p < 0.05$). This study correlated cephalometric, two-dimensional measures with a dynamic assessment of pharyngeal collapse, along the same lines of the current work.

Further epidemiological and biological studies are warranted to confirm this association and to provide further insight into biological mechanisms for purported association. The concept of measuring a dynamic soft tissue structure in a static cone beam CT is far from accurate. However, we attempted to standardize patient posture and use small scan time thus reducing chances of motion or multiple breathing cycles. We are aware of our small sample size, and the lack of polysomnographic data which prevents us from making any generalizable conclusions to the larger population, nor establishing a dose response relation. However, given this is an exploratory study, and the first to investigate the correlation between gonial angle, the static inclination of the epiglottis and dynamic TBC in children with SDB, findings are valuable for hypothesis generation for future larger scale studies.

Conclusions
The preliminary observation indicates that tongue base collapse is associated with a large gonial angle, which provides a hypothesis for a phenotypic marker that could explain persistence of SDB after traditional AT.

Abbreviations
CBCT: Cone beam computed tomography; DISE: Drug induced sleep endoscopy; MMD: Maxillo-mandibular disproportion; OSA: Obstructive sleep apnea; PSQ: Pediatric Sleep Questionnaire; SDB: Sleep disordered breathing; SNP: Sleep nasopharyngoscopy; TA: Adenotonsillectomy; TBC: Tongue base collapse

Authors' contributions
SM, NA and HE were responsible for the inception, planning / protocol, ERB application, data collection, analysis, writing and revision. MG and AI were responsible for the data collection, analysis and revision. All authors read and approved the final manuscript.

Competing interests
The authors declare that they have no competing interests.

Author details
[1]Department of Dentistry, Faculty of Medicine and Dentistry, University of Alberta, Edmonton, Canada. [2]Department of Oral Medicine and Diagnostic Sciences, College of Dentistry, King Saud University Division of Otolaryngology-Head and Neck Surgery Department of Surgery, Riyadh, Saudi Arabia. [3]University of Alberta, Edmonton, AB, Canada. [4]Division of Pediatric Surgery, Department of Surgery, Stollery Children's Hospital, Edmonton, AB, Canada. [5]Division of Otolaryngology-Head and Neck Surgery, Department of Surgery, University of Alberta, 2C3.57 Walter MacKenzie Centre, 8440 112 St NW, Edmonton, AB T6G 2R7, Canada.

References

1. American Academy of Otolaryngology - Head and Neck Surgery. Pediatric Sleep Disordered Breathing/Obstructive Sleep Apnea | American Academy of Otolaryngology-Head and Neck Surgery [Internet]. 2017 [cited 12 Apr 2017]. Available from: http://www.entnet.org/content/pediatric-sleep-disordered-breathingobstructive-sleep-apnea.
2. Huang Y-S, Guilleminault C, Li H-Y, Yang C-M, Wu Y-Y, Chen N-H. Attention-deficit/hyperactivity disorder with obstructive sleep apnea: A treatment outcome study. Sleep Med. 2007;8(1):18–30. [cited 23 Mar 2017]. Available from: http://linkinghub.elsevier.com/retrieve/pii/S1389945706001845
3. O'Brien LM, Tauman R, Gozal D, Weatherly RA, Dillon JE, Hodges EK, et al. Sleep pressure correlates of cognitive and behavioral morbidity in snoring children. Sleep. 2004;27(2):279–82. [cited 23 Mar 2017]. Available from: http://www.ncbi.nlm.nih.gov/pubmed/15124723
4. Gozal D, Capdevila OS, Kheirandish-Gozal L. Metabolic Alterations and Systemic Inflammation in Obstructive Sleep Apnea among Nonobese and Obese Prepubertal Children. Am J Respir Crit Care Med. 2008;177(10):1142–9. [cited 23 Mar 2017]. Available from: http://www.atsjournals.org/doi/abs/10.1164/rccm.200711-1670OC
5. Friedman M, Wilson M, Lin H-C, Chang H-W. Updated systematic review of tonsillectomy and adenoidectomy for treatment of pediatric obstructive sleep apnea/hypopnea syndrome. Otolaryngol Head Neck Surg. 2009;140(6):800–8.
6. Tarasiuk A, Greenberg-Dotan S, Simon-Tuval T, Freidman B, Goldbart AD, Tal A, et al. Elevated Morbidity and Health Care Use in Children with Obstructive Sleep Apnea Syndrome. [cited 12 Apr 2017]; Available from: http://www.atsjournals.org/doi/pdf/10.1164/rccm.200604-577OC.
7. Bixler EO, Vgontzas AN, Lin H-M, Liao D, Calhoun S, Vela-Bueno A, et al. Sleep disordered breathing in children in a general population sample: prevalence and risk factors. Sleep. 2009;32(6):731–6. [cited 7 Apr 2017]. Available from: http://www.ncbi.nlm.nih.gov/pubmed/19544748
8. Bhattacharjee R, Kheirandish-Gozal L, Spruyt K, Mitchell RB, Promchiarak J, Simakajornboon N, et al. Adenotonsillectomy outcomes in treatment of obstructive sleep apnea in children. Am J Respir Crit Care Med. 2010;182(5):676–83. [cited 12 Apr 2017]. Available from: http://www.ncbi.nlm.nih.gov/pubmed/20448096
9. Lumeng JC, Chervin RD. Epidemiology of pediatric obstructive sleep apnea. Proc Am Thorac Soc. 2008;5(2):242–52. [cited 12 Apr 2017]. Available from: http://www.ncbi.nlm.nih.gov/pubmed/18250218
10. Marcus CL, Brooks LJ, Draper KA, Gozal D, Halbower AC, Jones J, et al. Diagnosis and Management of Childhood Obstructive Sleep Apnea Syndrome. Pediatrics. 2012;130(3):576–84. [cited 12 Apr 2017]. Available from: http://www.ncbi.nlm.nih.gov/pubmed/22926173
11. Tauman R, Gulliver TE, Krishna J, Montgomery-Downs HE, O'Brien LM, Ivanenko A, et al. Persistence of obstructive sleep apnea syndrome in children after adenotonsillectomy. J Pediatr. 2006 ;149(6):803–808. [cited 12 Apr 2017]. Available from: http://www.sciencedirect.com.login.ezproxy.library.ualberta.ca/science/article/pii/S0022347606008201.
12. Lipton AJ, Gozal D. Treatment of obstructive sleep apnea in children: do we really know how? Sleep Med Rev. 2003 ;7(1):61–80. [cited 12 Apr 2017]. Available from: http://ac.els-cdn.com.login.ezproxy.library.ualberta.ca/S1087079201902564/1-s2.0-S1087079201902564-main.pdf?_tid=ccad79f0-2003-11e7-b753-00000aacb35e&acdnat=1492058815_3ea971f51febdd28fa670da7d0498f4a.
13. Alsufyani N, Isaac A, Witmans M, Major P, El-Hakim H. Predictors of failure of DISE-directed adenotonsillectomy in children with sleep disordered breathing.

J Otolaryngol Head Neck Surg. 2017;46(1):37. [cited 29 Nov 2017]. Available from: http://www.ncbi.nlm.nih.gov/pubmed/28476166
14. Tomes CS. The bearing of the development of the jaws on irregularities. Dent Cosm. 1873;115:292–6.
15. Linder-Aronson S, Woodside DG, Lundström A. Mandibular growth direction following adenoidectomy. Am J Orthod. 1986;89(4):273–84. [cited 16 Apr 2017]. Available from: http://www.ncbi.nlm.nih.gov/pubmed/3515955
16. Linder-Aronson S. Adenoids. Their effect on mode of breathing and nasal airflow and their relationship to characteristics of the facial skeleton and the denition. A biometric, rhino-manometric and cephalometro-radiographic study on children with and without adenoids. Acta Otolaryngol Suppl. 1970;265:1–132. [cited Apr 16 2017]. Available from: http://www.ncbi.nlm.nih.gov/pubmed/5272140
17. Ramji M, Biron VL, Jeffery CC, Côté DWJ, El-Hakim H. Validation of pharyngeal findings on sleep nasopharyngoscopy in children with snoring/sleep disordered breathing. J Otolaryngol Head Neck Surg. 2014;43(1):13. [cited 7 Jun 2017]. Available from: http://www.ncbi.nlm.nih.gov/pubmed/24919758
18. Alsufyani NA, Noga ML, Witmans M, Major PW. Upper airway imaging in sleep-disordered breathing: role of cone-beam computed tomography. Oral Radiol. https://doi.org/10.1007/s11282-017-0280-1.
19. Chervin RD, Hedger K, Dillon JE, Pituch KJ. Pediatric sleep questionnaire (PSQ): validity and reliability of scales for sleep-disordered breathing, snoring, sleepiness, and behavioral problems. Sleep Med. 2000;1(1):21–32. [cited 29 Nov 2017]. Available from: http://www.ncbi.nlm.nih.gov/pubmed/10733617
20. Nixon GM, Kermack AS, Davis GM, Manoukian JJ, Brown KA, Brouillette RT. Planning adenotonsillectomy in children with obstructive sleep apnea: the role of overnight oximetry. Pediatrics. 2004;113(1 Pt 1):e19–25. [cited 6 Dec 2017]. Available from: http://www.ncbi.nlm.nih.gov/pubmed/14702490
21. Upadhyay RB, Upadhyay J, Agrawal P, Rao NN. Analysis of gonial angle in relation to age, gender, and dentition status by radiological and anthropometric methods. J Forensic Dent Sci. 2012;4(1):29–33. [cited 6 Apr 2017]. Available from: http://www.ncbi.nlm.nih.gov/pubmed/23087579
22. Chen H, Aarab G, de Ruiter MHT, de Lange J, Lobbezoo F, van der Stelt PF. Three dimensional imaging of the upper airway anatomy in obstructive sleep apnea: a systematic review. Sleep Med. 2016;21:19–27.
23. Katyal V, Pamula Y, Martin AJ, Daynes CN, Kennedy JD, Sampsonf WJ. Craniofacial and upper airway morphology in pediatric sleep-disordered breathing: systematic review and meta-analysis. Am J Orthod Dentofac Orthop. 2013;143:20–30.
24. Finkelstein Y, Wexler D, Berger G, Nachmany A, Shapiro-Feinberg A, Ophir D. Anatomical basis of sleep related breathing abnormalities in children with nasal obstruction. Arch Otolaryngol Head Neck Surg. 2000;126:593–600.
25. Iwasaki T, Saitoh I, Takemoto Y, Inada E, Kakuno E, Kanomi R, Hayasaki H, Yamasakif Y. Tongue posture improvement and pharyngeal airway enlargement as secondary effects of rapid maxillary expansion: a cone-beam computed tomography study. Am J Orthod Dentofac Orthop. 2013;143:235–45.
26. Watanabe T, Isono S, Tanaka A, Tanzawa H, Nishino T. Contribution of body habitus and craniofacial characteristics to segmental closing pressures of the passive pharynx in patients with sleep-disordered breathing. Am J Respir Crit Care Med. 2002;165:260–5.

20

A prospective cohort study assessing the clinical utility of the Cottle maneuver in nasal septal surgery

James P. Bonaparte[1*] (iD) and Ross Campbell[2]

Abstract

Background: A nasal septal deviation can have a significant detrimental effect on a patient's quality of life. Nasal valve collapse (NVC) often co-exists with a septal deviation. The Cottle maneuver is one of the most common methods to diagnose NVC; however, no study has assessed the efficacy of this physical exam finding. This study tests the hypothesis that patients with nasal obstruction due to a septal deviation with a negative pre-operative Cottle maneuver will demonstrate a greater improvement in their Nasal Obstruction Symptom Evaluation (NOSE) score, compared to patients who demonstrate a positive pre-operative Cottle maneuver, when assessed at 12 months following a septoplasty with turbinate diathermy.

Methods: This was a prospective Cohort Study. The population was 141 patients with nasal obstruction due to a septal deviation with or without nasal valve collapse, excluding patients with bilateral complete nasal valve collapse. Patients were placed in cohorts according to the results of the Cottle maneuver (positive or negative). A NOSE questionnaire was administered at baseline and 12-months after a septoplasty with turbinate diathermy. Non-adjusted NOSE scores were used (score out of 20). An ANOVA was used to compare if there was a difference in outcomes between patient cohorts.

Results: One hundred and forty-one patients completed 12-month follow-up with 71.5% of patients demonstrating a positive Cottle maneuver at baseline. The mean (95% C.I.) difference in NOSE score at 12 months between patients with a positive Cottle versus a negative Cottle was 0.18 (− 1.6 to 1.92; $p = 0.38$).

Conclusion: In a univariate, single surgeon study, a positive Cottle Maneuver does not appear to influence outcomes in the described patient population compared to those with a negative Cottle Maneuver when undergoing a septoplasty.

Keywords: Septoplasty, Nasal obstruction, Nasal valve collapse, Cottle maneuver

Background

Nasal obstruction is the most common sinonasal complaint with which patients present to an otolaryngologist [1–3]. A nasal septal deviation, a common cause of nasal obstruction, can have a significant detrimental effect on a patient's quality of life [4]. Nasal valve collapse (NVC) often co-exists with a septal deviation [5–10]. Although physicians have studied objective measures to diagnose NVC, the vast majority rely on physical exam findings [5, 6, 11]. A systematic review by Speilmann et al. [6]

identified 43 papers assessing the treatment of nasal valve collapse. Of those, 24 papers utilized the Cottle maneuver to diagnose nasal valve collapse, 11 did not specify the method of diagnosis, while only one study utilized objective measures, specifically rhinomanometry. Of the studies that employed the Cottle maneuver, five utilized the Cottle maneuver as a single variable, while the remainder used a combination of the Cottle maneuver and a subjective assessment of intra-nasal support for their formal diagnosis of nasal valve collapse. Needless to say, the Cottle maneuver is a common component of the nasal examination [12, 13] and a common method to diagnose NVC.

To conduct the Cottle maneuver, the patient is required to inspire while the physician applies tension on the skin lateral to the nasolabial fold, thereby increasing nasal wall tension and widening of the nasal valve. In

* Correspondence: Drjames.bonaparte@gmail.com
Presented at the American Academy of Otolaryngology – Head and Neck Surgery Annual Meeting, Sept 29, 2015, Dallas, Texas, USA
[1]Department of Otolaryngology – Head and Neck Surgery Senior Clinical Investigator, The Ottawa Hospital Research Institute, University of Ottawa, 1919 Riverside Drive, Suite 308, Ottawa, Ontario K1H 7W9, Canada
Full list of author information is available at the end of the article

patients who have narrow or collapsing nasal valves, this maneuver improves nasal airflow, which constitutes a positive test. To many physicians, a positive test suggests that a functional rhinoplasty to specifically address the nasal valve may be necessary [6]. Indeed, in a clinical consensus statement published by the American Academy of Otolaryngology – Head and Neck Surgery (AAO-HNS), [13] the authors researched a consensus regarding the utility of certain physical exam findings in diagnosing NVC. These include: the subjective improvement in nasal airflow during a Cottle maneuver, the visible inspiratory collapse of the nasal wall and/or alar rim during inspiration, and the increased nasal obstruction during deep inspiration. Audible improvement in nasal airflow along with subjective improvement during the Cottle maneuver reached consensus; however, audible improvement alone did not. Interestingly, there was a consensus that there is no gold standard test to diagnose NVC.

As mentioned previously, results of a systematic review [6] noted that the Cottle maneuver is the most common method used to diagnose clinically relevant NVC that requires surgical repair. Of the studies reviewed, 55% of papers reviewed relied on the Cottle maneuver alone or in combination with a physical exam as the definition of clinically relevant NVC. Despite the widespread acceptance of the Cottle maneuver as a physical examination test to diagnose and define NVC, it has never been validated, nor has it been confirmed that all patients with a positive Cottle maneuver require repair of the nasal valve.

Based on our review, the majority of studies that assessed the effectiveness of a septoplasty in treating nasal obstruction secondary to a septal deviation have used the evidence of NVC as an exclusion criterion [14–21]. A number of other studies assessing the outcomes of septoplasty indicated that other causes of nasal obstruction were excluded, but made no specific reference to nasal valve collapse [14, 22–26]. We found only one study that assessed septoplasty outcomes in patients with a septal deviation along with evidence of NVC [7]. However, given that the nasal septum and inferior turbinates themselves constitute boundaries of the internal nasal valve, [5, 6, 11, 13, 27–32] a septoplasty with a reduction in the anterior edge of the inferior turbinate will theoretically have an effect on the internal nasal valve. Garcia et al. [33] assessed nasal resistance due to a septal deviation at different points of the nasal cavity. The authors noted that a septal deviation located at the level of the nasal valve (within 3 cm of the nasal opening) resulted in an increase in nasal resistance by 124%, while deviations in other areas of the nasal cavity increased resistance by no more than 30%. This increase in resistance could in itself alter the biomechanics of nasal airflow and thereby alter transnasal pressure and thereby result in alar or valve collapse.

Schalek and Hahn (2011) [7] noted that, in patients with an anterior septal deviation along with contralateral nasal valve collapse, a septoplasty led to resolution of both the nasal obstruction and nasal valve collapse. The authors noted that 91% of patients demonstrated an improvement on the side with nasal valve collapse. This study was limited by its small sample size of 12 patients, and the lack of a validated outcome measure. The clinical consensus statement published by Rhee et al. [13] noted that there was a strong consensus that procedures targeted to support the lateral nasal wall/alar rim are distinct entities from a septoplasty. However, there was moderate to strong agreement that, "in some cases" a septoplasty can treat NVC without other nasal wall procedures. The authors note that surgical procedures targeting the nasal wall are indicated when septal and/or turbinate surgery is not sufficient. Apart from the previously discussed study, there is little or no research specifically assessing the role of a septoplasty in patients with NVC. Therefore, the effectiveness of a septoplasty with inferior turbinate treatment alone in treating nasal obstruction secondary to a septal deviation with co-existing NVC has not been adequately studied.

Given the recommendations for diagnosing NVC as well as the frequency in which studies utilize the Cottle maneuver to diagnose it, one should question whether the test is clinically useful in patients with a septal deviation. If the Cottle maneuver accurately diagnoses NVC, and by extension, patients that also require surgery of the nasal valve, one can make the assumption that patients with a septal deviation and a positive Cottle maneuver may require specific treatment of the nasal valve. This is turn would suggest, that if patients require nasal valve surgery in addition to a septoplasty, not performing this required surgery might result in poorer outcomes compared to patients with a septal deviation who require only a septoplasty with or without inferior turbinate diathermy. However, this too has not been adequately studied.

The primary objective of this study was to test the hypothesis that patients with nasal obstruction due to a septal deviation who have a negative pre-operative Cottle maneuver will demonstrate a greater improvement in their Nasal Obstruction Symptom Evaluation (NOSE) score, compared to patients who have a positive pre-operative Cottle maneuver, when assessed at 12 months following a septoplasty with turbinate diathermy [15].

The secondary objective was to test the hypothesis that the odds of failure of a septoplasty, as defined by a published patient centered outcome [34] using the NOSE score, would be higher in patients with a positive pre-operative Cottle maneuver versus a negative Cottle maneuver.

Methods

Study design

This study was approved by our institutional ethics review board (20140735-01H). This was a prospective cohort study, consisting of two groups of patients with nasal obstruction. All patients were diagnosed with a septal deviation with or without visible evidence of NVC. Patients underwent a thorough standard pre-operative clinical evaluation of the nasal airway, including administration of the NOSE score. Patients were then placed in groups depending on the result of the Cottle maneuver, either positive or negative.

Population

All adult patients over the age of 18 years old, referred to the otolaryngology clinic of the senior author (JB) between Nov 1, 2014 and March 1, 2017 with nasal obstruction with a septal deviation were asked to enroll in the study. All patients had a minimum of a one-month trial on a topical intranasal corticosteroid prior to enrollment in the study.

Patients with bilateral partial NVC or unilateral complete NVC in addition to a septal deviation, either unilateral or bilateral (Grade 0–2 OVCS: Ottawa Valve Collapse Scale), [35] were included in the study. Partial collapse was defined as collapse of the internal and/or external valve during inspiration with the maintenance of nasal airway airflow; complete collapse was defined as total collapse of external nasal valve with the nasal ala contacting the caudal septum during inspiration, thereby completely occluding nasal airflow. Patients with complete bilateral collapse of the external nasal valve during inspiration were considered to have severe NVC and were excluded (Grade 3 OVCS). Patients were also excluded from the study if they previously had nasal structural surgery, static narrowing of the alar rim or external nasal valve (ie. a caudal septal deviation along the columellar edge, wide columella, statically collapsed alar rim), co-existing traumatic deviation of the nasal bones, allergic rhinitis, chronic rhinosinusitis with or without nasal polyposis, a neoplastic or autoimmune process.

Assessment of nasal airway

All patients had a thorough otolaryngological physical examination. Specifically, the external structure of the nose was assessed, and any deviation of the bony nasal pyramid or other deformities was documented. Visual inspection for collapse of the internal and/or nasal valves with both normal and deep inspiration was performed, and the presence or absence, laterally and severity of observed nasal collapse was recorded. A nasal speculum was used to perform anterior rhinoscopy and finding of a septal deviation and/or inferior turbinate hypertrophy were documented. Nasal decongestion was not utilized as all patients had a minimum of 1 month trial of topical nasal corticosteroids prior to inclusion. Flexible nasolaryngoscopy was performed in all patients to rule out non-septal causes of nasal obstruction.

All patients had the Cottle maneuver performed pre-operatively by the primary author (JB) as part of a general nasal examination. The examiner instructed the patient to breathe to breath in deeply through his or her nose two times. The first with no intervention, and the second time with the examiners' thumbs placed on the patients' cheeks, applying firm lateral pressure to stent open the nasal valves. A patient was defined as having a positive Cottle maneuver if he/she indicated his/her breathing improved compared to breathing without the Cottle maneuver. Finally, a baseline NOSE score was obtained for each patient.

Intervention

All patients had a septoplasty with bilateral inferior turbinate diathermy performed by the senior author in Ottawa, Ontario, Canada. The surgical approach was similar for all patients. A Killian incision, placed approximately 0.3–0.5 cm from the edge of the columella on the left side, was performed for all patients. A unilateral mucoperichondrial flap was raised on the left side. The deviated portion of the septum as well as the maxillary crest, if deviated, was removed. The surgery was individualized in accordance with the patient's individual anatomy and sites of obstruction. The L-strut of the septum was not altered according to standard practice. The mucoperichondrial flap was then closed using a 4–0 gut quilting suture followed by 4–0 gut closure of the Killian incision. No septal splints or packing were used in any patient [36]. The anterior edges of the inferior turbinates were reduced using needle-tip electrocautery set on 15 coagulation in a submucosal fashion. The turbinates were then lateralized by out-fracturing the bone. Follow-up for patients occurred between one and 2 weeks post-operatively for initial assessment, and again at 1 month, 6 months and 12 months.

Outcome measure

The primary outcome measure utilized for the study was the NOSE [15, 20] score at 12 months post-operatively. The relative change in NOSE score, defined as the percentage change as a function of baseline score, was not used as this would convert normally distributed data into non-normal distribution [37]. Instead, the NOSE score at 12 months was used as the primary outcome and the baseline NOSE score [22] was used as a covariate to correct for baseline differences in symptom severity in an ANOVA [37].

A secondary outcome measure, surgical failure, was defined as an improvement in the NOSE score of 40% or less at 12 months; this value has recently been shown to be the minimal important difference for patients, in a study of patient-defined outcomes following nasal airway surgery [34]. Using this definition, we were able to dichotomize outcomes into treatment success or treatment failure [34].

A physical exam was performed to document any complications at 12 months. In patients who did not meet the definition of a successful surgery, we attempted to identify the reason for failure. To identify dynamic internal or external nasal valve collapse post-operatively, the Modified Cottle maneuver [38] was used. Static collapse was assessed subjectively if patients appeared to have a narrow valve that did not improve with the Modified Cottle maneuver. Caudal septal deviations were defined as a septal deviation occurring within the area of the external nasal valve.

Statistical analysis

A pilot test of 25 patients without complaints of nasal obstruction resulted in an average NOSE score of 2.26 with a standard deviation of 3.06. while those with nasal obstruction had a mean score of 15.68 with a standard deviation of 2.96 [39]. Assuming a power of 95% and a p-value of 0.05, and significance difference between groups defined as 3 with a standard deviation of 3.5, a minimum of 37 patients per group would be required for the study. With this study, we aimed to enroll a minimum of 40 patients per group to ensure an analysis of covariates and subgroup analysis could be performed.

All summary data was presented as mean (standard deviation). An Anderson-Darling test was used to assess the NOSE score for a normal distribution. A general linear model ANOVA was used to compare patients with and without a positive Cottle maneuver. The outcome measure was NOSE score at 12 months. The pre-operative Cottle maneuver result (positive or negative) was used as the categorical variable. Gender was included as a potential variable. Age and baseline pre-operative baseline NOSE score were used as covariates. Statistical significance was defined as a $p < 0.05$.

To assess our secondary objective, a logistic binary regression was used to assess whether a positive Cottle maneuver increased the odds of a failure of a septoplasty. The definition of failure was based on a patient centered outcome [34]. Specifically, if a patient did not improve their NOSE score by 40% or more, patients were considered to have failed surgical intervention.

A chi-square test was used to determine if there was a relationship between patients with a positive Cottle maneuver and visible evidence of NVC.

Results

A total of 181 patients were screened for inclusion (Fig. 1). A total of 170 patients provided baseline data and completed the surgical treatment. One hundred and forty-one (141) patients completed the 12-month follow-up data collection, corresponding to a drop-out rate of 17%,; 21.1% in negative Cottle cohort and 15.2% in positive Cottle cohort.

The mean (standard deviation) age of patients who completed follow-up was 41.3 (13.4); 28.5% of patients were female. After a baseline screening exam, 67.4% of subjects had a positive Cottle maneuver. Summary data for all patients are presented in Table 1. The NOSE data at 12 months did not differ from a normal distribution ($p = 0.23$).

Of those with a negative Cottle maneuver, 56.5% had no evidence of visible valve collapse while 43.5% had visible evidence of valve collapse on exam. For those with a positive Cottle maneuver, 41.0% had no visible evidence of valve collapse while 58.9% had visible evidence of valve collapse on physical exam ($p = 0.084$) (Table 2).

The results of the ANOVA are presented in Table 3. Assessment of residuals versus fits appeared to be random and fit the model. There were 10 outliers in the model. The ANOVA was tested a second time with the outliers removed and there was no change in the results. There was no statistically significant difference in the NOSE score at 12 months between those patients with and without a positive pre-operative Cottle maneuver ($p = 0.38$, R-squared = 56.29%). The mean (95% C.I.) difference in NOSE score at 12 months between patients with a positive Cottle versus a negative Cottle was 0.18 (– 1.6 to 1.92).

Performing the same ANOVA model with the presence of absence of visible valve collapse on exam did not reach significance ($p = 0.27$).

Of the 141 patients who completed the one-year follow-up, 14 did not meet the definition of surgical success. The causes of failure, as assessed by the primary author are listed in Table 4. In those patients that failed the surgery, the most common cause was a persistent caudal septal deviation (33%) followed by static nasal valve narrowing (27%). Dynamic collapse was the cause of only one surgical failure in our population. One patient failed due to nasal polyps that were not appreciated during the pre-operative evaluation.

Results of the logistic regression failed to demonstrate the usefulness of the Cottle maneuver as a predictor of surgical failure in this population ($p = 0.99$). Specifically, a positive Cottle maneuver increased the odds of surgical failure by an odds ratio (95% C.I.) of 0.79 (0.22–2.8).

Discussion

The diagnosis and treatment of nasal valve collapse in the context of a septal deviation can be challenging

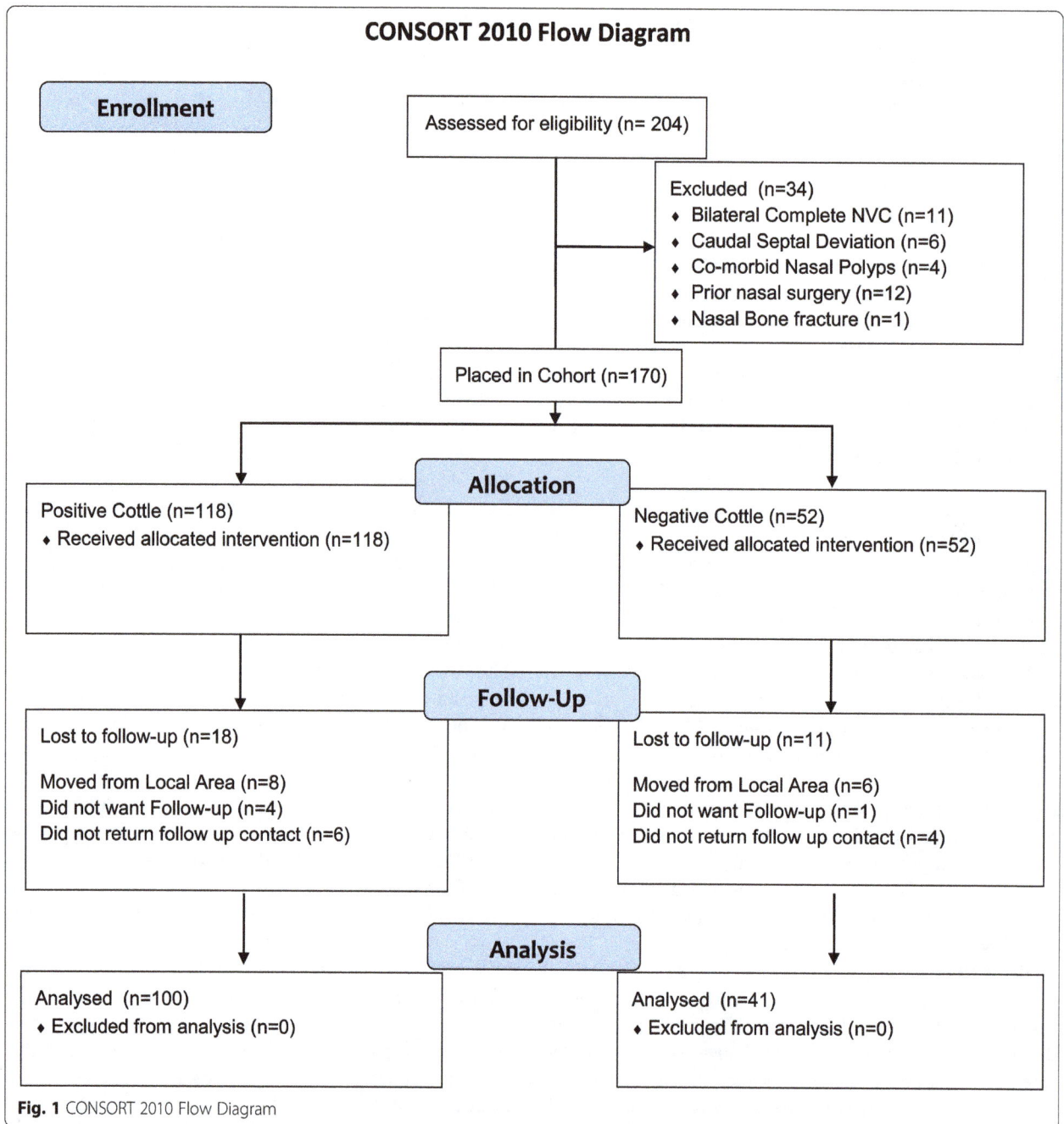

Fig. 1 CONSORT 2010 Flow Diagram

surgical and diagnostically. Published expert consensus states that there is no gold standard test to diagnose NVC [13]. Given the limited availability of objective measures to diagnose NVC, clinicians and surgeons utilize their history and physical exam. Understanding the efficacy of individual components of the physical exam and their relationship to nasal obstructive will provide a better understanding of the utility of these measures. This study provides evidence that as a single diagnostic measure, the Cottle maneuver has limited clinical utility in predicting which patients with nasal

obstruction secondary to a septal deviation will fail a septoplasty and inferior turbinate reduction. One key assumption with this reasoning, however, is that those patients with a positive Cottle maneuver also have nasal valve collapse. Although this is not always the case, the Cottle maneuver is the most commonly utilized physical examination for excluding [14–21] and including [6] NVC in previous studies.

The results of this study provide evidence that many patients with a positive Cottle maneuver who undergo a septoplasty and turbinate reduction will demonstrate an

Table 1 Summary of demographics and baseline outcome measures. Although scores for the change in NOSE and the percentage change in NOSE relative to baseline are presented, this data has not been controlled for the covariates included in the ANOVA model

Variable		All Patients	Positive Cottle	Negative Cottle	p-value
Patient Count	N	141	95	46	n/a
Age	Mean	41.3	40.4	43.4	0.17[a]
	SD	13.4	12	16.3	
Gender	% Female	28.5	23.1	41.9	0.007[b]
Baseline NOSE	Mean	13.3	13.1	13.7	0.43[a]
	SD	4.06	4.1	3.9	
12 Month NOSE	Mean	4.1	4.2	4.2	0.57[a]
	SD	4.6	4.6	4.5	
Change in NOSE	Mean	9.1	8.9	9.5	0.78[a]
	SD	5.7	5.8	5.6	
% Change in NOSE	Mean	67.5	66.8	68.8	0.81[a]
	SD	35.8	36.9	33.5	
Surgical Failure	n	14	9	5	0.99[b]
	% of Total	9.9	9.5	10.5	

N number of patients, SD standard deviation, NOSE nasal obstruction symptom index, n/a not applicable
[a] two-sample t-test, [b] Chi-square test

equivalent improvement in their symptoms to those patients with a negative Cottle maneuver. The reduction in the NOSE score after a septoplasty in both positive and negative Cottle maneuver patients were similar to those in other published papers assessing patients without evidence of nasal valve collapse [16–18, 20, 40]. To our knowledge, there is no published study that provides evidence demonstrating the usefulness of nasal valve lateralization techniques or lateral nasal sidewall strengthening over a standard septoplasty with turbinate reduction in patients with mild to moderate valve collapse based on the Cottle maneuver. One important consideration, however, is that this study was an assessment of a single examination. It is likely that multiple factors predict the failure of a septoplasty, and several examinations considered together may be more appropriate than a single assessment using a single test. The goal of this study is to provide the basis of future studies assessing a multivariate assessment of nasal examinations of surgical outcomes.

Two recent systematic reviews evaluated the surgical treatment of NVC [6, 11]. None of the studies captured in the review compared the use of a septoplasty (with or without turbinate reduction) alone versus other methods of nasal valve repair (with or without a septoplasty) [6, 11]. In many of the reported studies a septoplasty was

performed at the time of the nasal sidewall (nasal valve) surgical procedure; however, in no cases was this quantified or controlled as a confounding variable. A recent meta-analysis by Floyd et al. [10] noted that the NOSE score in patients with nasal obstruction due to NVC was significantly reduced following a functional rhinoplasty, with or without a cosmetic component. Although it was noted that a septoplasty is part of a functional rhinoplasty and performed for nearly all patients, the efficacy of this alone was not controlled nor accounted for in the statistical methods. In fact, the authors excluded any paper that included patients who had a septoplasty alone. In addition, in their series of 12 patients with a septal deviation and contralateral alar valve collapse, Schalek and Hahn reported that 11 of 12 patients reported significant improvement of nasal breathing following a septoplasty, without additional procedures to address the nasal valve [7]. Certainly, there is a role for functional rhinoplasty in many patients with nasal obstruction with NVC; however, an evidence-based approach to identify these patients, and to identify which patients will experience sufficient improvement with a septoplasty and inferior turbinate reduction alone, is currently lacking.

Considering surgical failure, dynamic NVC represented a surprisingly small number of surgical failures.

Table 2 Summary of Patients with and without subjective evidence of nasal valve collapse on exam

Subjective NVC	N	NOSE (mean)	NOSE (SD)	Positive Cottle	Negative Cottle
Negative	65	14.78	3.9	39	26
Positive	76	11.79	4.1	56	20

Table 3 Summary of ANOVA for the primary outcome measure

Source of Variation	df	Sum of Squares	Mean Square	f-value	p-value
Baseline Score	1	1536.24	1536.24	147.72	< 0.001
Age	1	117.44	117.44	11.29	0.001
Cottle	1	7.96	7.96	0.77	0.383
Gender	1	1.58	1.58	0.15	0.697
Error	124	1289.54	10.4		
Total	128	3027.67			

df degrees of freedom

The results of our study identify a caudal septal deviation followed by static nasal valve narrowing as the two most common causes of failure. Previous studies have noted that failure to recognize dynamic NVC pre-operatively is the most common cause of septoplasty failure [9, 32, 41, 42]. Chambers et al. (2015) [43] performed a retrospective assessment of patients who did not demonstrate clinical improvement after a septoplasty. Due to the lack of baseline population numbers, overall the rate of failure is not possible to calculate; however, the cause of failure appeared to be multifactorial. Further complicating the analysis of the results, the authors did not provide information on what tests were used to define specific causes failure causes.

Another unexpected finding in this study was that age was a significant covariate in the ANOVA model. When reviewing this outcome, although statistically significant, the relationship was weak and did not add any clinically meaningful predictive benefit. Prior studies failed to demonstrate any correlation between age and improvements after a septoplasty [22, 23], and therefore it is possible that the positive results in this study are due to being over-powered; it may in fact be a false positive outcome.

Although this study represents a high quality, prospective assessment of patients with nasal obstruction, there are some limitations. One limitation of the study design was that patients could not be randomized to undergo septoplasty and inferior turbinate reduction versus functional rhinoplasty and have post-operative

results compared. Given the heterogeneity in both type and location of septal deviation, no specific data was collected with respect to the location of the septal deviation in our patients; this could have been of interest for a more detailed understanding of the etiology of individual patients' NVC, and should occur in future studies. Similarly, we did not prospectively record other commonly utilized assessments of NVC pre-operatively, such as the modified Cottle maneuver. Specific findings in nasal endoscopy was not recorded in our pre-operative evaluation, apart from using it to rule out other causes of nasal obstruction. However, the authors of the AAO-HNS clinical consensus statement indicate that anterior rhinoscopy can be sufficient for an intra-nasal examination of the nasal valve [13] and therefore we did not include specific endoscopy information. We selected the NOSE score as our primary outcome measure, as the AAO-HNS clinical consensus statement indicates that a NOSE score is valid for the purpose of assessing the outcome of surgical interventions and that the NOSE scale was the most common outcome measure used in a systematic review of studies evaluation the surgical treatment of internal NVC [11, 13]. However, additional outcome measures such as visual analogue scales for nasal breathing could also have been of value, given that nasal breathing is subjective and not a dichotomous variable.

Another limitation of this study is that a single surgeon performed all assessments. Given a lack of a validated grading scheme, a general assessment of NVC is

Table 4 Causes of surgical failure

Reason for Surgical Failure	Positive Cottle Count	% Total	Negative Cottle Count	% Total	All Patients Count	% Total
Caudal Septal Deviation	4	4.2	1	2.2	5	3.5
Narrow External Nasal Valve (Static)	3	3.2	1	2.2	4	2.8
Valve Collapse (Dynamic)	0	0.0	1	2.2	1	0.7
Perforation	0	0.0	1	2.2	1	0.7
Untreated allergy	2	2.1	0	0.0	2	1.4
Nasal Polyps	0	0.0	1	2.2	1	0.7
TOTAL	9	9.5	5	10.9	14	9.9

therefore subjective. Finally, biases can occur in assessment of surgical failure, and therefore a more robust and preferably blinded assessment would be optimal to validate these findings studies. However, we chose to use a patient centered definition of surgical failure, therefore limiting this bias.

The findings of this study have considerable applicability in terms of patient safety and health care resource utilization. Potential complications, as well as morbidity of more advanced surgical procedures are likely greater for a functional rhinoplasty than for a standard septoplasty, particularly if grafting is required from sites other than the nasal septum. With respect to health economics, in the practice of the primary author, a septoplasty and turbinate reduction can be performed rapidly, resulting in less time in the operating room and less post-operative care compared to more advanced functional rhinoplasty techniques specific for nasal valve collapse. The reduction in operative time, healing time and complications likely all contribute to lower health care costs, both direct and indirect. Future studies will be required to assess these questions.

In summary, this study demonstrated that there is no difference in patients with and without a positive Cottle maneuver when used as a single univariate assessment tool. In these patients, it should be used cautiously as a single outcome measure when predicting which patients may require nasal valve surgery and as an exclusion or inclusion criteria in research studies. However, it remains unclear if the test plays a role in a multivariable predictive model for detecting clinically relevant NVC. The results of this study could potentially influence practice, by encouraging clinicians to consider multiple factors when assessing the cause of nasal obstruction, as well as the need for advanced nasal surgery in addition to a septoplasty, and not simply relying on the Cottle maneuver as a dichotomous indicator of nasal valve collapse. Consequently, the accurate diagnoses of clinically relevant NVC requiring nasal sidewall repair continues to remains a challenge [44].

Conclusion

The Cottle maneuver offers limited clinical utility to predict symptom improvement following septoplasty with inferior turbinate reduction in patients with nasal obstruction due to a septal deviation, with or without NVC. This study also suggests that a large proportion of patients with clinical evidence of NVC, based on the Cottle maneuver and physical examination, may not require advanced nasal valve procedures in addition to a septoplasty and turbinate reduction.

To date, there is no evidence-based outcome measure, or combination of outcome measures that predicts which patients will require more advanced nasal valve

surgery. Certainly there remains a role for functional rhinoplasty to address the nasal valve; however, future studies are necessary to determine the variables that predict which patients are at a high risk of surgical failure, and to more accurately determine which patients with nasal obstruction and NVC require a functional rhinoplasty.

Abbreviations
AAO-HNS: American Academy of Otolaryngology – Head and Neck Surgery; ANOVA: Analysis of variance; NOSE: Nasal obstruction symptom evaluation; NVC: Nasal valve collapse; OVCS: Ottawa Valve Collapse Scale

Authors' contributions
JPB Project design, data collection, analysis and writing. RC Analysis and writing. Both authors read and approved the final manuscript.

Competing interests
The authors declare that they have no competing interests.

Author details
[1]Department of Otolaryngology – Head and Neck Surgery Senior Clinical Investigator, The Ottawa Hospital Research Institute, University of Ottawa, 1919 Riverside Drive, Suite 308, Ottawa, Ontario K1H 7W9, Canada. [2]Department of Otolaryngology – Head and Neck Surgery, The University of Ottawa, Ottawa, Canada.

References
1. Baumann I. Quality of life before and after septoplasty and rhinoplasty. GMS Curr Top Otorhinolaryngol Head Neck Surg. 2010;9:Doc06.
2. Kim CS, Moon BK, Jung DH, Min YG. Correlation between nasal obstruction symptoms and objective parameters of acoustic rhinometry and rhinomanometry. Auris Nasus Larynx. 1998;25:45–8.
3. Simon P, Sidle D. Augmenting the nasal airway: beyond septoplasty. Am J Rhinol Allergy. 2012;26:326–31.
4. Naraghi M, Amirzargar B, Meysamie A. Quality of life comparison in common rhinologic surgeries. Allergy Rhinol (Providence). 2012;3:e1–7.
5. Bloching MB. Disorders of the nasal valve area. GMS Curr Top Otorhinolaryngol Head Neck Surg. 2007;6:Doc07.
6. Spielmann PM, White PS, Hussain SS. Surgical techniques for the treatment of nasal valve collapse: a systematic review. Laryngoscope. 2009;119:1281–90.
7. Schalek P, Hahn A. Anterior septal deviation and contralateral alar collapse. B-ENT. 2011;7:185–8.
8. Goudakos JK, Daskalakis D, Patel K. Revision rhinoplasty: retrospective chart review analysis of deformities and surgical maneuvers in patients with nasal airway obstruction-five years of experience. Facial Plast Surg. 2017;33:334–8.
9. Nouraei SA, Virk JS, Kanona H, Zatonski M, Koury EF, Chatrath P. Non-invasive Assessment and Symptomatic improvement of the obstructed nose (NASION): a physiology-based patient-centred approach to treatment selection and outcomes assessment in nasal obstruction. Clin Otolaryngol. 2016;41:327–40.
10. Floyd EM, Ho S, Patel P, Rosenfeld RM, Gordin E. Systematic review and meta-analysis of studies evaluating functional rhinoplasty outcomes with the NOSE score. Otolaryngol Head Neck Surg. 2017;156:809–15.
11. Goudakos J, Fishman J, Patel K. A systematic review of the surgical techniques for the treatment of internal nasal valve collapse: where do we stand? Clin Otolaryngol. 2017;42:60–70.
12. Murrell GL. Components of the nasal examination. Aesthet Surg J. 2013; 33:38–42.
13. Rhee JS, Weaver EM, Park SS, Baker SR, Hilger PA, Kriet JD, Murakami C, Senior BA, Rosenfeld RM, DiVittorio D. Clinical consensus statement:

diagnosis and management of nasal valve compromise. Otolaryngol Head Neck Surg. 2010;143:48–59.

14. Manestar D, Braut T, Kujundzic M, Malvic G, Velepic M, Donadic Manestar I, Matanic Lender D, Starcevic R. The effects of disclosure of sequential rhinomanometry scores on post-septoplasty subjective scores of nasal obstruction: a randomised controlled trial. Clin Otolaryngol. 2012;37:176–80.

15. Stewart MG, Witsell DL, Smith TL, Weaver EM, Yueh B, Hannley MT. Development and validation of the nasal obstruction symptom evaluation (NOSE) scale. Otolaryngol Head Neck Surg. 2004;130:157–63.

16. Gillman GS, Egloff AM, Rivera-Serrano CM. Revision septoplasty: a prospective disease-specific outcome study. Laryngoscope. 2014;124:1290–5.

17. Mondina M, Marro M, Maurice S, Stoll D, de Gabory L. Assessment of nasal septoplasty using NOSE and RhinoQoL questionnaires. Eur Arch Otorhinolaryngol. 2012;269:2189–95.

18. Kahveci OK, Miman MC, Yucel A, Yucedag F, Okur E, Altuntas A. The efficiency of NOSE obstruction symptom evaluation (NOSE) scale on patients with nasal septal deviation. Auris Nasus Larynx. 2012;39:275–9.

19. Dinesh Kumar R, Rajashekar M. Comparative study of improvement of nasal symptoms following septoplasty with partial inferior Turbinectomy versus septoplasty alone in adults by NOSE scale: a prospective study. Indian J Otolaryngol Head Neck Surg. 2016;68:275–84.

20. Stewart MG, Smith TL, Weaver EM, Witsell DL, Yueh B, Hannley MT, Johnson JT. Outcomes after nasal septoplasty: results from the nasal obstruction septoplasty effectiveness (NOSE) study. Otolaryngol Head Neck Surg. 2004; 130:283–90.

21. Umihanic S, Brkic F, Osmic M, Umihanic S, Imamovic S, Kamenjakovic S, Hodzic S. The discrepancy between subjective and objective findings after septoplasty. Med Arch. 2016;70:336–8.

22. Hong SD, Lee NJ, Cho HJ, Jang MS, Jung TY, Kim HY, Chung SK, Dhong HJ. Predictive factors of subjective outcomes after septoplasty with and without turbinoplasty: can individual perceptual differences of the air passage be a main factor? Int Forum Allergy Rhinol. 2015;5:616–21.

23. Habesoglu M, Kilic O, Caypinar B, Onder S. Aging as the impact factor on septoplasty success. J Craniofac Surg. 2015;26:e419–22.

24. Aziz T, Biron VL, Ansari K, Flores-Mir C. Measurement tools for the diagnosis of nasal septal deviation: a systematic review. J Otolaryngol Head Neck Surg. 2014;43:11.

25. Shiryaeva O, Tarangen M, Gay C, Dosen LK, Haye R. Preoperative signs and symptoms as prognostic markers in nasal septoplasty. Int J Otolaryngol. 2017;2017:4718108.

26. Bugten V, Nilsen AH, Thorstensen WM, Moxness MH, Amundsen MF, Nordgard S. Quality of life and symptoms before and after nasal septoplasty compared with healthy individuals. BMC Ear Nose Throat Disord. 2016;16:13.

27. Haight JS, Cole P. The site and function of the nasal valve. Laryngoscope. 1983;93:49–55.

28. Hamilton GS 3rd. The external nasal valve. Facial Plast Surg Clin North Am. 2017;25:179–94.

29. Motamedi KK, Stephan SJ, Ries WR. Innovations in nasal valve surgery. Curr Opin Otolaryngol Head Neck Surg. 2016;24:31–6.

30. Nigro CE, Nigro JF, Mion O, Mello JF Jr. Nasal valve: anatomy and physiology. Braz J Otorhinolaryngol. 2009;75:305–10.

31. Sclafani AP, Victor W, Sclafani MS. Geometric modeling of the nasal valve. Facial Plast Surg. 2017;33:444–50.

32. Wittkopf M, Wittkopf J, Ries WR. The diagnosis and treatment of nasal valve collapse. Curr Opin Otolaryngol Head Neck Surg. 2008;16:10–3.

33. Garcia GJ, Rhee JS, Senior BA, Kimbell JS. Septal deviation and nasal resistance: an investigation using virtual surgery and computational fluid dynamics. Am J Rhinol Allergy. 2010;24:e46–53.

34. Ziai H, Bonaparte JP. Determining a successful nasal airway surgery: calculation of the patient-centered minimum important difference. Otolaryngol Head Neck Surg. 2017;157(2):325–30.

35. Ziai H, Bonaparte JP. Reliability and construct validity of the Ottawa valve collapse scale when assessing external nasal valve collapse. J Otolaryngol Head Neck Surg. 2018;47:15.

36. Quinn JG, Bonaparte JP, Kilty SJ. Postoperative management in the prevention of complications after septoplasty: a systematic review. Laryngoscope. 2013;123:1328–33.

37. Vickers AJ. The use of percentage change from baseline as an outcome in a controlled trial is statistically inefficient: a simulation study. BMC Med Res Methodol. 2001;1:6.

38. Fung E, Hong P, Moore C, Taylor SM. The effectiveness of modified cottle maneuver in predicting outcomes in functional rhinoplasty. Plast Surg Int. 2014;2014:618313.

39. Lodder WL, Leong SC. What are the clinically important outcome measures in the surgical management of nasal obstruction? Clin Otolaryngol. 2018; 43(2):567–71.

40. Bakshi SS, Coumare VN, Priya M, Kumar S. Long-term complications of button batteries in the nose. J Emerg Med. 2016;50:485–7.

41. Ricci E, Palonta F, Preti G, Vione N, Nazionale G, Albera R, Staffieri A, Cortesina G, Cavalot AL. Role of nasal valve in the surgically corrected nasal respiratory obstruction: evaluation through rhinomanometry. Am J Rhinol. 2001;15:307–10.

42. Rhee JS, Poetker DM, Smith TL, Bustillo A, Burzynski M, Davis RE. Nasal valve surgery improves disease-specific quality of life. Laryngoscope. 2005;115:437–40.

43. Chambers KJ, Horstkotte KA, Shanley K, Lindsay RW. Evaluation of improvement in nasal obstruction following nasal valve correction in patients with a history of failed septoplasty. JAMA Facial Plast Surg. 2015;17:347–50.

44. Han JK, Stringer SP, Rosenfeld RM, Archer SM, Baker DP, Brown SM, Edelstein DR, Gray ST, Lian TS, Ross EJ, et al. Clinical consensus statement: septoplasty with or without inferior turbinate reduction. Otolaryngol Head Neck Surg. 2015;153:708–20.

21

Analytic and clinical validity of thyroid nodule mutational profiling using droplet digital polymerase chain reaction

Vincent L. Biron[1,2,4*] (iD), Ashlee Matkin[2,3], Morris Kostiuk[2,4], Jordana Williams[4], David W. Cote[1], Jeffrey Harris[1,2], Hadi Seikaly[1,2] and Daniel A. O'Connell[1,2]

Abstract

Background: Recent guidelines for the management of thyroid nodules incorporate mutation testing as an adjunct for surgical decision-making, however current tests are costly with limited accuracy. Droplet digital PCR (ddPCR) is an ultrasensitive method of nucleic acid detection that is particularly useful for identifying gene mutations. This study aimed to assess the analytic and clinical validity of RAS and BRAF ddPCR mutational testing as a diagnostic tool for thyroid fine needle aspirate biopsy (FNAB).

Methods: Patients with thyroid nodules meeting indication for FNAB were prospectively enrolled from March 2015 to September 2017. In addition to clinical protocol, an additional FNAB was obtained for ddPCR. Optimized ddPCR probes were used to detect mutations including HRASG12 V, HRASQ61K, HRASQ61R, NRASQ61R, NRASQ61K and BRAFV600E. The diagnostic performance of *BRAF* and *RAS* mutations was assessed individually or in combination with Bethesda classification against final surgical pathology.

Results: A total of 208 patients underwent FNAB and mutational testing with the following Bethesda cytologic classification: 26.9% non-diagnostic, 55.2% benign, 5.3% FLUS/AUS, 2.9% FN/SPN, 2.4% SFM and 7.2% malignant. Adequate RNA was obtained from 91.3% (190) FNABs from which mutations were identified in 21.1% of HRAS, 11.5% of NRAS and 7.4% of BRAF. Malignant cytology or BRAFV600E was 100% specific for malignancy. Combining cytology with ddPCR BRAF600E mutations testing increased the sensitivity of Bethesda classification from 41.7 to 75%. Combined BRAFV600E and Bethesda results had a positive predictive value (PPV) of 100% and negative predictive value (NPV) of 89.7% for thyroid malignancy in our cohort.

Conclusions: DdPCR offers a novel and ultrasensitive method of detecting RAS and BRAF mutations from thyroid FNABs. BRAFV600E mutation testing by ddPCR may serve as a useful adjunct to increase sensitivity and specificity of thyroid FNAB.

Background

The incidence of thyroid nodules may be as high as 70% in the adult population. Based on clinical and sonographic features, further diagnostic work-up is largely based on cytologic analysis of fine needle aspirate biopsy (FNAB). Unfortunately, up to 30% of FNABs are inconclusive and as a result of inaccurate pre-operative diagnosis, many patients with thyroid nodules undergo unnecessary surgery [1, 2]. Molecular analysis of thyroid FNABs has been shown to improve diagnostic accuracy [3]. Incorporating these findings, recent American and European guidelines support the use of mutation testing of genes associated with thyroid cancer (*BRAF, RAS, RET/PTC, PAX8/PPARG*) in order to improve surgical decision making [3, 4].

The most common mutation associated with thyroid cancer involves *BRAF* codon V600, followed by mutations in *RAS* [5]. The *BRAF* activating V600E mutation (BRAFV600E) is found in 29–83% of papillary thyroid cancers (PTC), and is associated with more aggressive

* Correspondence: vbiron@ualberta.ca
[1]Division of Otolaryngology-Head and Neck Surgery, University of Alberta, 8440-112 st, 1E4 Walter Mackenzie Centre, Edmonton, AB T6G 2B7, Canada
[2]Alberta Head and Neck Centre for Oncology and Reconstruction, Walter MacKenzie Health Sciences Centre, Edmonton, AB, Canada
Full list of author information is available at the end of the article

disease [4, 6–8]. A number of *RAS* mutations have been associated with thyroid cancer, with variable diagnostic utility [5]. Mutations in codon 61 of *HRAS* and *NRAS* are thought to have the highest positive predictive value for malignancy (85–87%) [5, 9]. Data from The Cancer Genome Atlas demonstrates that alterations in *BRAF* and *RAS* enable molecular classification of PTC subtypes that is more representative of their differences in tumor biology than histopathologic classification [10]. Recent exploration of the mutational landscape of follicular thyroid cancers (FTCs) has suggested that perhaps well differentiated thyroid cancers could best be classified in three molecular subtypes: BRAF-like, RAS-like and Non-BRAF-Non-RAS [10]. Yet numerous genetic alterations have been identified as potential diagnostic markers for thyroid cancer, many of which are used in commercial tests with inconsistent clinical performance [4].

A major limitation of current molecular tests for thyroid cancer is these assays require large volumes of high quality RNA, often lacking from FNABs. This amount of genetic material is required for amplification of low copy mutations attributed with thyroid cancers. Recent advancements in nucleic acid detection using digital droplet PCR (ddPCR) can circumvent these limitations [11, 12]. DdPCR is a rapid and ultrasensitive method of detecting nucleic acid targets, shown to be particularly useful for the identification of mutant alleles in a variety of cancers [6, 12–14]. This technology has recently been employed for the rapid and accurate detection of BRAFV600E in colorectal cancer and melanoma [6, 15]. Given the precision of ddPCR for mutation detection, especially with nucleic acids of low abundance, it is an ideal molecular diagnostic tool for FNAB that has not yet been utilized for this purpose. We describe the first use of ddPCR for the detection of *RAS* and *BRAF* mutations in thyroid nodules.

Methods
Patients
Patients presenting to the University of Alberta Head and Neck Clinic for consultation regarding a thyroid nodule were prospectively recruited and consented for enrolment in this study from March 2015 to September 2017, in keeping with approved health research ethics board protocols (Pro00062302 and Pro00016426) . An ultrasound-guided fine needle aspirate biopsy (FNAB) was performed as standard of care for cytology, with an additional needle pass taken for ddPCR analysis immediately transferred to a 1.5 mL tube containing 200 ul RNA*later*™ (Thermofisher AM7021). FNA samples suspended in RNAlater were kept at room temperature < 24 h and at 4°C for < 7 days until processed for RNA extraction. Determination of mutation status by ddPCR was performed by MK, who was

blinded to clinical and pathologic characteristics associated with FNAB samples. Decision to treat patients surgically followed 2015 American Thyroid Association (ATA) guidelines [3] and was not influenced by ddPCR mutation results.

RNA extraction and cDNA synthesis
RNA was extracted using the RNeasy PlusMini Kit (Qiagen Cat No./ID: 79656). 550 ul of Buffer RLT, 40 mM DTT was added directly to the tube containing the FNA and the tube was vortexed extensively. The sample was loaded onto a QIAshredder (Qiagen Cat No./ID: 79656) and centrifuged at 8000 x g for 30 s at room temperature. The resulting flow through was loaded onto a gDNA Eliminator mini Spin Column and centrifuged 30 s at 8000 x g. An equal volume of 70% ethanol was added to the flow through, mixed by pipetting, and the mixture was transferred to an RNeasy Mini spin column and centrifuged for 15 s at 8000 x g. Following RNA binding, the Mini column was washed as per manufacturer's instructions and the RNA was eluted with 50 ul RNase free H2O. RNA concentration was quantified using the Qubit RNA HS assay kit on a Qubit 2.0 fluorometer as per manufacturer's instructions. The RNA was either stored at -80° C or immediately used to carry out cDNA synthesis.

RNA (5–500 ng) was used to synthesize cDNA using the iScriptTM Reverse Transcription Supermix for RT-qPCR (BIO-RAD) as per the manufacturer's protocol. Following the reaction, the cDNA was diluted with nuclease free H_2O to a final concentration of 1 ng/ul (if initial RNA concentration was high enough) or, in some cases, 2 ng/ul. Newly synthesized cDNA was either stored at -20° C or used directly for ddPCR.

ddPCR reactions
Reactions were set up following the manufacturer's protocols using 12 ul/reaction of 2× ddPCR Supermix for Probes (No dUTP), 1.2 ul/reaction of 20× mutant primers/probe (FAM BIO-RAD), 1.2 ul/reaction 20× wildtype primers/probe (HEX, BIO-RAD), 2.4 ul cDNA (at up to 2 ng/ul) and 7.2 ul H2O. ddPCR was carried out using the ddPCRTM Supermix for Probes (No dUTP) (BIO-RAD), the QX200TM Droplet Generator (catalog #186–4002 BIO-RAD), the QX200 Droplet Reader (catalog #186–4003 BIO-RAD) the C1000 TouchTM Thermal Cycler (catalog #185–1197 BIO-RAD) and the PX1TM PCR Plate Sealer (catalog #181-40well plate, mixed using a Mixmate Vortex Shaker (Eppendorf) and 20 ul of the reaction mixture was transferred to DG8TM Cartridge for QX200/QX100 Droplet Generator (catalog #186–4008 BIO-RAD) followed by 70 μl of Droplet Generation Oil for Probes (catalog #186–3005 BIO-RAD) into the oil wells,

according to the QX200 Droplet Generator Instruction Manual (#10031907 BIO-RAD). Following droplet generation, 40 ul of the reaction was transferred to wells of a 96 well plate and the reactions were carried out in the thermocycler using the following parameters: Step 1) 95° C for 10 min, Step 2) 94° C for 30 s and 60° C for 1 min (Step 2 repeat 39 times for a total of 40), Step 3) 98° C for 10 min and Step 4) 4° C infinite hold. All steps had a ramp rate of 3° C/second. Following thermocycling the reactions were read in the QX200 Droplet Reader and the RNA targets were quantified using the QuantaSoftTM Software (BIO-RAD).

BIO-RAD proprietary ddPCR Primers and probes used were as follows: Unique Assay ID dHsaCP2000026 PrimePCR ddPCR Mutation Assay HRAS WT for p.G12 V Human, Unique Assay ID dHsaCP2000025 PrimePCR ddPCR Mutation Assay HRAS p.G12 V Human, Unique Assay ID dHsaCP2506815 PrimePCR ddPCR Mutation Assay HRAS WT for p.Q61K Human, Unique Assay ID dHsaCP2506814 PrimePCR ddPCR Mutation Assay HRAS p.Q61K Human, Unique Assay ID dHsaCP2500577 PrimePCR ddPCR Mutation Assay HRAS WT for p.Q61R Human, Unique Assay ID dHsaCP2500576 PrimePCR ddPCR Mutation Assay HRAS p.Q61R Human, Unique Assay ID dHsaCP2000068 PrimePCR ddPCR Mutation Assay NRAS WT for p.Q61K Human, Unique Assay ID dHsaCP2000067 PrimePCR ddPCR Mutation Assay NRAS p.Q61K Human, Unique Assay ID dHsaCP2000072 PrimePCR ddPCR Mutation Assay NRAS WT for p.Q61R Human, Unique Assay ID dHsaCP2000071 PrimePCR ddPCR Mutation Assay NRAS p.Q61R Human, Unique Assay ID dHsaCP2000028 PrimePCR ddPCR Mutation Assay BRAF WT for p.V600E Human, Unique Assay ID dHsaCP2000037 PrimePCR ddPCR Mutation Assay BRAF p.V600R Human. Determination of mutant versus wild type RAS and BRAF samples was based on the presence or absence of mutant droplets in the expected regions in two-dimensional data output plots determined using Quantasoft (Additional file 1: Figure S1). The first 98 collected FNA samples were repeated 2 or more times and demonstrated completely reproducible results for the detection of mutations.

Statistics

Statistical calculations were completed using SPSS version 25 (IBM, Chicago, IL) and MedCalc 12.2 where appropriate. Bayesian statistics were used to calculate means, Pearson correlation and Loglinear regression. The performance of standard pathology (Bethesda classification) and ddPCR mutation profiling was estimated using Bayes theorem. Where appropriate, 95% confidence intervals were calculated using Clopper-Pearson for sensitivity and specificity, the Log method for positive likelihood ratios (PLR) and negative likelihood ratios (NLR) [16], and standard logit for positive predictive value (PPV) and negative predictive value (NPV) [17].

Results

A total of 208 patients with thyroid nodules were prospectively enrolled for participation in this study. FNAB results from standard of care cytology yielded the following distribution in Bethesda classification: 26.9% (56) non-diagnostic, 55.2% (115) benign, 5.3% (11) AUS/FLUS, 2.9% (6) FN/SFN, 2.4% (5) SFM and 7.2% (15) malignant (Fig. 1). Based on clinical, sonographic and cytologic characteristics, thyroid surgery was performed on 44.2% (92) of patients in this cohort (Table 1 and Fig. 1). Of patients who were classified as Bethesda III-VI (17.8%), only 1 patient, who was Bethesda V, did not receive surgical intervention. All patients with Bethesda V or VI (9.1%) were found to have papillary thyroid cancer (PTC) on final surgical pathology (Fig. 1 and Additional file 2: Table S1). Seven patients (12.5%) had thyroid cancer (6 PTC, 1 FTC) with pre-operative cytology that was benign or non-diagnostic. Four patients (36.3%) had thyroid cancer (2 PTC, 2 FTC) with pre-operative cytology classified as AUS/FLUS.

An additional FNA sample for ddPCR analysis was obtained for all patients enrolled in this study. Following RNA extraction, mean concentration of nucleic acid obtained per sample was 11.6 µg/ml (3.48 µg total). Nineteen (9.1%) FNA samples did not have adequate amounts of RNA (< 0.001 µg) for ddPCR analysis (Table 2). Of patients who had non-diagnostic pathology (N = 56, 26.9%), 91% (51/56) of samples contained

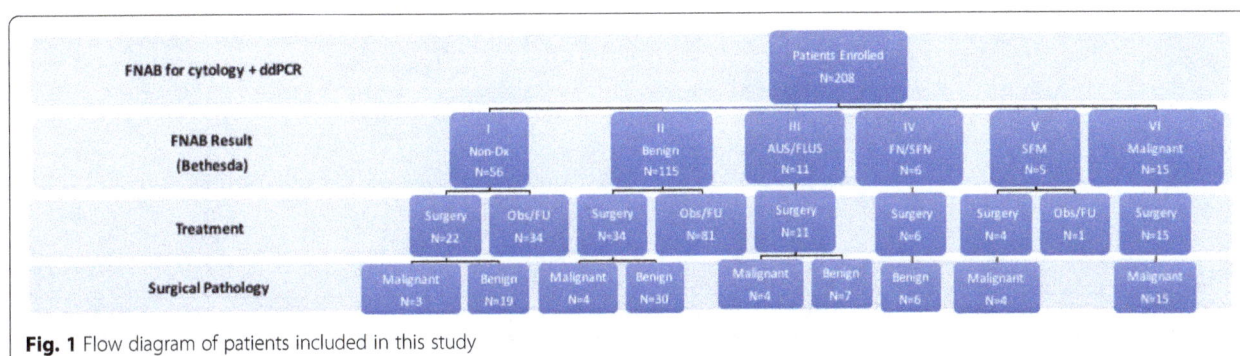

Fig. 1 Flow diagram of patients included in this study

Table 1 Clinicopathologic characteristics of patients with thyroid nodules enrolled in this study

Variable	All (%) N = 208	Bethesda Categories (%)					
		I (non-dx) N = 56	II (benign) N = 115	III (AUS/FLUS) N = 11	IV (FN/SFN) N = 6	V (SFM) N = 5	IV (malignant) N = 15
Age							
Mean	54.8	55.6	54.2	51.2	67.3	52.8	55.5
< 45	22.1	19.6	24.3	27.2	16.7	0	20.0
> 45	77.9	81.8	75.6	72.3	83.3	100.0	80.0
Sex (female)	67.8	23.6	46.2	81.8	50.0	80.0	66.7
Nodule size							
1.0–3.9 cm	90.4	100	86.1	100	66.7	100	86.7
≥4.0 cm	9.6	0	13.9	0	33.3	0	13.3
Sonographic Risk Features							
High	11.3	3.8	8.4	11.1	0	40.0	61.5
Intermediate	25.2	19.2	28.4	44.4	16.7	40.0	7.7
Low	39.7	48.1	38.5	22.2	83.3	0	23.1
Very low	18.0	21.2	18.3	22.2	0	20.0	7.7
Benign	5.6	7.7	6.4	0	0	0	0
Surgery Performed (%)	92 (44.2)	22 (39.2)	34 (29.6)	11 (100)	6 (100)	4 (80)	15 (100)

AUS/FLUS atypia of uncertain significance/follicular lesion of undetermined significance, *FN/SFN* follicular neoplasm/suspicious for follicular neoplasm, *SFM* suspicious for malignancy

sufficient high-quality RNA for ddPCR. Overall, HRASQ61R was the most common mutation identified (19.7%), followed by HRASG12 V (17.3%), NRASQ61R (8.2%), HRASQ61K (6.7%), BRAFV600E (6.7%) and NRASQ61K (1.9%). All patients with SFM or malignant cytology (Bethesda V or VI) harbored at least one mutation in *RAS* or *BRAF*.

In patients who received thyroid surgery, a higher percentage of BRAFV600E mutations was found compared to the entire cohort (15.2% vs 6.7%). All patients with a BRAFV600E mutation were found to have PTC on final pathology (Table 3 and Additional file 2: Table S2). Of these patients, 36% (5/14) also harbored a HRAS mutation (1 HRASG12 V, 4 HRASQR1R). In patients with FTC, 2 *RAS* mutations and no *BRAF* mutations were identified (Additional file 2: Table S2). A lower number of *RAS* mutations was found in patients with thyroid cancer compared to benign pathology (19.5% vs 50.0%). Only 3.2% of patients who received surgery did not have adequate RNA for

Table 2 Distribution of RAS and BRAF mutations identified by ddPCR according to Bethesda classification

Bethesda	Low RNA	HRAS G12 V	HRAS Q61R	HRAS Q61K	NRAS Q61R	NRAS Q61K	BRAF V600E
1-Non Dx N = 56 (26.9)	5	9	6	6	2	1	1
2-Benign N = 115 (55.2)	11	20	28	6	11	2	1
3-FLUS/AUS N = 11 (5.3)	2	2	2	2	1	1	1
4-FN/SFN N = 6 (2.9)	0	1	1	0	1	0	0
5-SFM N = 5 (2.4)	1	1	1	0	1	0	2
6-Malignant N = 15 (7.2)	0	3	3	0	2	0	9
Total (%)	19 (9.1)	36 (17.3)	41 (19.7)	14 (6.7)	18 (8.2)	4 (1.9)	14 (6.7)

Low RNA column indicates FNAB samples with RNA/nucleic acid < 1 ng, not used for ddPCR analysis

Dx diagnostic, *AUS/FLUS* atypia of uncertain significance/follicular lesion of undetermined significance, *FN/SFN* follicular neoplasm/suspicious for follicular neoplasm, *SFM* suspicious for malignancy

Table 3 Distribution of pre-operative fine needle aspirate cytology and ddPCR mutation results in surgical specimen

	Surgical Pathology		
	Benign (%)	Malignant (%)	Total (%)
Cytology (Bethesday)			
I –Non- diagnostic	19 (20.7)	3 (3.2)	22 (23.9)
II - Benign	30 (32.6)	4 (4.3)	34 (40.0)
III – AUS/FLUS	7 (7.6)	4 (4.3)	11 (12.0)
IV – FN/SFN	6 (6.5)	0	6 (6.5)
V - SFM	0	4 (4.3)	4 (6.5)
VI- Malignant	0	15 (16.3)	15 (16.3)
Mutations			
Low RNA	2 (2.2)	1 (1.1)	3 (3.2)
HRASG12 V	14 (15.2)	6 (6.5)	20 (21.7)
HRASQ61R	14 (15.2)	5 (5.4)	19 (20.7)
HRASQ61K	8 (8.7)	1 (1.1)	9 (9.8)
NRASQ61R	6 (6.5)	5 (5.4)	11 (12.0)
NRASQ61K	3 (3.2)	0	3 (3.2)
BRAFV600E	0	14 (15.2)	14 (15.2)

Low RNA column indicates FNAB samples with RNA/nucleic acid < 1 ng, not used for ddPCR analysis
AUS/FLUS atypia of uncertain significance/follicular lesion of undetermined significance, *FN/SFN* follicular neoplasm/suspicious for follicular neoplasm, *SFM* suspicious for malignancy

ddPCR, whereas 23.9% of patients had non-diagnostic cytology (Bethesda I).

Correlative analysis between pre-operative Bethesda classification, RAS/BRAF mutations and final surgical pathology was performed (Fig. 2). The Bethesda classification showed statistically significant correlation with malignant vs benign pathology (0.57, 95% CI 0.41–0.70). BRAFV600E mutation had a slightly higher but similar correlation with surgical pathology results (0.59, 95% CI 0.43–0.71). Individual *RAS* mutations had no significant correlation with pathology, however, combined N/HRASQ61K was negatively correlated with thyroid cancer (– 0.17, 95% CI -0.37 - 0.03, 90% CI -0.34 - -0.004).

The diagnostic performance of Bethesda classification and RAS/BRAF mutation testing is shown in Table 4. Bethesda V/VI was 100% specific and 41.7% sensitive for thyroid cancer. When including all Bethesda categories that could recommend surgical intervention (Bethesda III-VI), specificity is lowered to 70.7% for a 3% improvement in sensitivity (44.7%). BRAFV600E testing provided 100% specificity and 50% sensitivity for the diagnosis of thyroid cancer. Combining the Bethesda system with BRAFV600E, higher sensitivity is achieved (75%) while maintaining 100% specificity. The addition of H/NRASQ61K mutations results in minimal increase in sensitivity (77.8%) and decrease in specificity (98.4%).

Discussion

We describe the first use of ddPCR for the identification of *RAS* and *BRAF* mutations from thyroid FNAB samples. With the addition of a single needle sample taken as part of standard of care FNAB, adequate material for ddPCR mutation analysis was obtained in > 90% of cases. In contrast, 26.9% of FNAB were cytologically non-diagnostic. Consistent with other studies [18], the identification of

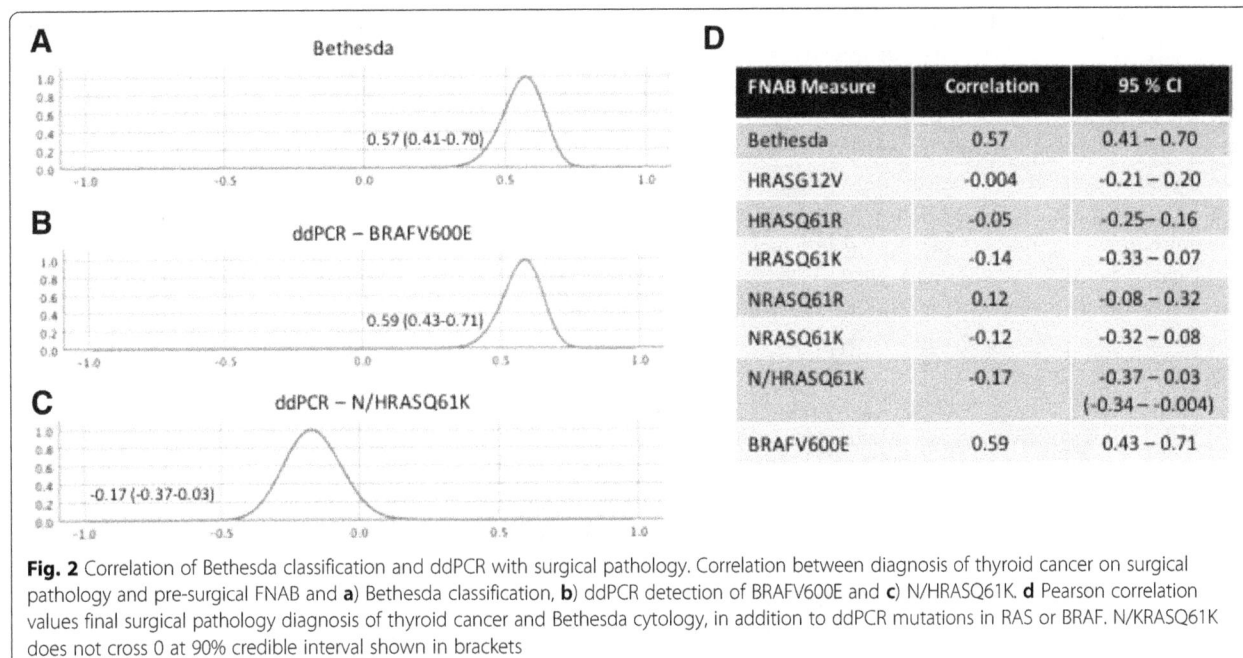

Fig. 2 Correlation of Bethesda classification and ddPCR with surgical pathology. Correlation between diagnosis of thyroid cancer on surgical pathology and pre-surgical FNAB and **a**) Bethesda classification, **b**) ddPCR detection of BRAFV600E and **c**) N/HRASQ61K. **d** Pearson correlation values final surgical pathology diagnosis of thyroid cancer and Bethesda cytology, in addition to ddPCR mutations in RAS or BRAF. N/KRASQ61K does not cross 0 at 90% credible interval shown in brackets

Table 4 Comparative diagnostic performance of pre-operative standard cytology and ddPCR mutation testing

MEASURE	Bethesda III-VI	Bethesda V/VI	BRAFV600E	BRAFV600E + BETHESDA V/VI[b]	BRAFV600E + H/NRASQ61K + Bethesda V/VI
Sensitivity	44.7 (30.2–59.9)	41.7 (27.6–56.8)	50 (30.7–69.4)	75.0 (55.1–89.3)	77.8 (57.7–91.4)
Specificity	70.7 (54.5–83.9)	100 (92.6–100)	100 (94.1–100)	100 (94.1–100)	98.4 (91.3–100)
PPV[a]	63.6 (49.7–75.6)	100	100	100	95.5 (74.8–99.3)
NPV[a]	52.7 (44.6–60.6)	60 (54.1–65.6)	81.3 (75.1–86.3)	89.7 (82.1–94.3)	91 (83.4–95.4)
PLR	1.53 (0.86–2.71)	–	–	–	48.2 (6.8–340.5)
NLR	0.78 (0.6–1.1)	0.6 (0.5–0.8)	0.5 (0.4–0.7)	0.25 (0.1–0.5)	0.2 (0.11–0.5)

NLR negative likelihood ratio, *NPV* negative predictive value, *PLR* positive likelihood ratio, *PPV* positive predictive value
[a]Because the sample sizes in disease positive and disease negative groups may not reflect the true population prevalence of the disease, PPV and NPV may be inaccurate [9]. 95% confidence interval is shown in brackets where appropriate
[b]Combined BRAF and Bethesda V/VI classifies test as positive if BRAFV600E and/or Bethesda V/VI is present

BRAFV600E alone in our cohort was 100% specific for thyroid cancer, with sensitivity comparable to standard cytology. By combining the Bethesda system with BRAFV600E ddPCR testing, the sensitivity of FNAB diagnosis markedly increased while maintaining high specificity. As shown by our group and others, ddPCR analysis can provide rapid results (< 24 h) that are highly reproducible and accurate, requires minimal nucleic acid sample and can be performed at lower cost than standard pathology [6, 11, 13, 14]. BRAFV600E testing by ddPCR circumvents limitations of other currently available molecular tests and therefore has the potential to be of clinical utility. Recent studies in melanoma and colorectal cancer have demonstrated the clinical potential of BRAFV600E testing by ddPCR as a highly accurate and low-cost molecular test [6, 15].

This study aimed to identify somatic mutations most commonly found in well differentiated thyroid cancers, which includes *BRAF* and *RAS*. Using a PCR based approach in a large cohort, Moses et al. suggested *BRAF* and *RAS* mutation testing of FNAB could improve the rate of definitive surgical management [2]. An independent study suggested improved diagnostic accuracy of FNABs could be obtained by molecular profiling of *N/HRAS* and *BRAF* [18]. A more recent study evaluated use of next generation sequencing (NGS) analysis of thyroid nodules compared to surgical pathology in 63 patients (10/63 malignant) [19]. Consistent with our data, *RAS* mutations were commonly found but had low PPV (9%), whereas BRAFV600E had 100% PPV for malignancy. However, given the amount of nucleic acid required and cost of NGS, ddPCR analysis may be a preferred method for FNAB [6].

RAS mutations are the second most common genetic alteration in thyroid cancer, yet their role remains unclear for clinical management. A recent meta-analysis pooling 1025 patients found that *RAS* mutations were 34.3% sensitive and 93.5% specific for the detection of malignancy in indeterminate thyroid FNABs [5]. This study only included Bethesda III-V lesions, excluding thyroid adenomas (Bethesda II, benign) known to harbor *RAS* mutations in 20% to 40% of cases [20]. A literature review of 36 molecular markers used to increase the diagnostic accuracy of thyroid FNAB found that *RAS* mutations had the lowest sensitivity among these [21]. The most recent European Thyroid Association Guidelines state that *RAS* mutations are associated with a higher risk of malignancy but should not be used to dictate more aggressive surgical intervention. Our data are consistent with the literature, identifying a high number of *RAS* mutations in benign disease, with low correlation to malignancy. In our surgical cohort only 10% of malignancies were FTCs, more commonly associated with *RAS* mutations, with the remaining 90% consisting of PTCs, known to have a low association with *RAS*. Given the higher number of follicular adenomas vs carcinomas in our cohort, *RAS* mutations were expectedly higher in the benign vs malignant group. It is possible that in a larger cohort of indeterminate nodules (excluding benign), *RAS* mutation testing by ddPCR could be of predictive value as suggested by others [5].

The Bethesda system for reporting FNA cytology is currently the most widely adopted classification scheme [4]. The 2017 revision confirms this system to be robust, maintaining *status quo* in the six diagnostic categories [22]. For lesions in category V and VI (suspicious for malignancy and malignant), high specificity for malignancy warrants surgical intervention in most cases. Nevertheless, up to 30% of cases may be classified in an "indeterminate" category (III/IV) that requires diagnostic surgery. An estimated 70% to 80% of these cases will be found to have benign pathology following surgery. This is a diagnostic limitation that is associated with a tremendous burden on healthcare utilization and costs. In our study cohort, 76.5% of patients who had indeterminate (III/IV) cytology were found to have benign pathology. In addition, malignant pathology was found in 11.7% of patients who were classified as having benign disease. Although ddPCR results were not used for treatment decisions in this study, our results suggest that BRAFV600E mutation testing could have triaged patients to expedite appropriate surgical care.

In response to the increasing incidence of thyroid nodules and the significant, potentially avoidable, healthcare costs associated with diagnostic thyroid surgery a number of commercial molecular tests have been developed. Among the most commonly utilized tests include the Afirma Gene Expression Classifier (GEC) ($4875, $475 for *BRAF* only), ThyGenX ($1675), ThyraMIR ($3300) and ThyroSeq ($3200) [23]. The Afirma GEC and ThyroSeq have high NPV but low PPV, whereas ThyGenX is thought to have high PPV with low NPV [19, 24]. ThyMIR (when combined with ThyGenX) may provide good NPV and PPV but validation data is limited [23]. The 2015 ATA guidelines suggest the use of molecular testing in specific instances for nodules with Bethesda class III-V, however the level of quality evidence is currently weak to moderate [3, 9]. In terms of heathcare savings, it has been suggested that at a cost of $3200/test, $1453 could be saved on total cost of care. This calculation is based on an assumed number of diagnostic surgeries avoided [4, 23]. In an economic model based on patients with a single indeterminate FNA, it has been estimated that healthcare savings could be obtained if the cost of molecular testing is less than $870/test [25]. Data from our study suggests combining ddPCR BRAFV600E testing with Bethesda cytology results can achieve high PPV (100%) and NPV (89.7%), comparable to other commercially available tests [9, 23]. The estimated cost for ddPCR of BRAFV600E is $20.45/FNAB [14] in addition to standard of care cytologic analysis (Bethesda), which is varies between health care regions. For certain thyroid nodules, ddPCR testing combined with Bethesda grading may be economically advantageous over currently available commercial assays, however further analysis in the context of a clinical utility study would be required.

With the goal of improving FNA diagnostics, research efforts have been predominantly focused on the molecular classification of indeterminate cytology, with little attention paid to the resolution of non-diagnostic (Bethesda I) results [4]. The rate of non-diagnostic FNAB ranges from 2 to 36%, depending on several factors including the sonographic characteristics of a nodule, the technique and experience of the physician obtaining the biopsy, and the experience of the cytopathologist [1, 26, 27]. The rate of non-diagnostic FNAB in our study cohort was 26.9%, similar to an earlier study with a cohort from the same institution (23%) [1]. RNA of sufficient quality was obtained in 91% of non-diagnostic specimen, of which one BRAFV600E mutation was identified in one PTC. Given the known ultrasensitive properties of ddPCR, this may be a useful clinical tool to triage non-diagnostic cytology.

As the first study to investigate the use of ddPCR mutation testing of FNABs, a number of limitations require consideration to address the potential clinical utility of this this test. This is a single centre experience in a tertiary referral clinic consisting of head and neck oncologic surgeons, therefore creating an inherent bias toward patients who are more likely to require surgical intervention. A single centre study is limited in the generalizability of results given that differences in the diagnostic yield of FNAB cytology and molecular testing are known to vary between centres [28]. The sensitivity and specificity calculated in our cohort may be affected by disease prevalence, however unlike PPV and NPV these measures of test performance are most often not affected by prevalence [29]. The performance of ddPCR mutation analysis from FNAB is measured against surgical pathology, however, ddPCR was not done on surgical pathology specimen for comparison. This places some limitation on our understanding of the true performance of ddPCR from an FNA especially in genetically heterogenous tumors where results could be dependent on where the biopsy is being taken. Comparison of pre- and post-surgical samples would be required to further define the analytic validity of ddPCR mutation testing in FNAB. Although this study was conducted over the course of 30 months, the follow-up time may not have been adequate to determine if some patients with *RAS* mutations go on to develop malignancy. In addition, only somatic mutations thought to provide the highest-yield information were included in this study. Given that ddPCR has been shown to be superior to other techniques for the identification of point mutations, primers and/or probes can be designed to develop a multiplex assay that uncovers other mutations as has been done by others. Re-analysis of FNAB samples processed for ddPCR with a larger panel of mutations and long-term follow-up may provide further insight. A larger, multi-institutional study would be an important step in assessing the clinical utility of ddPCR mutation testing as a diagnostic tool for FNAB.

Conclusions

DdPCR offers a novel and ultrasensitive method of detecting *RAS* and *BRAF* mutations from thyroid FNABs. BRAFV600E mutation testing by ddPCR may serve as a useful adjunct to increase sensitivity and specificity thyroid FNAB. Further studies are required to determine the diagnostic utility of ddPCR mutational testing of thyroid FNABs.

Additional files

Additional file 1: Figure S1. Identification of BRAF and RAS mutations by ddPCR. Two-dimensional data outputs showing an example of a A) BRAF^{V600E} positive FNAB sample demonstrating BRAF^{V600E} mutant (FAM+, blue) and BRAF^{WT} (HEX+, green) copies and B) a FNAB sample harboring a NRASQ61K (FAM+, blue, 44 copies), shown compared to NRAS^{WT} (HEX +, green). Only samples containing droplets with clear separation from the baseline and directly vertical to the baseline were considered as positive for the mutation in question. Distribution of mutant probes was as expected, correlating with BIO-RAD data from proprietary assays. Samples only containing droplets at a 45° angle to the baseline (suggestive of containing both mutant and wildtype) were considered as false positives in this study. ddPCR, droplet digital PCR; HEX, hexachloro-fluorescein; FAM, 6-carboxyfluorescein; FNAB, fine needle aspirate biopsy.

Additional file 2: Table S1. Distribution of pre-operative fine needle aspirate cytology results in surgical specimen. **Table S2.** ddPCR mutational profile according to final surgical pathology.

Abbreviations

ATA: American Thyroid Association; AUS/FLUS: Atypia of uncertain significance/follicular lesion of undetermined significance; BRAFV600E: BRAF valine to glutamic acid mutation at residue 600; cDNA: complementary deoxyribonucleic acid; ddPCR: droplet digital polymerase chain reaction; DNA: Deoxyribonucleic acid; DTT: 1,4-dithiothreitol; FAM: 6-carboxyfluorescein; FN/SFN: Follicular neoplasm/suspicious for follicular neoplasm; FTC: Follicular thyroid carcinoma; HEX: Hexachloro-fluorescein; miFTC: minimally invasive follicular thyroid carcinoma; NGS: Next generation sequencing; NLR: Negative likelihood ratio; NPV: Negative predictive value; PLR: Positive likelihood ratio; PPV: Positive predictive value; PTC: Papillary thyroid cancer; RNA: Ribonucleic acid; SFM: Suspicious for malignant cells; WT: Wild type

Funding

Funding for this study was obtained from the Alberta Head and Neck Centre for Oncology and Reconstruction Foundation.

Authors' contributions

VLB was involved in all aspects of experimental design, data collection, data analysis and the primary contributor in manuscript preparation. AM and MK participated in data collection and data analysis. JW participated in data collection. DWC, JH, HS and DAO were involved in data collection and manuscript preparation. All authors read and approved the final manuscript.

Competing interests

The authors declare that they have no competing interests.

Author details

[1]Division of Otolaryngology-Head and Neck Surgery, University of Alberta, 8440-112 st, 1E4 Walter Mackenzie Centre, Edmonton, AB T6G 2B7, Canada. [2]Alberta Head and Neck Centre for Oncology and Reconstruction, Walter MacKenzie Health Sciences Centre, Edmonton, AB, Canada. [3]Faculty of Medicine and Dentistry, Undergraduate Medical Education, University of Alberta, Edmonton, AB, Canada. [4]Otolaryngology-Head and Neck Surgery Research Laboratory of Alberta, University of Alberta, Edmonton, AB, Canada.

References

1. Isaac A, Jeffery CC, Seikaly H, Al-Marzouki H, Harris JR, O'Connell DA. Predictors of non-diagnostic cytology in surgeon-performed ultrasound guided fine needle aspiration of thyroid nodules. J Otolaryngol Head Neck Surg. 2014;43:48. BioMed Central

2. Moses W, Weng J, Sansano I, Peng M, Khanafshar E, Ljung B-M, et al. Molecular testing for somatic mutations improves the accuracy of thyroid fine-needle aspiration biopsy. World J Surg. 2010;34:2589–94. Springer-Verlag

3. Haugen BR, Alexander EK, Bible KC, Doherty GM, Mandel SJ, Nikiforov YE, et al. 2015 American Thyroid Association management guidelines for adult

4. Paschke R, Cantara S, Crescenzi A, Jarzab B, Musholt TJ, Sobrinho SM. European thyroid association guidelines regarding thyroid nodule molecular fine-needle aspiration cytology diagnostics. Eur Thyroid J. 2017;6:115–29. Karger Publishers

5. Clinkscales W, Ong A, Nguyen S, Harruff EE, Gillespie MB. Diagnostic value of RAS mutations in indeterminate thyroid nodules. Otolaryngol Head Neck Surg. 2017;156:472–9.

6. Bidshahri R, Attali D, Fakhfakh K, McNeil K, Karsan A, Won JR, et al. Quantitative detection and resolution of BRAF V600 status in colorectal Cancer using droplet digital PCR and a novel wild-type negative assay. J Mol Diagn. 2016;18:190–204.

7. Lu H-Z, Qiu T, Ying J-M, Lyn N. Association between BRAFV600E mutation and the clinicopathological features of solitary papillary thyroid microcarcinoma. Oncol Lett. 2017;13:1595–600. Spandidos Publications

8. Haugen BR, Sawka AM, Alexander EK, Bible KC, Caturegli P, Doherty GM, et al. American Thyroid Association guidelines on the Management of Thyroid Nodules and Differentiated Thyroid Cancer Task Force Review and recommendation on the proposed renaming of encapsulated follicular variant papillary thyroid carcinoma without invasion to noninvasive follicular thyroid neoplasm with papillary-like nuclear features. Thyroid. 2017;27:481–3. Mary Ann Liebert, Inc. 140 Huguenot Street, 3rd Floor New Rochelle, NY 10801 USA

9. Ferris RL, Baloch Z, Bernet V, Chen A, Fahey TJ, Ganly I, et al. American Thyroid Association statement on surgical application of molecular profiling for thyroid nodules: current impact on perioperative decision making. Thyroid. 2015;25:760–8. Mary Ann Liebert, Inc. 140 Huguenot Street, 3rd Floor New Rochelle, NY 10801 USA

10. Yoo S-K, Lee S, Kim S-J, Jee H-G, Kim B-A, Cho H, et al. Comprehensive analysis of the transcriptional and mutational landscape of follicular and papillary thyroid cancers. PLoS Genet. 2016;12:e1006239. Public Library of Science

11. Bishop JA, Ha PK. Human papillomavirus detection in a "digital" age. Cancer. 2016;122:1502–4.

12. Perkins G, Lu H, Garlan F, Taly V, Droplet-Based Digital PCR. Application in Cancer research. Adv Clin Chem. 2017;79:43–91. Elsevier

13. Biron VL, Kostiuk M, Isaac A, Puttagunta L, O'Connell DA, Harris J, et al. Detection of human papillomavirus type 16 in oropharyngeal squamous cell carcinoma using droplet digital polymerase chain reaction. Cancer. 2016;122:1544–51.

14. Isaac A, Kostiuk M, Zhang H, Lindsay C, Makki F, O'Connell DA, et al. Ultrasensitive detection of oncogenic human papillomavirus in oropharyngeal tissue swabs. J Otolaryngol Head Neck Surg. 2017;46:5. BioMed Central

15. Garlan F, Blanchet B, Kramkimel N, Puszkiel A, Golmard J-L, Noe G, et al. Circulating tumor DNA measurement by Picoliter droplet-based digital PCR and Vemurafenib plasma concentrations in patients with advanced BRAF-mutated melanoma. Target Oncol. 2017;12:365–71.

16. Altman D, Machin D, Bryant T, Gardner M. Statistics with confidence. Hoboken: Wiley; 2013.

17. Mercaldo ND, Lau KF, Zhou XH. Confidence intervals for predictive values with an emphasis to case-control studies. Stat Med. 2007;26:2170–83. John Wiley & Sons, Ltd

18. Decaussin-Petrucci M, Descotes F, Depaepe L, Lapras V, Denier M-L, Borson-Chazot F, et al. Molecular testing of BRAF, RAS and TERT on thyroid FNAs with indeterminate cytology improves diagnostic accuracy. Cytopathology. 2017;28:482–7.

19. Taye A, Gurciullo D, Miles BA, Gupta A, Owen RP, Inabnet WB, et al. Clinical performance of a next-generation sequencing assay (ThyroSeq v2) in the evaluation of indeterminate thyroid nodules. Surgery. 2017;163(1):97–103

20. Gupta N, Dasyam AK, Carty SE, Nikiforova MN, Ohori NP, Armstrong M, et al. RAS mutations in thyroid FNA specimens are highly predictive of predominantly low-risk follicular-pattern cancers. J Clin Endocrinol Metab. 2013;98:E914–22.

21. Rodrigues HGC, DE Pontes AAN, Adan LFF. Use of molecular markers in samples obtained from preoperative aspiration of thyroid. Endocr J. 2012;59:417–24.

22. Cibas ES, Ali SZ. The 2017 Bethesda System for Reporting Thyroid

patients with thyroid nodules and differentiated thyroid Cancer: the American Thyroid Association guidelines task force on thyroid nodules and differentiated thyroid Cancer. Thyroid. 2016;26:1–133. Mary Ann Liebert, Inc. 140 Huguenot Street, 3rd Floor New Rochelle, NY 10801 USA

Cytopathology. Thyroid. 2017;27:1341–6. Mary Ann Liebert, Inc. 140 Huguenot Street, 3rd Floor New Rochelle, NY 10801 USA

23. Zhang M, Lin O. Molecular testing of thyroid nodules: a review of current available tests for fine-needle aspiration specimens. Arch Pathol Lab Med. 2016;140:1338–44. the College of American Pathologists

24. Zhang H-H, Zhang Y, Cheng Y-N, Gong F-L, Cao Z-Q, Yu L-G, et al. Metformin incombination with curcumin inhibits the growth, metastasis, and angiogenesis of hepatocellular carcinoma in vitro and in vivo. Mol Carcinog. 2017;65:87.

25. Yip L, Farris C, Kabaker AS, Hodak SP, Nikiforova MN, McCoy KL, et al. Cost impact of molecular testing for indeterminate thyroid nodule fine-needle aspiration biopsies. J Clin Endocrinol Metab. 2012;97:1905–12.

26. Gill AS, Amdur R, Joshi AS. Importance of FNA technique for decreasing non-diagnostic rates in thyroid nodules. Head Neck Pathol. 2017;19:1167.

27. Poller DN. Value of cytopathologist review of ultrasound examinations in non-diagnostic/unsatisfactory thyroid FNA. Diagn Cytopathol. 2017;45:1084–7.

28. Kay-Rivest E, Tibbo J, Bouhabel S, Tamilia M, Leboeuf R, Forest V-I, et al. The first Canadian experience with the Afirma® gene expression classifier test. J Otolaryngol Head Neck Surg. 2017;46:25. BioMed Central

29. ALTMAN DG. ROC curves and confidence intervals: getting them right. Heart. 2000;83:236–6. Publishing Group Ltd.

22

Multi-dimensional analysis of oral cavity and oropharyngeal defects following cancer extirpation surgery, a cadaveric study

Sherif Idris[1]*[iD], Alex M. Mlynarek[2], Khalid Ansari[1], Jeffrey R. Harris[1], Nabil Rizk[1], David Cote[1], Daniel A. O'Connell[1], Heather Allen[1], Peter Dziegielewski[3] and Hadi Seikaly[1]

Abstract

Background: Defects following resection of tumors in the head and neck region are complex; more detailed and defect-specific reconstruction would likely result in better functional and cosmetic outcomes. The objectives of our study were: 1) to improve the understanding of the two- and three-dimensional nature of oral cavity and oropharyngeal defects following oncological resection and 2) to assess the geometric dimensions and the shapes of fasciocutaneous free flaps and locoregional tissue flaps required for reconstruction of these defects.

Methods: This study was an anatomic cadaveric study which involved creating defects in the oral cavity and oropharynx in two cadaveric specimens. Specifically, partial and total glossectomies, floor of mouth excisions, and base of tongue excisions were carried out. These subsites were subsequently geometrically analyzed and their volumes measured. The two-dimensional (2D) assessment of these three-dimensional (3D) structures included measures of surface area and assessment of tissue contours and shapes.

Results: The resected specimens all demonstrated unique dimensional geometry for the various anatomic sites. Using 2D analysis, hemiglossectomy defects revealed right triangle geometry, whereas total glossectomy geometry was a square. Finally, the base of tongue defects exhibited a trapezoid shape.

Conclusions: Customizing the geometry and dimensions of fasciocutaneous free flaps so that they are specific to the confronted head and neck defects will likely result in better functional and cosmetic outcomes.

Keywords: Oral cavity, Oropharynx, Head and neck, Reconstructive surgery

Background

Fasciocutaneous free flaps, such as radial forearm and anterolateral thigh, are commonly used to reconstruct oral and oropharyngeal anatomy following cancer extirpation surgery [1–7]. Most reconstructive surgeons design these free flaps by visually estimating the size of the defect and using basic geometric shapes, such as rectangles, squares or fusiform shapes, to translate the soft tissue flap into the desired form. However, defects following resection of tumors in the head and neck region are considerably more complex. A more detailed and defect-specific reconstruction would likely result in better functional and cosmetic outcomes.

This study endeavors to improve the understanding of the two-dimensional (2D) and three-dimensional (3D) geometric nature of oral cavity and oropharyngeal defects. An enhanced understanding of the dimensional geometry of surgical defects following

---
* Correspondence: sherif@ualberta.ca
[1]Division of Otolaryngology—Head and Neck Surgery, University of Alberta, 1E4 Walter Mackenzie Center, 8440 112 Street, Edmonton, AB T6G 2B7, Canada
Full list of author information is available at the end of the article

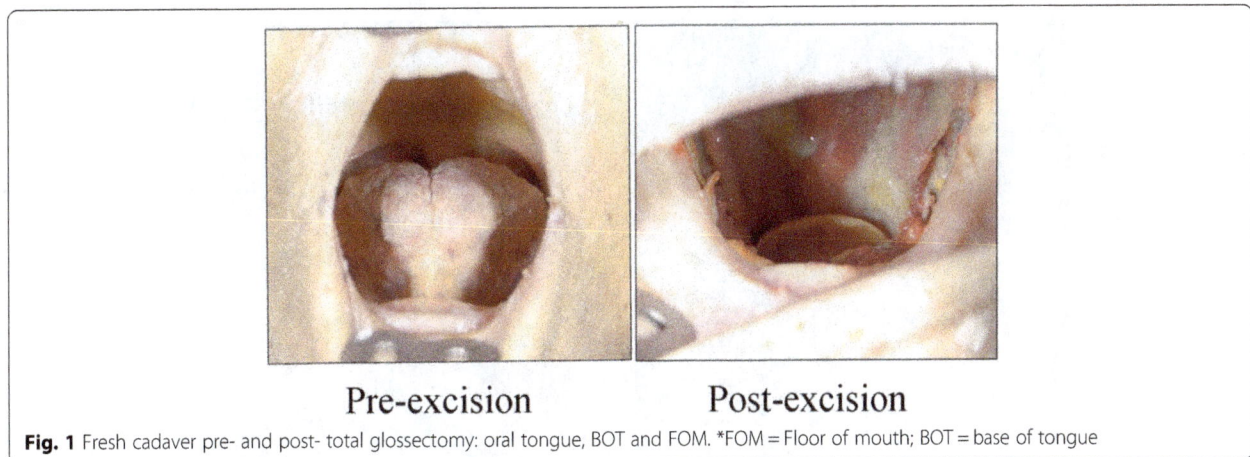

Fig. 1 Fresh cadaver pre- and post- total glossectomy: oral tongue, BOT and FOM. *FOM = Floor of mouth; BOT = base of tongue

cancer extirpation surgery will undoubtedly benefit the reconstructive efforts that utilize free and locoregional tissue transfer.

Methods

Institutional Research Ethics Board approval was obtained prior to commencement of the project. This study was conducted at a tertiary-care centre, the University of Alberta Hospital. Two fresh cadavers, one being an 82-year old, 72 kg male and the other being a 90-year old, 60 kg female underwent total glossectomies (Fig. 1). The specimens were then sectioned into specific subsites: floor of mouth, anterior tongue, and base of tongue. Each specimen was subsequently measured for dimensions, volume, and surface area. De-mucosalizing the tissues and spreading them out on a corkboard allowed us to analyze the 2D shape of each specimen (Fig. 2). The component lengths for each resultant geometric shape were measured (Fig. 3). The volume of each subsite was estimated by placing the specimen in a container filled with water and measuring the amount of displaced liquid (Fig. 4).

Results

The post-excision anterior total glossectomy defect revealed a square shape measuring 8–8 cm, with a volume of about 50 mL. Hemiglossectomy specimens exhibited right triangle geometry, measuring 12–8-8 cm with a volume of 25 mL on average. Hemi-

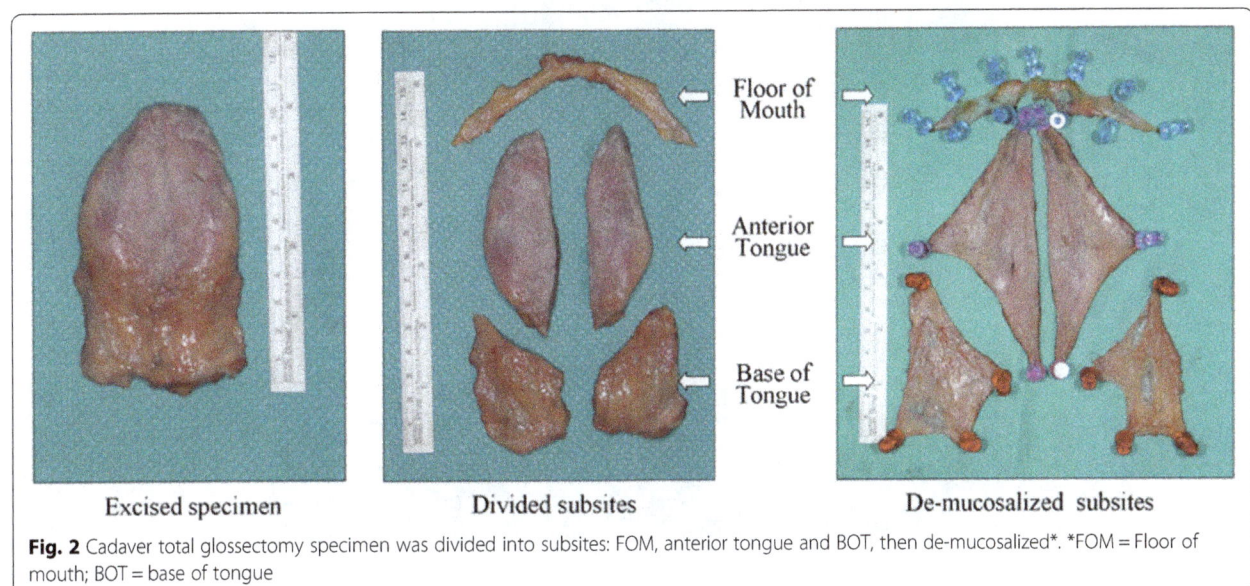

Fig. 2 Cadaver total glossectomy specimen was divided into subsites: FOM, anterior tongue and BOT, then de-mucosalized*. *FOM = Floor of mouth; BOT = base of tongue

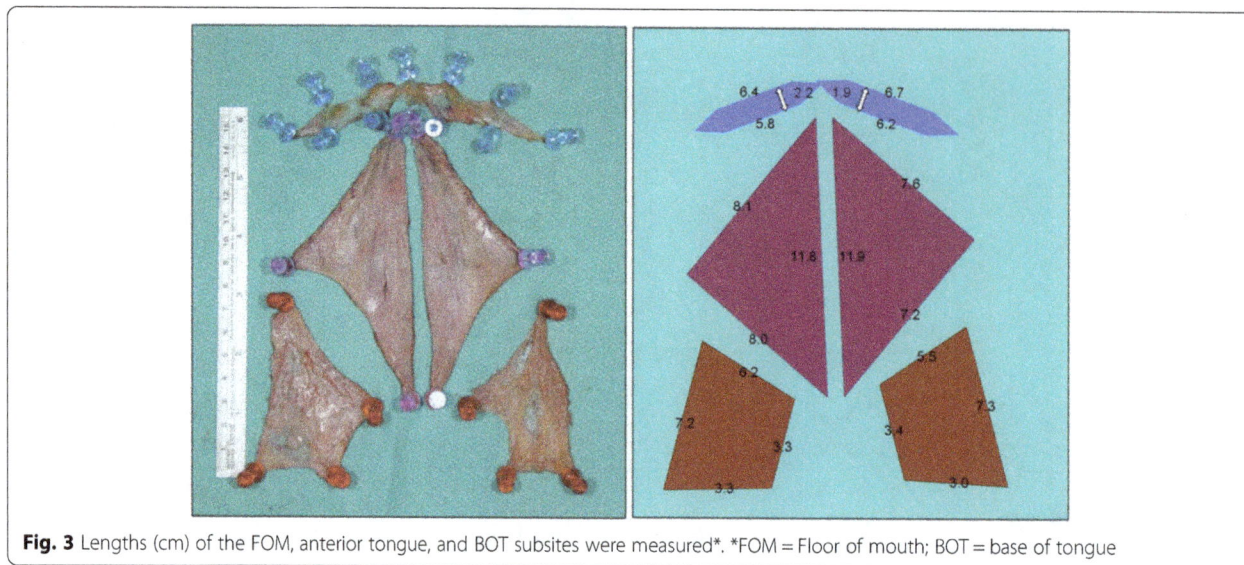

Fig. 3 Lengths (cm) of the FOM, anterior tongue, and BOT subsites were measured*. *FOM = Floor of mouth; BOT = base of tongue

base of tongue specimens revealed a trapezoid shape, measuring an average of 3–3-6-7 cm. There was a high degree of variability in the volume of the base of the tongue, with one cadaver measuring 8 mL and 6 mL for each hemi-base while the other measured 29 mL and 15 mL for each hemi-base. The hemi-floor of mouth specimens were hexagonal in shape, measuring an average of 7 cm in length and

2 cm in width, with a volume of 8.5 mL (Fig. 3). Measurements of specific anatomic structures for each cadaver are highlighted in Tables 1 and 2.

Discussion
Reconstruction of head and neck defects following oncologic resection can be challenging. The surgeon must consider both functional and cosmetic outcomes

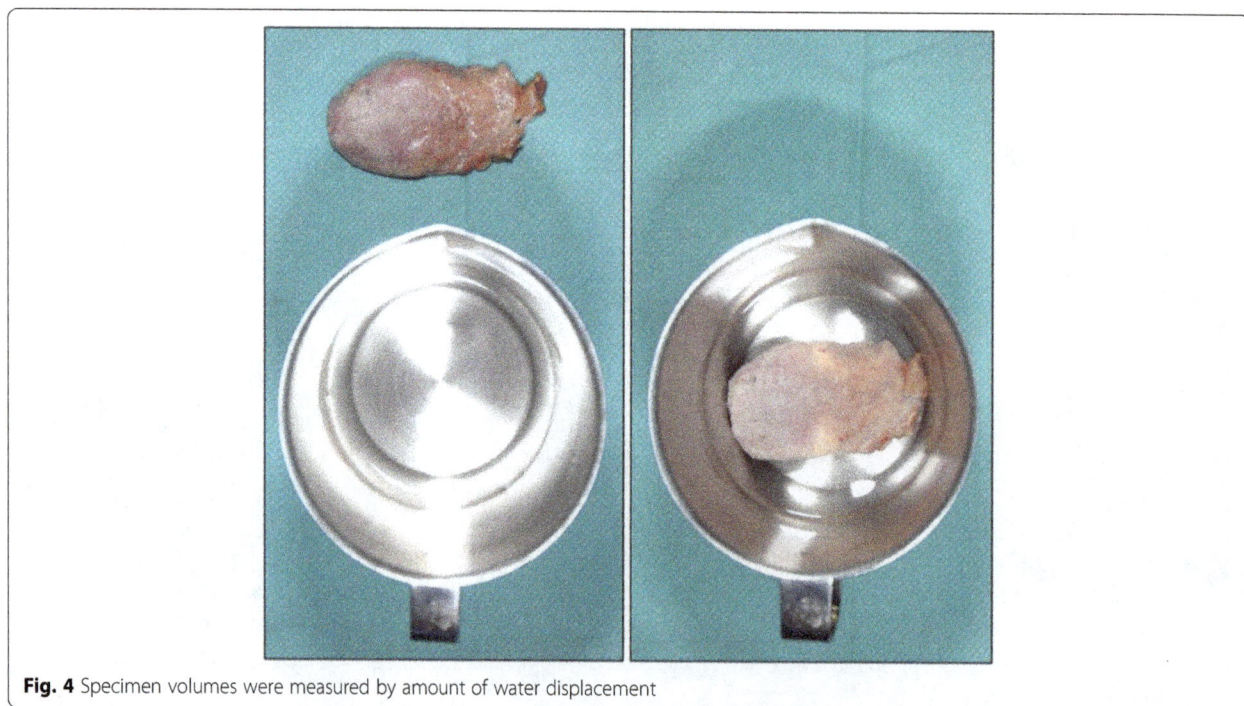

Fig. 4 Specimen volumes were measured by amount of water displacement

Table 2 Measurements from cadaver #2

	Volume (ml)	Height (cm)	Length (cm)	Width (cm)
Tot gloss + BOT + FOM	98	1.75	10.5	6
Tot gloss + BOT	89	1.5	10.5	6
Tot gloss	54	1.5	8	6
Hemi gloss (R)	24	1.5	8	2.5
Hemi gloss (L)	30	1.5	8	3.5
Hemi gloss + BOT (R)	43	1.5	10.5	2.4
Hemi gloss + BOT (L)	46	1.5	10.5	3.2
FOM	9	0.5	7	2
Hemi BOT (R)	29	1.5	2.5	2.8
Hemi BOT (L)	15	1.5	2.5	2.7

Tot gloss total glossectomy, *BOT* base of tongue, *FOM* floor of mouth, *Hemi gloss* hemiglossectomy, *L* left, *R* right

when planning the reconstruction. Swallowing and speech are the chief physiological functions affected by oral and oropharyngeal defects [1, 2, 4, 5, 8, 9]. Numerous reports have been published describing various techniques available to reconstruct these defects [1–3, 10, 11]. Most authors agree that the transfer of a fasciocutaneous free flap is the optimal method for oral cavity and oropharyngeal defect reconstruction. However, considerable debate remains regarding the choice of the donor site and the shape of the flap required for optimal reconstruction. To our knowledge, there are no published anatomical studies that investigate the shape and size of defects and resected tissue following oral and oropharyngeal cancer extirpation surgery.

The results of our study support the practice of creating customized, defect-specific, shaped flaps for oral cavity and oropharyngeal reconstruction after cancer extirpation surgery. For example, the ideal shape to reconstruct a hemiglossectomy defect is a triangle, as we

have shown that the 2D defect with this resection is a right triangle. Similarly, a total glossectomy defect would ideally involve the use of a square free flap, and a base of tongue defect would employ a trapezoid-shaped flap for optimal reconstruction. This study is limited by its study size, involving only two cadavers; it is difficult to draw definitive conclusions regarding exact measurements and volumes necessary for these reconstructions. This should be evaluated on a case-by-case basis, depending largely on amount of tissue resected and the size and weight of the patient. Creation of enough bulk and volume for propulsion of the food bolus, while simultaneously protecting the airway, remains of utmost importance when planning the reconstruction of oral and oropharyngeal defects.

Conclusion

Designing customized fasciocutaneous free flaps that are specifically tailored for the different defects of the oral cavity and oropharynx would likely results in better

Table 1 Measurements from cadaver #1

	Volume (ml)	Height (cm)	Length (cm)	Width (cm)
Tot gloss + BOT + FOM	72	1.75	10.5	6
Tot gloss + BOT	64	1.5	10.5	6
Tot gloss	50	1.5	8	6
Hemi gloss (R)	23	1.5	8	2.5
Hemi gloss (L)	27	1.5	8	3.5
Hemi gloss + BOT (R)	31	1.5	10.5	2.4
Hemi gloss + BOT (L)	33	1.5	10.5	3.2
FOM	8	0.5	7	2
Hemi BOT (R)	8	1.5	2.5	2.8
Hemi BOT (L)	6	1.5	2.5	2.7

Tot gloss total glossectomy, *BOT* base of tongue, *FOM* floor of mouth, *Hemi gloss* hemiglossectomy, *L* left, *R* right

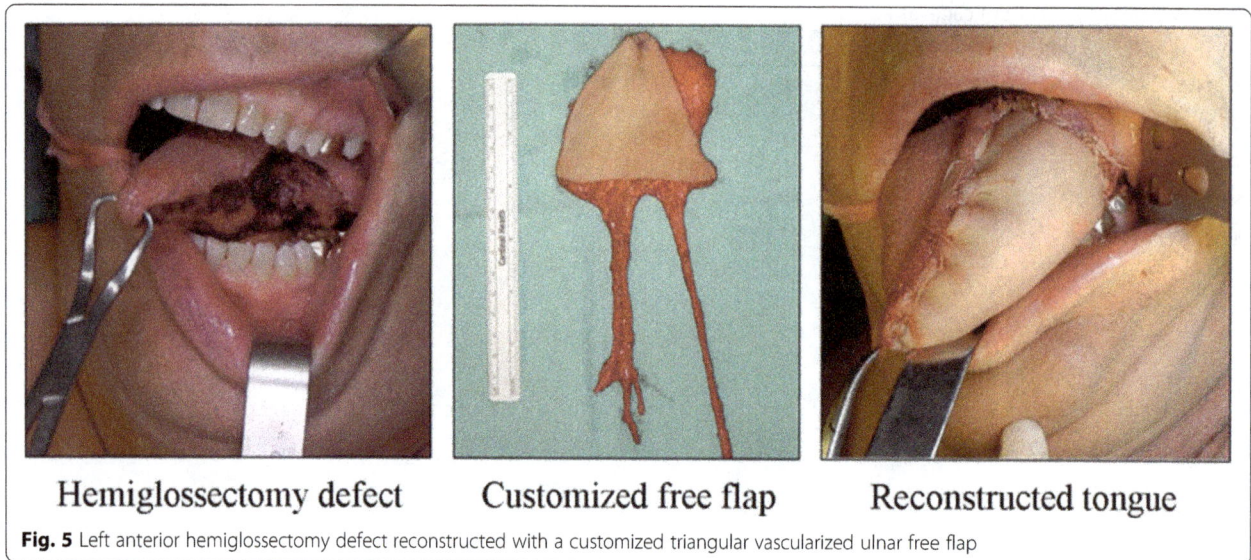

Hemiglossectomy defect   Customized free flap   Reconstructed tongue

Fig. 5 Left anterior hemiglossectomy defect reconstructed with a customized triangular vascularized ulnar free flap

functional and cosmetic outcomes after reconstruction. For example, an anterior hemiglossectomy defect should be reconstructed with a triangular shaped free flap, such as shown in Fig. 5.

Authors' contributions

SI, designed the project idea and protocol, contributed to the data acquisition, analysis and interpretation, drafted the manuscript and reviewed the final version, approved the final version of the manuscript, agreed to be accountable to all aspects of the project; AMM, KA, JRH, NR, DC, DAO, HA, PD and HS, designed the project idea and protocol, contributed to the data acquisition, contributed to the manuscript revision, approved the final manuscript, agreed to be accountable for all aspects of the project.

Competing interests

The authors declare that they have no competing interests.

Author details

[1]Division of Otolaryngology—Head and Neck Surgery, University of Alberta, 1E4 Walter Mackenzie Center, 8440 112 Street, Edmonton, AB T6G 2B7, Canada. [2]Department of Otolaryngology—Head and Neck Surgery, McGill University, Montréal, Quebec, Canada. [3]Department of Otolaryngology—Head and Neck Surgery, University of Florida, Gainesville, Florida, USA.

References

1. Uwiera T, Seikaly H, Rieger J, Chau J, Harris JR. Functional outcomes after Hemiglossectomy and reconstruction with a Bilobed radial forearm free flap. J Otolaryngol. 2004;33:356.
2. Seikaly H, Rieger J, O'Connell D, Ansari K, AlQahtani K, Harris J. Beavertail modification of the radial forearm free flap in base of tongue reconstruction: technique and functional outcomes. Head Neck. 2009;31:213–9.
3. Urken ML, Biller HFA. New Bilobed Design for the Sensate Radial Forearm Flap to preserve tongue mobility following significant Glossectomy. Arch Otolaryngol Head Neck Surg. 1994;120:26–31.
4. Hsiao H-T, Leu Y-S, Liu C-J, Tung K-Y, Lin C-C. Radial forearm versus anterolateral thigh flap reconstruction after Hemiglossectomy: functional assessment of swallowing and speech. J Reconstr Microsurg. 2008;24:85–8.
5. de Vicente JC, de Villalaín L, Torre A, Peña I. Microvascular free tissue transfer for tongue reconstruction after Hemiglossectomy: a functional assessment of radial forearm versus anterolateral thigh flap. J Oral Maxillofac Surg. 2008;66:2270–5.
6. Biron VL, O'Connell DA, Barber B, et al. Transoral robotic surgery with radial forearm free flap reconstruction: case control analysis. J Otolaryngol Head Neck Surg. 2017;46:56–63.
7. Orlik JR, Horwich P, Bartlett C, Trites J, Hart R, Taylor S. Long-term functional donor site morbidity of the free radial forearm flap in head and neck cancer survivors. J Otolaryngol Head Neck Surg. 2014;43:20–7.
8. Kimata Y, Sakuraba M, Hishinuma S, et al. Analysis of the relations between the shape of the reconstructed tongue and postoperative functions after subtotal or Total Glossectomy. Laryngoscope. 2003;113:905–9.
9. Dzioba A, Aalto D, Papadopoulos-Nydam G, et al. Functional and quality of life outcomes after partial glossectomy: a multi- institutional longitudinal study of the head and neck research network. J Otolaryngol Head Neck Surg. 2017;46:59–11.
10. Sakuraba M, Asano T, Miyamoto S, et al. A new flap design for tongue reconstruction after total or subtotal glossectomy in thin patients. J Plast Reconstr Aesthet Surg. 2009;62:795–9.
11. Chepeha DB, Teknos TN, Shargorodsky J, et al. Rectangle tongue template for reconstruction of the Hemiglossectomy defect. Arch Otolaryngol Head Neck Surg. 2008;134:993–8.

23

Effectiveness of skull X-RAY to determine cochlear implant insertion depth

Vinay Fernandes[1†], Yiqiao Wang[2*†] (iD), Robert Yeung[3], Sean Symons[3] and Vincent Lin[1]

Abstract

Background: Cochlear implant (CI) insertion depth can affect residual hearing preservation, tonotopic range coverage, and Mapping. Therefore, determining insertion depth has the potential to maximize CI performance. A post-op skull X-RAY is commonly used to assess insertion depth, however its effectiveness has not been well established. Our primary objective was to assess the accuracy of post-op skull X-RAYs to determine insertion depth, compared to CT as the gold standard. Secondary objectives were to compare experience level of raters and different skull X-RAY views.

Methods: Thirteen patients with Advanced Bionic HiRes 90 K implants, and post-operative temporal bone CT scans were selected from the CI database at Sunnybrook Health Sciences Centre. Medical students, otology fellows, and CI surgeons evaluated insertion depths on post-op skull X-RAYs, while neuroradiologists evaluated CT scans. Descriptive statistics, regression analysis, and paired t-tests were used to compare the two types of imaging.

Results: X-RAYs and CTs provided an equivalent mean insertion depth of 337 degrees ($p = 0.93$), a mean difference of − 0.9 degrees and a standard deviation of paired differences of 43 degrees. Although means were similar across rater groups, CI surgeons (45 degrees) had the lowest standard deviation of paired differences. Comparing X-RAY views, Caldwell (29 degrees) had less variation than Towne (59 degrees) for standard deviation of paired differences.

Conclusions: Skull X-RAYs provide accurate and reliable measurements for CI insertion depth. The Caldwell view alone may be sufficient for evaluations of insertion depth, and experience has a minor impact on the variability of estimates.

Keywords: Cochlear implant, Insertion depth, CT, X-RAY

Background

The cochlear implant (CI) converts acoustic energy into electrical stimuli, bypassing hair cells to directly stimulate spiral ganglion neurons using a series of platinum electrodes [1]. CIs with longer electrode arrays that are inserted deeper and closer to the apex of the cochlea can potentially increase tonal range [2]. With greater insertion depth, hearing perception, including Hearing In Noise and Consonant Nucleus Consonant test scores appear to improve in some studies [3–5]. Conversely, deeper insertion can also increase iatrogenic injury to the cochlea, leading to decreased hearing preservation [6]. Although "soft surgery" techniques involving use of corticosteroids, and scala tympani insertion can minimize this damage, shallower insertion depths are still associated with a lower rate of iatrogenic injury [6–9].

Previously it was believed that CI surgery would destroy all residual hearing. It is now accepted that hearing preservation is possible, and should be maximized [6, 10].

Imaging post-operatively to determine CI electrode insertion depth and placement may vary greatly and include Computerized Topography (CT) or skull X-RAY [11–13]. CT is a highly accurate technique physicians currently utilize and can be reconstructed to yield 3D high-resolution data to determine electrode position [12, 14–16]. More commonly, immediate post-operative skull X-RAYs are performed following CI surgery at implant centres. At Sunnybrook Health Sciences Centre (SHSC), our patients undergo a routine three-view series of X-RAYs often the night of their surgery, or occasionally the day afterwards. These X-RAYs help confirm appropriate electrode placement within the cochlea including insertion depth, as well as identify kinking, squeeze, and integrity of the electrode [12].

* Correspondence: Dwang101@uottawa.ca
†Vinay Fernandes and Yiqiao Wang contributed equally to this work.
²Faculty of Medicine, University of Ottawa, Ottawa, Canada
Full list of author information is available at the end of the article

Although skull X-RAYs are commonly used in practice for CIs, and many studies have used X-RAYs to determine insertion depth, accuracy of skull X-RAYs have not been fully established. Furthermore, few studies have compared skull X-RAYs to other modalities for insertion depth estimates [13, 17]. Our primary objective was to evaluate the accuracy of post-op skull X-RAYs to determine insertion depth when compared to CT. Comparison of insertion depths by experience level, and by different X-RAY views were assessed in a secondary analysis.

Methods

Study population

Institutional Research Ethics Board approval was obtained. Patients from 2003 to 2009 were selected from an existing database of CIs at SHSC. We included adults (≥18 years old) who had a post-operative CT scan of their temporal bones. CT scans were only provided for the unique circumstance of being considered for a second contralateral CI. Only Advanced Bionic HiRes 90 K implants were included; this eliminated the potential variable of more than one type of electrode being studied [18]. Patients were excluded if they already had other types of CIs, or were missing a postoperative skull Caldwell or Towne view in their X-RAY series. The Stenvers view was not available for most patients and was therefore not assessed.

Skull X-RAY imaging

Skull X-RAYs were obtained from the SHSC system. All skull X-RAYs were performed within 24 h of surgery. The Caldwell and Towne views were optimized in the radiology suite by the principle investigator to provide best face value images of the implants. De-identified images were presented on PowerPoint (Microsoft ©) and all images were randomized using a random number generator. Rater participants included medical students, otology fellows, and CI surgeons. All groups were instructed to estimate CI insertion depth in degrees based on post-op skull X-RAYs. We used the round window as the zero degree standard [16].

CT imaging

Two experienced neuroradiologists at our institution interpreted the actual degree of insertion using CTs. CT images of temporal bones were reviewed in sequence. Degree of insertion was rated on a 360° scale. Neuroradiologists were blinded to previous CT reports, and patient IDs were removed to eliminate detection bias.

Statistical analysis

Statistical analysis was performed using SPSS software ©. Inter-rater reliability between neuroradiologists as well as between-rater groups was determined using intra-class correlations (ICC). Skull X-RAY insertion depth estimates were compared to CT using descriptive statistics, regression analysis, and paired t-tests. A p-value of < 0.05 was used for statistical significance.

Results

Demographics

In total, we selected 13 patients who underwent CT scans of their temporal bones following cochlear

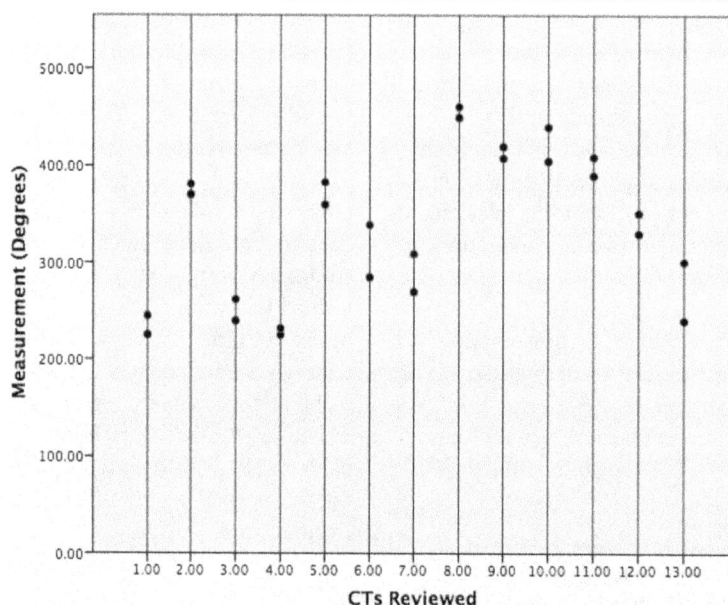

Fig. 1 Dot plot of neuroradiologist agreement. Intra-Class Coefficient = 0.962, 95% confidence interval is between 0.549 and 0.990

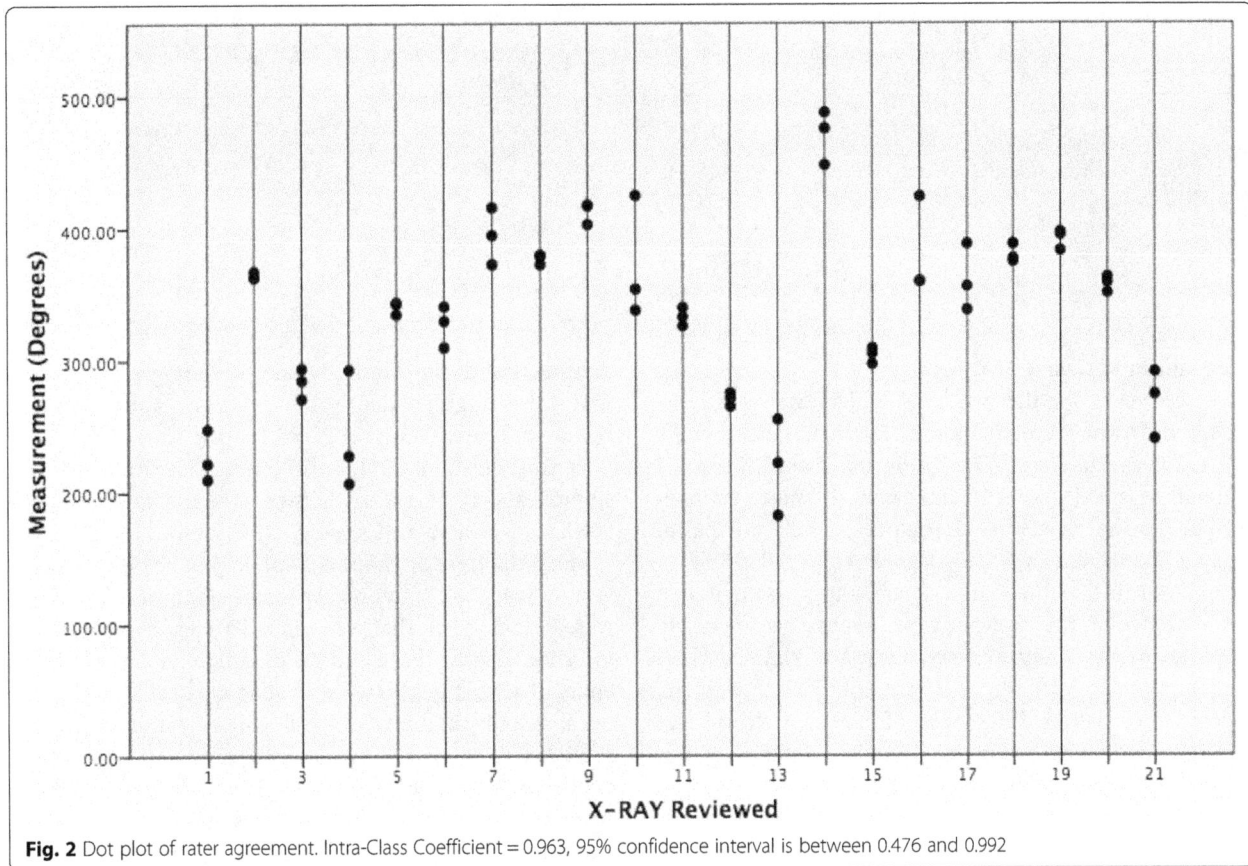

Fig. 2 Dot plot of rater agreement. Intra-Class Coefficient = 0.963, 95% confidence interval is between 0.476 and 0.992

implantation. These patients had 21 skull X-RAYs, including 12 Caldwell views and 9 Towne views available for comparison. Two CI surgeons, four otology fellows, and seven medical students participated in skull X-RAY insertion depth estimations, providing a total of 273 X-RAY estimates.

Comparison of skull X-RAY to CT

ICC Coefficients showed a high reliability of estimates between neuroradiologists (ICC = 0.962, Fig. 1) and between raters (ICC = 0.963, Fig. 2). Mean X-RAY insertion depth estimates were equivalent to mean CT insertion depth estimates at 337 degrees. Mean difference was – 0.9° (95% confidence interval – 20.6 to 18.8) and the standard deviation of paired differences was 43° (Tables 1 and 2). The estimated X-RAY insertion depths correlate with CT without significant differences between estimations (p = 0.93). The linear regression was inversely proportional, representing an underestimation on skull X-RAY for insertions higher than 360°, and an overestimation for insertions lower than 360° (Fig. 3).

Impact of rater experience

The three rater groups, medical students, otology fellows, and CI surgeons, were analyzed individually for the correlation of their skull X-RAY estimates to CTs. Estimations from the seven medical students resulted in a mean of 335° (p = 0.83), a mean difference of – 2.2° and standard deviation of paired differences of 47° (Tables 1 and 2). Estimations from the four fellows resulted in a mean of 341° (p = 0.76), a mean difference of 3.2°, and a standard deviation of paired differences of 49° (Tables 1 and 2). Similarly, the six CI surgeons had a mean of 335° (p = 0.84), a mean difference of – 2.0 degrees, and a standard deviation of paired differences of 45° (Tables 1 and 2). Paired differences of the rater groups were represented on box plots (Fig. 4).

Table 1 Group means and standard deviations

Group	Mean (degrees)	Standard deviation (degrees)
CI surgeons	335	65
Fellows	341	63
Medical students	335	76
All raters	337	67
Caldwell	323	70
Towne	351	86
CT	337	79

Table 2 X-RAY versus CT insertion depth estimates

Group	Standard deviation of paired differences (degrees)	Mean difference (degrees)	Maximum difference (degrees)	Minimum difference (degrees)	P-value
CI surgeons	45	−2.0	99	−68	0.84
Fellows	49	3.2	112	−83	0.76
Medical students	47	−2.2	100	−78	0.83
All raters	43	−0.9	93	−75	0.93
Caldwell	29	−5.8	40	−57	0.51
Towne	59	5.7	93	−75	0.78

Comparison of skull X-RAY views

Rater estimates for the two skull X-RAY views of Caldwell and Towne were compared. The mean estimate for the Caldwell view was 323°, while the paired mean CT estimate was 333° ($p = 0.51$). Likewise, the mean estimate for the Towne view was 351 degrees, while the paired mean CT estimate was 343 degrees ($p = 0.78$, Table 1). Compared to CT, the Caldwell view appears to underestimate while the Towne view appears to overestimate. Although mean differences are similar, there was a sizeable difference when comparing standard deviation of paired differences (Table 2). Caldwell (29 degrees) provided a more precise estimate than Towne view (59°) (Table 3).

Discussion

CI insertion depth has become an important metric to quantify in cochlear implant patients. Accurate determination may potentially impact on implant performance including mapping parameters. However, few studies have discussed the effectiveness of X-RAYs post-operatively. One study by Syrakic et al.,

demonstrated the strength of the radiograph to estimate the angular depth of insertion, and used CT scans to assess error on X-RAY. Our study adds support to their findings for the efficacy of skull X-RAYs, shows validity at a Canadian centre, and evaluates differences by rater and skull X-RAY views [13, 17].

Mean differences showed skull X-RAY estimates to be very similar to CT, and no statistical significant differences were found. Given that we used a 360-degree scale to rate insertion depth, the standard deviation of paired differences of 43 degrees between the two types of imaging supports a low variability of skull X-RAY estimations. Our skull X-RAY estimates were less accurate as CI insertion depths move further from 360 degrees. Therefore, skull X-RAYs may not be as useful for insertion depths that are extremely deep or shallow. This may become problematic, as the extremes in insertion depth likely have the greatest impact on CI performance.

At our centre, Caldwell and Towne skull X-RAY views are commonly used for patients post CI surgery. Our study suggests the Caldwell view is less variable than the Towne view for estimating electrode insertion depth,

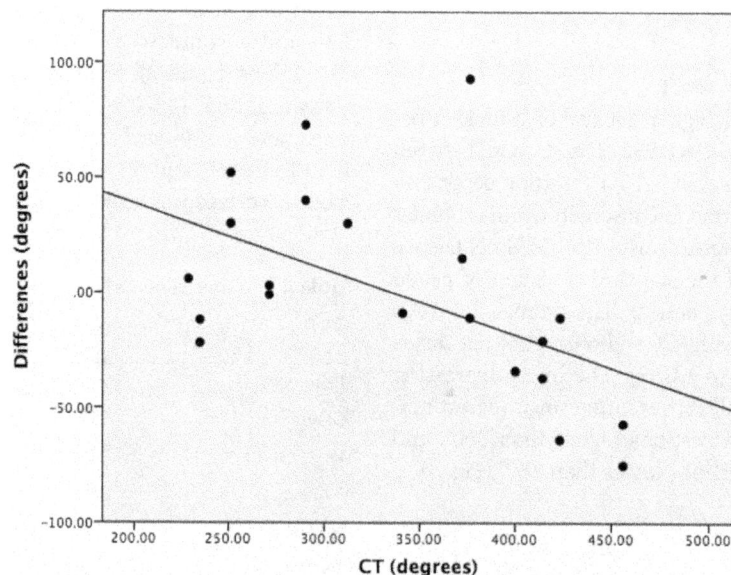

Fig. 3 Differences between X-RAY and CT insertion depths. Absolute differences increase as insertion depth deviates from 360 degrees

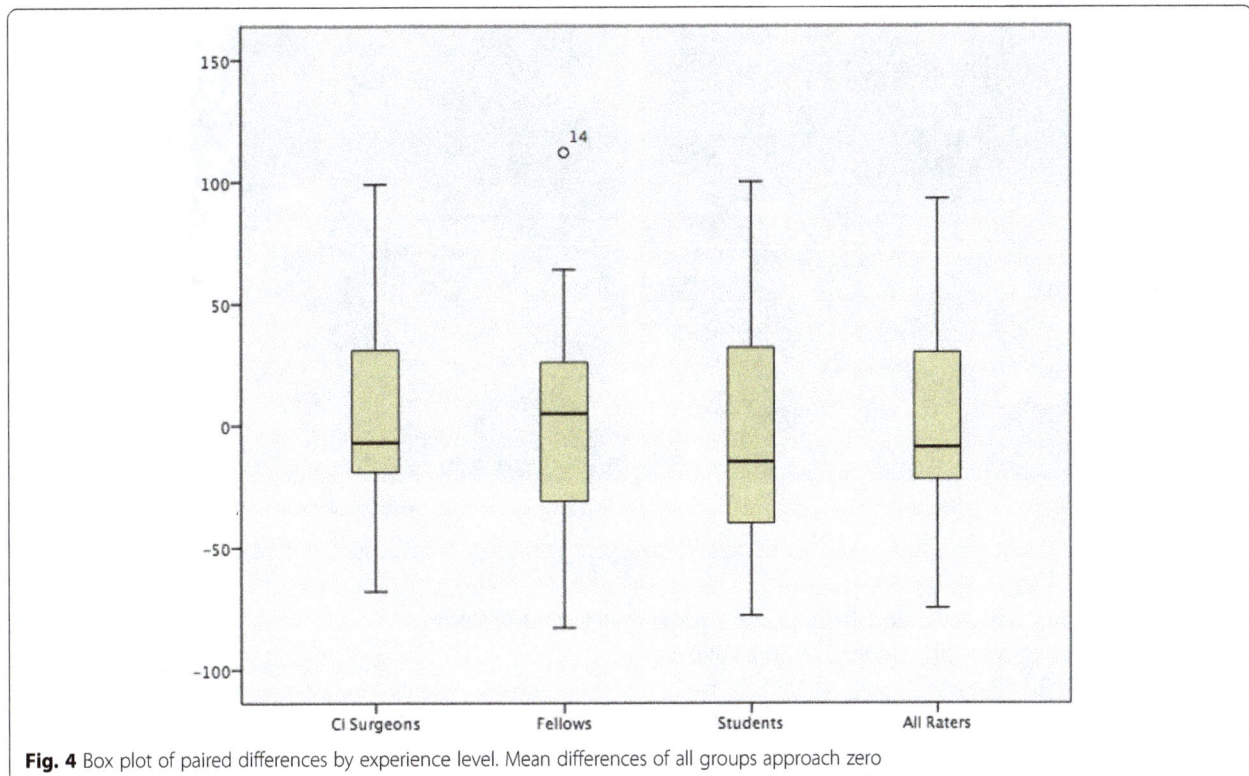

Fig. 4 Box plot of paired differences by experience level. Mean differences of all groups approach zero

and therefore the Towne view may not be required post-op. Caldwell is a less angled anteroposterior view, allowing for easier visualization of the cochlear spiral, facilitating identification of 360°. If 360° can be identified, raters can easily add or subtract from that value (Fig. 5). A decrease in the number of skull X-RAYs used would decrease radiation and time, as well as lower hospital costs [19].

Rater experience may have a minor influence on the variability of skull X-RAY estimates. Although mean differences are similar, CI surgeons provided slightly lower standard deviation of paired differences than the other groups. However, their ratings were not much different from medical students when examining the Caldwell view alone (Table 3). This may be due to our low sample size for the specific skull X-RAY views. Due to the high accuracy of our rater estimates, this study brings into question the need for insertion depth estimates by radiologists. A post-hoc analysis of neuroradiologist insertion depth estimates on skull X-RAY demonstrated a mean of 343°, and a p-value of 0.79 when compared to CT. These values are highly comparable to our rater estimates.

Our results have important implications practically as skull X-RAYs provide many advantages compared to CTs. X-RAYs are less costly for institutions, easier to access, more comfortable for patients, and provide substantially less radiation. However, one disadvantage is the inability of skull X-RAYs to demonstrate intracompartmental placement.

There were a few limitations to this study. Firstly, only 13 patients with post-op CTs were included. At our centre, patients are typically given skull X-RAYs alone post-operatively to assess electrode insertion depth. In addition, CTs were only provided to patients who required a second contralateral CI, which may be a source of selection bias. There was also a delay between taking X-RAY and CT images for several patients of 1 to 2 years. During this time, the electrode may have migrated affecting the accuracy of direct comparisons [20]. Lastly, the Stenvers view was not routinely available for our patients and was not assessed. However, this view is commonly used in cochlear implantation studies to assess insertion depth [12, 21, 22].

Due to the recent influx of studies evaluating the impact of insertion depth, revision surgery for insertion depth may be an important area of future study. There is no indication in the literature that post-op imaging of CIs significantly alters management. Coombs et al. reported no immediate revisions after 220 CI cases [11]. However, in our experience revision surgery is

Table 3 Standard deviation of paired differences (Degrees)

X-RAY view	Surgeons	Fellows	Students	All raters
Caldwell	33	38	30	29
Towne	58	63	64	58

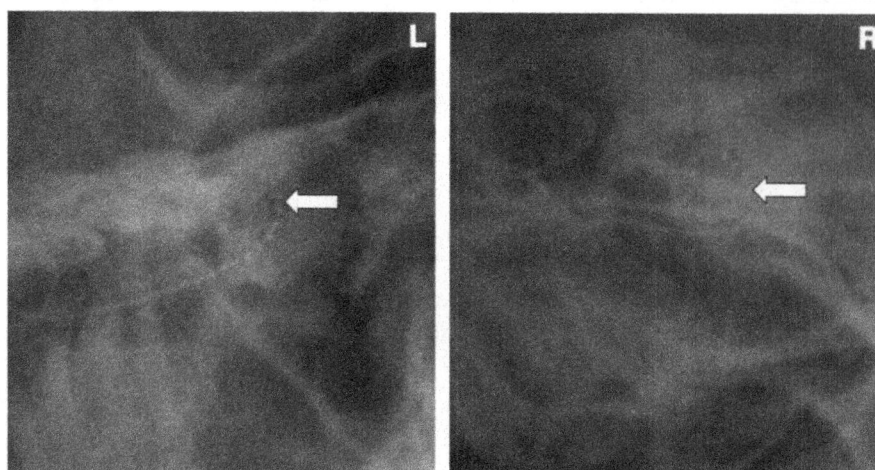

Fig. 5 Left Caldwell and right Towne views. Arrows are pointing to electrode position. Notice an easier visualization of the electrode spiral on the Caldwell view

usually required prior to activation if there were gross abnormalities in electrode placement (i.e. tip rollover, insertion into vestibule, significant electrode extrusion), and insertion depth has the potential to be included as well.

Further studies should include prospective trials to evaluate insertion depth, and also focus on determining optimal CI insertion depths to maximize hearing preservation. Pelliccia et al. suggested an insertion depth of 270° to optimize sound perception while minimizing cochlear trauma. Similarly, Nayak et al. suggested in the pediatric population, optimal hearing outcomes are observed with insertion depths of 270° to 360° [21, 23]. Once optimal insertion depths are determined, techniques to intra-operatively assess and change electrode depth will become important. This can be achieved by using landmarks on the array, which can then be monitored with post-operative X-RAY [23].

Conclusions

Skull X-RAYs provide accurate measurements of CI insertion depth, supporting their use in the post-operative setting. In addition, the Caldwell view alone may be sufficient for evaluations of insertion depth, and experience has a minor impact on the variability of estimates.

Abbreviations
CI: Cochlear Implant; CT: Computerized Topography; ICC: intra-class correlation; SHSC: Sunnybrook Health Sciences Centre

Funding
Sunnybrook Health Sciences Centre provided the necessary funding, and no additional sources of funding were required.

Author's contributions
VF created objectives and study design, collected data, interpreted results, wrote part of manuscript. YW wrote manuscript, analyzed data, and interpreted the results. RY Analyzed the CTs and X-RAYs. SS Analyzed the CTs and X-RAYs. VL determined study objectives and was the content expert. All authors read and approved the final manuscript.

Competing interests
The authors declare that they have no competing interests.

Author details
[1]Division of Otolaryngology – Head and Neck Surgery, Faculty of Medicine, University of Toronto, Toronto, Canada. [2]Faculty of Medicine, University of Ottawa, Ottawa, Canada. [3]Division of Radiology, Faculty of Medicine, University of Toronto, Toronto, Canada.

References
1. Yawn R, Hunter JB, Sweeney AD, Bennett ML. Cochlear implantation: a biomechanical prosthesis for hearing loss. F1000Prime Rep. 2015;7:45.
2. Roy AT, Penninger RT, Pearl MS, Wuerfel W, Jiradejvong P, Carver C, Buechner A, Limb CJ. Deeper Cochlear implant electrode insertion angle improves detection of musical sound quality deterioration related to bass frequency removal. Otol Neurotol. 2016;37(2):146–51.
3. Hamzavi J, Arnoldner C. Effect of deep insertion of the cochlear implant electrode array on pitch estimation and speech perception. Acta Otolaryngol. 2006;126(11):1182–7.
4. Hilly O, Smith L, Hwang E, Shipp D, Symons S, Nedzelski JM, Chen JM, Lin VY. Depth of Cochlear implant Array within the cochlea and performance outcome. Ann Otol Rhinol Laryngol. 2016;125(11):886–92.
5. O'Connell BP, Hunter JB, Haynes DS, Holder JT, Dedmon MM, Noble JH, Dawant BM, Wanna GB. Insertion depth impacts speech perception and hearing preservation for lateral wall electrodes. Laryngoscope. 2017;127(10):2352–7.
6. Suhling MC, Majdani O, Salcher R, Leifholz M, Buchner A, Lesinski-Schiedat A, Lenarz T. The impact of electrode Array length on hearing preservation in Cochlear implantation. Otol Neurotol. 2016;37(8):1006–15.
7. Bruce IA, Bates JE, Melling C, Mawman D, Green KM. Hearing preservation via a cochleostomy approach and deep insertion of a standard length cochlear implant electrode. Otol Neurotol. 2011;32(9):1444–7.
8. Gifford RH, Dorman MF, Skarzynski H, Lorens A, Polak M, Driscoll CL, Roland P, Buchman CA. Cochlear implantation with hearing preservation yields

significant benefit for speech recognition in complex listening environments. Ear Hear. 2013;34(4):413–25.

9. Hochmair I, Hochmair E, Nopp P, Waller M, Jolly C. Deep electrode insertion and sound coding in cochlear implants. Hear Res. 2015;322:14–23.

10. Carlson ML, Driscoll CL, Gifford RH, Service GJ, Tombers NM, Hughes-Borst BJ, Neff BA, Beatty CW. Implications of minimizing trauma during conventional cochlear implantation. Otol Neurotol. 2011;32(6):962–8.

11. Coombs A, Clamp PJ, Armstrong S, Robinson PJ, Hajioff D. The role of post-operative imaging in cochlear implant surgery: a review of 220 adult cases. Cochlear Implants Int. 2014;15(5):264–71.

12. Vogl TJ, Tawfik A, Emam A, Naguib NN, Nour-Eldin A, Burck I, Stover T. Pre-, intra- and post-operative imaging of Cochlear implants. Rofo. 2015;187(11):980–9.

13. Aschendorff A. Imaging in cochlear implant patients. GMS Curr Top Otorhinolaryngol Head Neck Surg. 2011;10:Doc07.

14. Schuman TA, Noble JH, Wright CG, Wanna GB, Dawant B, Labadie RF. Anatomic verification of a novel method for precise intrascalar localization of cochlear implant electrodes in adult temporal bones using clinically available computed tomography. Laryngoscope. 2010;120(11):2277–83.

15. Trieger A, Schulze A, Schneider M, Zahnert T, Murbe D. In vivo measurements of the insertion depth of cochlear implant arrays using flat-panel volume computed tomography. Otol Neurotol. 2011;32(1):152–7.

16. Colby CC, Todd NW, Harnsberger HR, Hudgins PA. Standardization of CT depiction of cochlear implant insertion depth. AJNR Am J Neuroradiol. 2015;36(2):368–71.

17. Svrakic M, Friedmann DR, Berman PM, Davis AJ, Roland JT, Svirsky MA. Measurement of Cochlear implant electrode position from intraoperative post-insertion skull radiographs: a validation study. Otol Neurotol. 2015; 36(9):1486–91.

18. Kos MI, Boex C, Sigrist A, Guyot JP, Pelizzone M. Measurements of electrode position inside the cochlea for different cochlear implant systems. Acta Otolaryngol. 2005;125(5):474–80.

19. Hassan AM, Patel R, Redleaf M. Intra-operative skull X-ray for misdirection of the cochlear implant array into the vestibular labyrinth. J Laryngol Otol. 2015;129(9):923–7.

20. van der Marel KS, Verbist BM, Briaire JJ, Joemai RM, Frijns JH. Electrode migration in cochlear implant patients: not an exception. Audiol Neurootol. 2012;17(5):275–81.

21. Nayak G, Panda NK, Banumathy N, Munjal S, Khandelwal N, Saxena A. Deeper insertion of electrode array result in better rehabilitation outcomes - do we have evidence? Int J Pediatr Otorhinolaryngol. 2016;82:47–53.

22. Louza J, Mertes L, Braun T, Gurkov R, Krause E. Influence of insertion depth in cochlear implantation on vertigo symptoms and vestibular function. Am J Otolaryngol. 2015;36(2):254–8.

23. Pelliccia P, Venail F, Bonafe A, Makeieff M, Iannetti G, Bartolomeo M, Mondain M. Cochlea size variability and implications in clinical practice. Acta Otorhinolaryngol Ital. 2014;34(1):42–9.

24

Re-visiting the ATA 2015 sonographic guidelines - who are we missing?

D. S. Chan[1]*[iD], K. Gong[2], M. G. Roskies[1], V. I. Forest[1], M. P. Hier[1] and R. J. Payne[1]

Abstract

Background: The American Thyroid Association published revised guidelines in 2015 on the management of differentiated thyroid cancer in adults. One of the key changes introduced in the revision proposes that diagnostic biopsy be based on ultrasound findings (i.e. size and nodule characteristics). The overall effect of these changes results in fewer nodules requiring biopsy. This study was conducted to determine if the changes to the guidelines will result in overlooked thyroid cancers, specifically malignancies with aggressive characteristics measuring between 1 and 1.49 cm.

Methods: Patients ($n = 2083$) with thyroid nodules who underwent total or subtotal/hemi thyroidectomy with or without neck dissection by a single surgeon between 2006 and 2016 were retrospectively enrolled. Demographic information and nodule characteristics were collected for all patients. Ultrasonography and final pathology reports were reviewed for patients with thyroid nodules between the sizes of 1–1.49 cm ($n = 155$).

Results: 45% ($n = 70$) of patients with nodules between 1 and 1.49 cm were "low suspicion" nodules according to ultrasound. 47 of these nodules contained malignancies on final histopathological examination, 100% of which were of the papillary subtype. 21% ($n = 10$) of these malignant nodules demonstrated extrathyroidal extension and 34% ($n = 16$) were associated with regional metastases.

Conclusions: Reliance on sonographic patterns alone could result in missed cancer diagnoses in patients with thyroid nodules measuring between 1 and 1.49 cm. Moreover, a portion of these malignancies may be associated with aggressive features. The effect of this finding on long-term outcomes is unclear.

Keywords: Thyroid nodule, Thyroid Cancer, FNAB, Ultrasound

Background

Thyroid nodules are a common presenting problem, detectable in up to 68% of the general population [1, 2]. Recent epidemiological studies show that the incidence of true thyroid cancer diagnoses is on the rise, nearly tripling in the last thirty years [3]. Thyroid sonography is an inexpensive and noninvasive test that is performed in patients with thyroid nodules. Certain ultrasound characteristics have been well-established as predictors of malignancy, including the presence of microcalcifications, nodule hypoechogenicity, irregular nodule borders,

and a taller-than-wider shape [4]. These findings are then used to stratify the risk of malignancy and aid in decision-making regarding the necessity for more invasive investigations like ultrasound fine needle aspiration (USFNA).

The American Thyroid Association (ATA) published revised guidelines for the management of differentiated thyroid cancer in 2015 [4]. One of the key changes introduced in the revision proposes that diagnostic biopsy be based on ultrasound findings (i.e. size and nodule characteristics). The diversion from recommendations made in 2009 [5] come after review of evidence that sensitivity and specificity of sonographic characteristics predictive of malignancy improve when looking at a constellation of features, rather than individual ones [6, 7]. Thus, the

* Correspondence: david.chanchunkong@mail.mcgill.ca
[1]Department of Otolaryngology Head and Neck Surgery, Jewish General Hospital, McGill University, 3755 Côte-Ste-Catherine Road, Montreal H3T 1E2, Canada
Full list of author information is available at the end of the article

2015 ATA guidelines stratify thyroid nodules based on sonographic patterns into five levels of suspicion from "benign" to "high suspicion"; recommendations for or against USFNA are then given based on nodule size. The overall effect of these changes ultimately results in fewer nodules requiring biopsy [8].

Given the imperfect sensitivities of sonographic characteristics for predicting malignancy, it is possible that the exclusive reliance on these characteristics will lead to missed diagnoses. This study was conducted to determine if the changes to the guidelines will result in overlooked thyroid cancers, specifically malignancies with aggressive characteristics measuring between 1 and 1.49 cm.

Methods
Ethics approval was obtained from the Research Ethics Board at a single academic institution. All patient information was anonymized and stored in a password-encrypted database.

Patient selection
Between August 2006 and June 2016, 2382 patients with thyroid nodules underwent thyroid surgery by a single surgeon at our institution. Patients who underwent total or subtotal/hemi-thyroidectomy for thyroid nodules were included. Patients without a pre-operative ultrasound report, patients undergoing completion thyroidectomies, and patients undergoing thyroid surgery for reasons other than thyroid nodules were excluded. A total of 2083 patients were included in our analyses.

Clinical data collected
Clinical data for all patients were collected from outpatient and inpatient charts, ultrasound and pathology reports. Data collected from all patients included age, sex, number of thyroid nodules, largest nodule size and tumor type based on final histopathology. For patients with the largest nodule between 1 and 1.49 cm, pre-operative ultrasound reports were also reviewed. This group selection was based on the 2015 ATA guidelines, which categorize thyroid nodules first based on ultrasonography findings, and then on size. For nodules of "low" suspicion (i.e. hyperechoic, partially cystic, regular margins without microcalcifications), the guidelines recommend performing USFNA on nodules ≥1.5 cm. Given this recommendation, nodules between 1 and 1.49 cm with low suspicion ultrasound patterns represent a group of potentially missed or delayed malignancy diagnoses. Final pathology, lymph node involvement, staging and tumor status were recorded for nodules in this group to determine the proportion of small nodules that would be missed if the decision to proceed to USFNA were based on sonography patterns of the 2015 ATA guidelines alone. Note that in our group of patients with thyroid nodules between 1 and

1.49 cm, the decision to operate was based on pre-op USFNA results which reflects the 2009 ATA guidelines.

Statistical analysis
Statistical analysis was performed using "MedCalc" version 17.4. Simple descriptive statistics including means and standard deviations for continuous variables and percentages for categorical data were used. Unpaired T-tests and chi-square tests were used to compare malignancies that were included in analysis and those that were excluded, as well as potentially missed/delayed diagnoses and detected malignancies.

Results
A total of 2083 patient charts were retrospectively reviewed for the purposes of this study. Females comprised 80.8% of our sample and the average age was 50 years old (SD 13.8). Demographic data are summarized in Table 1. The majority of the patients were operated on for a single thyroid nodule, 1208 (58%), with the mean largest nodule size being 3.02 cm (SD 1.44).

One thousand eight hundred sixty (89.3%) of patients had a largest thyroid nodule identified on ultrasound of ≥1.5 cm in size (Table 2). On pathological examination, 625 (30%) thyroid glands contained benign histology, 793 (38%) had evidence of micropapillary carcinoma, 991 (48%) of papillary cancer, 23 (2.8%) of follicular cancer, 23 of medullary (1.1%), 1 (0.04%) anaplastic thyroid cancer and 6 (0.3%) that were classified as "Other" (Table 3). The cancers classified as "Other" included lymphoma, metastatic colorectal carcinoma, neuroendocrine carcinoma, sclerosing mucoepidermoid carcinoma and insular carcinoma. It is important to note, for these results, that some thyroid glands operated on had more than one type of cancer histology found in the pathological specimen, that micropapillary was considered separate from papillary cancer, and that the size of the nodule was based on ultrasound reports.

There were 179 patients with the largest nodule size between 1 and 1.49 cm. 24 patients were excluded from further analyses based on a lack of pre-operative ultrasound report and age. Of the remaining 155 patients, 70 (45%) had nodules without hypoechogenicity or microcalcifications, making them "low suspicion" nodules, and

Table 1 Demographic information

	N (%)
Total patients	2083
Females	1683 (81%)
Age	
Mean	50
Range	11–91
Total Thyroidectomy	1316 (63%)

Table 2 Largest nodule size

Largest Nodule Size	N (%)
< 1 cm	44 (2%)
1–1.49 cm	179 (9%)
≥1.5 cm	1860 (89%)

Table 4 T-Staging of potentially missed malignant nodules between 1 and 1.49 cm

T Stage	N (%)
T1	36 (77%)
T2	1 (2%)
T3	10 (21%)
T4	0

thus would not have met criteria for biopsy using the 2015 ATA guidelines (Fig. 1).

Fourty-seven "low suspicion" nodules contained malignancy on final histopathology. 10 (21%) nodules were staged as T3 based on extra thyroidal extension (Table 4), 16 (34%) demonstrated lymph node involvement (3 with extranodal extension), 7 (15%) with lymphovascular invasion, and 1 (2%) displaying a tall cell variant histology (Table 5). Staging information is summarized in Table 6. All 47 tumours were papillary or micropapillary carcinomas on final histopathological examination. Nodules classified as "micropapillary" carcinomas were only included if the size of the largest nodule on pathology was within 2 mm of the size of the largest nodule identified on ultrasound. A micropapillary carcinoma on final pathology with a > 2 mm difference was considered an incidental finding and was excluded. This cut off was chosen as there can be discrepancies of 2 mm between thyroid ultrasound and gross pathological size of carcinomas [9].

Patient and tumor characteristics for nodules with suspicious ultrasound findings (and thus would have been "detected") and those without ("potentially missed" nodules) were not significantly different (Table 7).

Discussion

This study demonstrates that the changes to the ATA 2015 guidelines regarding which thyroid nodules require USFNA will likely result in delayed or potentially missed cancer diagnoses in patients at our institution. Moreover, a number of these missed malignancies are associated with aggressive features.

Sonographic characteristics of thyroid nodules have been widely studied for their value in predicting malignancy. Reported sensitivities and specificities for individual characteristics vary widely between studies [10–12], but a recent meta-analysis of over 18,000 thyroid nodules found that hypoechogenicity has a sensitivity of 73% and specificity of 56%, whereas the sensitivity and specificity

for internal calcifications were 54% and 81% respectively [13]. When ultrasonography findings are combined into patterns, as presented in the 2015 ATA Guidelines, specificity and positive predictive values increase, while sensitivities are diminished. Taken together, the combination of hypoechogenicity, microcalcification, and margin irregularity has the most predictive power, but a sensitivity between 41 and 65% [13]. However, negative predictive values are reportedly high, between 97 and 98% for varying combinations of features [13]; this is most likely due to the low rate of malignancy in this group, cited to be between 5 and 10% [4]. Given these findings then, it is unsurprising that the 2015 ATA guidelines makes only a *weak recommendation* on nodules with a low suspicion sonographic pattern, emphasizing the need for further data collection.

Small thyroid nodules between the sizes of 1-2 cm present an especially interesting diagnostic question, due to their increasing prevalence and varying clinical prognosis. It has been estimated that tumors smaller than 2 cm account for 87% of the increase in thyroid cancer incidence in the United States [14]. Although the ATA guidelines provide size cutoffs for indications to proceed with USFNA, nodule size has a somewhat unclear relationship to thyroid cancer risk. Whereas one research group found that nodules greater than 2 cm had a moderately increased risk of malignancy versus nodules less than 2 cm (15% vs. 10.9%) [15], meta-analysis found that thyroid nodule size was not an accurate predictor of thyroid cancer [12]. Moreover, the cutoff of 1.5 cm for low suspicion nodules is not based on unanimous consensus. In fact, a comparison of six different guidelines for thyroid nodules describes that, the guidelines that did not apply this size cutoff (TIRADS and Kim criteria) had similar or higher performances than those that did [16].

Justification for the higher size cutoff of low suspicion nodules relies on the finding that iso- or hyper-echoic

Table 3 Distribution by largest nodule size on ultrasound and any histology identified on pathology

	Benign	Micropapillary	Papillary	Medullary	Follicular	Anaplastic	Other
< 1 cm	2	37	0	7	0	0	0
1–1.49 cm	34	83	108	1	1	0	0
≥1.5 cm	589	694	862	15	58	1	6
Total	625	793	991	23	59	1	6

Table 5 Aggressive features of potentially missed malignant nodules between 1 and 1.49 cm

Aggressive Feature	N (%)
Positive lymph node	16 (34%)
Extra-nodal extension	3 (6%)
Extra-thyroidal extension	10 (21%)
Lymphovascular invasion	7 (15%)
Tall Cell Variant	1 (2%)

nodules without calcification are more likely to be follicular thyroid cancers (FTC) or follicular variants of papillary thyroid cancer (PTC) [17]. It has been reported that distant metastases are rarely observed from FTC < 2 cm in diameter [18], thereby explaining why observation may be warranted when the nodule is < 1.5 cm in size. In our patient population, however, 100% of detected malignancies with low suspicion ultrasound features contained papillary carcinoma, which has earlier progression to extra-thyroidal extension and lymph node metastases as compared with FTC [18].

This study has enumerated the number of delayed or potentially missed diagnoses of thyroid malignancies in patients presenting with small low suspicion nodules. The effect on long-term patient outcomes is less clear. Since the ATA guidelines do suggest repeated ultrasounds for low suspicion nodules, it is uncertain if delaying treatment for these nodules would have any impact on patient morbidity or mortality. Recent studies have aimed at demonstrating the indolent nature of papillary thyroid cancers - especially microcarcinomas, defined as tumors 1 cm or less in size. It has been reported that only 7–8% of patients with papillary thyroid microcarcinomas show tumor enlargement at 5 and 10-year follow-ups without intervention [19, 20]. Here, despite the lack of outcome measures, we have shown that the thyroid cancers that could have potentially been missed or have had a delay in diagnosis are not only of significant size (> 1 cm), but also associated with aggressive features, such as lymph node metastasis, extranodal extension, extra-thyroidal extension and tall-cell variant histology. These features have been reported by multiple studies to be independent prognostic factors associated with poorer patient outcomes and increased disease-specific mortality [21–23]. As such, future directions of research must answer the question:

Table 6 Staging of potentially missed malignant nodules between 1 and 1.49 cm

Stage	N (%)
1	34 (72%)
2	1 (2%)
3	10 (21%)
4	2 (4%)

Table 7 Comparison of potentially missed and detected malignant nodules between 1 and 1.5 cm

	Detected N = 74		Potentially Missed N = 47		χ^2	p
	n	%	n	%		
Age (years)						
< 45	31	42	20	43	0.005	0.943
≥45	43	58	27	57		
Sex						
Male	11	15	11	23	1.397	0.2372
Female	63	85	36	77		
Tumor type						
Micropapillary	19	26	4	9	7.156	0.0671
Papillary	53	72	43	92		
Medullary	1	1	0	0		
Follicular	1	1	0	0		
T stage						
1	57	77	36	77	0.755	0.8603
2	1	1	1	2		
3	15	20	10	21		
4	1	1	0	0		
Stage						
1	62	84	34	72	4.409	0.2206
2	1	1	1	2		
3	11	15	10	21		
4	0	0	2	4		
ETE						
+	16	22	10	21	0.002	0.9642
−	58	78	37	79		
LN						
+	21	72	16	34	0.431	0.5116
−	53	28	31	66		

what are the consequences of these delayed or potentially missed cancer diagnoses on patient survival?.

Furthermore, given the uncertainties surrounding the predictive values of sonographic findings and nodule size, clinical information obtained on history and physical exam should not be ignored when making decisions regarding clinical investigations. Accordingly, the 2015 ATA Guidelines suggest that since clinical risk factors have not been included in multivariate analyses of sonographic features and thyroid malignancy risk, USFNA can be considered at lower size cutoffs for all nodules in the presence of these risk factors [4]. Future directions of research should aim to identify patient factors that predict malignancy in otherwise unsuspicious nodules, allowing for the use of the complete clinical picture in decision making.

Limitations of this study include its retrospective nature and selection bias, as only nodules that underwent surgical removal were included in our database. However, the use of this surgical database does not overestimate the absolute number of potentially missed malignancies and thus should not affect the validity of our findings. Also, the long-term outcome of these patients is unknown. In other words, if an aggressive malignancy goes undetected for a longer period of time, is the patient's outcome affected.

Conclusions

This study shows that although the pattern of sonographic features associated with a thyroid nodule confers a risk of malignancy, the exclusive reliance on these features could lead to delayed or missed cancer diagnoses. Furthermore, a proportion of these missed malignancies contain aggressive features associated with poorer patient prognosis. Although the exact effect on long-term patient survival is still unclear, our data provide novel insight into a diagnostic gray-zone and demonstrate the need for further evaluation of this patient population for optimal patient care and resource management.

Abbreviations

ATA: American Thyroid Association; FTC: Follicular Thyroid Carcinoma; PTC: Papillary Thyroid Carcinoma; SD: Standard Deviation; USFNA: Ultrasound fine needle aspiration

Funding

There was no funding for this project.

Authors' contributions

DC collected data and contributed to writing manuscript. KG collected data and contributed to writing the manuscript. MR analyzed and interpreted the patient data.WF analyzed and interpreted the patient data. MH analyzed and interpreted the patient data. RP is the supervisor of the project, analyzed and interpreted data. All authors read and approved the final manuscript.

Competing interests

The authors declare that they have no competing interests.

Author details

[1]Department of Otolaryngology Head and Neck Surgery, Jewish General Hospital, McGill University, 3755 Côte-Ste-Catherine Road, Montreal H3T 1E2, Canada. [2]Faculty of Medicine, McGill University, Montreal, Canada.

References

1. Tan GH, Gharib H. Thyroid incidentalomas: management approaches to nonpalpable nodules discovered incidentally on thyroid imaging. Ann Intern Med. 1997;126:226–31.
2. Guth S, Theune U, Aberle J, Galach A, Bamberger CM. Very high prevalence of thyroid nodules detected by high frequency (13 MHz) ultrasound examination. Eur J Clin Investig. 2009;39:699–706.
3. Davies L, Welch HG. Current thyroid cancer trends in the United States. JAMA Otolaryngol Head Neck Surg. 2014;140:317–22.
4. Haugen BR, Alexander EK, Bible KC, Doherty GM, Mandel SJ, Nikiforov YE, Pacini F, Randolph GW, Sawka AM, Schlumberger M, et al. 2015 American Thyroid Association management guidelines for adult patients with thyroid nodules and differentiated thyroid Cancer: the American Thyroid Association guidelines task force on thyroid nodules and differentiated thyroid Cancer. Thyroid. 2016;26:1–133.
5. American Thyroid Association Guidelines Taskforce on Thyroid N, Differentiated thyroid C, Cooper DS, Doherty GM, Haugen BR, Kloos RT, Lee SL, Mandel SJ, Mazzaferri EL, McIver B, et al. Revised American Thyroid Association management guidelines for patients with thyroid nodules and differentiated thyroid cancer. Thyroid. 2009;19:1167–214.
6. Horvath E, Majlis S, Rossi R, Franco C, Niedmann JP, Castro A, Dominguez M. An ultrasonogram reporting system for thyroid nodules stratifying cancer risk for clinical management. J Clin Endocrinol Metab. 2009;94:1748–51.
7. Tae HJ, Lim DJ, Baek KH, Park WC, Lee YS, Choi JE, Lee JM, Kang MI, Cha BY, Son HY, et al. Diagnostic value of ultrasonography to distinguish between benign and malignant lesions in the management of thyroid nodules. Thyroid. 2007;17:461–6.
8. Haugen BR. American Thyroid Association management guidelines for adult patients with thyroid nodules and differentiated thyroid Cancer: what is new and what has changed? Cancer. 2015;2017(123):372–81.
9. Hahn SY, Shin JH, Oh YL, Son YI. Discrepancies between the ultrasonographic and gross pathological size of papillary thyroid carcinomas. Ultrasonography. 2016;35:220–5.
10. Papini E, Guglielmi R, Bianchini A, Crescenzi A, Taccogna S, Nardi F, Panunzi C, Rinaldi R, Toscano V, Pacella CM. Risk of malignancy in nonpalpable thyroid nodules: predictive value of ultrasound and color-Doppler features. J Clin Endocrinol Metab. 2002;87:1941–6.
11. Cappelli C, Castellano M, Pirola I, Cumetti D, Agosti B, Gandossi E, Agabiti Rosei E. The predictive value of ultrasound findings in the management of thyroid nodules. QJM. 2007;100:29–35.
12. Remonti LR, Kramer CK, Leitao CB, Pinto LC, Gross JL. Thyroid ultrasound features and risk of carcinoma: a systematic review and meta-analysis of observational studies. Thyroid. 2015;25:538–50.
13. Brito JP, Gionfriddo MR, Al Nofal A, Boehmer KR, Leppin AL, Reading C, Callstrom M, Elraiyah TA, Prokop LJ, Stan MN, et al. The accuracy of thyroid nodule ultrasound to predict thyroid cancer: systematic review and meta-analysis. J Clin Endocrinol Metab. 2014;99:1253–63.
14. Davies L, Welch HG. Increasing incidence of thyroid cancer in the United States, 1973-2002. JAMA. 2006;295:2164–7.
15. Kamran SC, Marqusee E, Kim MI, Frates MC, Ritner J, Peters H, Benson CB, Doubilet PM, Cibas ES, Barletta J, et al. Thyroid nodule size and prediction of cancer. J Clin Endocrinol Metab. 2013;98:564–70.
16. Yoon JH, Han K, Kim EK, Moon HJ, Kwak JY. Diagnosis and Management of Small Thyroid Nodules: a comparative study with six guidelines for thyroid nodules. Radiology. 2017;283:560–9.
17. Moon WJ, Jung SL, Lee JH, Na DG, Baek JH, Lee YH, Kim J, Kim HS, Byun JS, Lee DH, et al. Benign and malignant thyroid nodules: US differentiation--multicenter retrospective study. Radiology. 2008;247:762–70.
18. Machens A, Holzhausen HJ, Dralle H. The prognostic value of primary tumor size in papillary and follicular thyroid carcinoma. Cancer. 2005;103:2269–73.
19. Ito Y, Miyauchi A, Kihara M, Higashiyama T, Kobayashi K, Miya A. Patient age is significantly related to the progression of papillary microcarcinoma of the thyroid under observation. Thyroid. 2014;24:27–34.
20. Mazzaferri EL. Management of low-risk differentiated thyroid cancer. Endocr Pract. 2007;13:498–512.
21. Randolph GW, Duh QY, Heller KS, LiVolsi VA, Mandel SJ, Steward DL, Tufano RP, Tuttle RM. American Thyroid Association surgical affairs Committee's taskforce on thyroid Cancer nodal S: the prognostic significance of nodal metastases from papillary thyroid carcinoma can be stratified based on the size and number of metastatic lymph nodes, as well as the presence of extranodal extension. Thyroid. 2012;22:1144–52.

25

Validation of a novel method for localization of parathyroid adenomas using SPECT/CT

Rachelle A. LeBlanc[1] ⓘ, Andre Isaac[1], Jonathan Abele[2], Vincent L. Biron[1], David W. J. Côté[1], Matthew Hearn[1], Daniel A. O'Connell[1], Hadi Seikaly[1] and Jeffrey R. Harris[1]*

Abstract

Background: Accurate localization of parathyroid adenomas is of critical importance in surgical planning for minimally invasive parathyroidectomy. SPECT/CT is considered the investigation of choice but has limitations regarding localization of superior versus inferior adenomas. We proposed a novel method for localization using SPECT/CT by determining the anterior-posterior relationship of the adenoma to a horizontal line in the coronal plane through the tracheoesophageal groove. Our objective was to determine the accuracy, validity, and inter-rater reliability of this method.

Method: This was a retrospective review of patients who underwent parathyroidectomy for a single adenoma between 2010-2017. SPECT/CT images were reviewed by two staff Otolaryngologists, a Radiologist, an Otolaryngology fellow and Otolaryngology resident. Results were compared using intra-operative report as the gold standard.
Overall accuracy in determining superior/inferior and right/left adenomas was calculated, as well as Cohen's Kappa to determine agreement with operative report and inter-rater reliability. The performance was compared to that of the original radiology report.

Results: One hundred thirty patients met criteria and were included. Our method correctly identified the location of the adenoma in terms of both side and superior/inferior position in 80.4% [76 - 84%] of patients, which considerably outperformed the original radiology report at 48.5% [4-78%] accuracy. The agreement level between our method and operative report was high (Kappa=0.717 [0.691-0.743]), as was the inter-rater reliability (Kappa=0.706 [0.674-0.738]).

Conclusion: We report a novel method for localization of parathyroid adenomas using SPECT/CT which outperforms standard radiology reporting. This tool can be used by surgeons and radiologists to better inform and plan for minimally invasive parathyroidectomy.

Background

Primary hyperparathyroidism (PHPT) is characterized by hypercalcemia and elevated levels of parathyroid hormone (PTH) and is most commonly caused by a single glandular enlargement, or adenoma. Parathyroid adenoma may occur in any of the four glands but tends to involve the inferior glands more commonly than superior glands [1].

The definitive management of primary hyperparathyroidism is surgical.

Although the number and position of parathyroid glands can vary, the most common arrangement involves four glands, two superior and two inferior glands [2]. The superior glands originate embryologically from the fourth pharyngeal pouch, whereas the inferior glands originate from the third pharyngeal pouch. As a result of their embryological migration patterns, the glands tend to have a predictable position with relation to the thyroid, thymus, and recurrent laryngeal nerve. Superior glands tend to be more intimately related to the recurrent laryngeal nerve and lie deep to the plane of the

* Correspondence: Jeffrey.Harris@albertahealthservices.ca
[1]Division of Otolaryngology—Head and Neck Surgery, University of Alberta, 1E4 Walter Mackenzie Center, 8440 112 Street, Edmonton, AB T6G 2B7, Canada
Full list of author information is available at the end of the article

nerve. Inferior glands in contrast tend to lie in a more superficial plane than the nerve and more inferiorly, between the thyroid and thymus [3–6].

Accurate pre-operative localization of parathyroid adenomas is critical for operative planning and the facilitation of minimally invasive surgery. In recent years, there has been development of more effective imaging methods to localize parathyroid adenomas, rather than the previous gold standard of surgical four-gland exploration. Non-invasive preoperative methods for localization of parathyroid adenomas include: ultrasonography, radioiodine or technetium scintigraphy, technetium 99 m sestamibi scintigraphy, computed tomography scan, and magnetic resonance imaging [1, 2, 7, 8]. Recently published studies have shown high utility in the use of single-photon emission CT (SPECT) using sestamibi radionucleotide imaging in combination with CT scanning (SPECT/CT). SPECT/CT has been found to have improved anatomic detail when compared with traditional sestamibi imaging [9].

Determining whether a parathyroid adenoma represents an inferior or superior adenoma can be difficult on imaging. This is preoperative localization is, however, paramount to successful excision, as superior and inferior glands are approached differently during surgery. Inaccurate localization seen in some traditional methods can result in more extensive or revision surgery. We have developed a novel method, known as the Harris method, of localizing parathyroid adenoma as inferior or superior based on SPECT/CT imaging. This method is based on the embryological origin and migration pathway of the parathyroid glands, as opposed to the traditional radiological method of their relation to the thyroid gland only. The technique consists of drawing a horizontal (coronal) line on axial cuts of SPECT/CT, bisecting the tracheoesophageal groove at the level of the cricoid cartilage. Adenomas that are anterior to this line on axial cuts are deemed inferior, while adenomas that are posterior to this line are superior. The aim of our study is to determine the validity and accuracy of this novel method for localization of parathyroid adenomas when compared to traditional radiological reporting, against the gold standard of intra-operative localization.

Methods

Study design

Institutional review board approval was obtained from the Human Research Ethics Board at the University of Alberta (Pro00077058). This was a retrospective diagnostic validation study evaluating the use of a novel

method of determining the location of a parathyroid adenoma using axial cuts of SPECT/CT.

Participants who underwent parathyroidectomy for a single parathyroid adenoma between November 1, 2010 until November 30, 2017 within the Division of Otolaryngology - Head and Neck Surgery in Edmonton, Alberta were recruited. Eligible patients were those aged > 18 years with a clinical diagnosis of primary hyperparathyroidism. Patients were excluded if they had previous head and neck surgery, greater than one identified parathyroid adenoma, or if radiology reports, SPECT/CT images and/or operative reports were unavailable. Patients were also excluded if there was a failure to identify whether the adenoma was superior or inferior intraoperatively.

Using SPECT/CT images, two staff Otolaryngologist – Head and Neck Surgeons, a Nuclear Medicine Radiologist, an Otolaryngology – Head and Neck Surgery fellow and resident performed the novel method, blinded to the operative findings, on eligible patients that met the inclusion and exclusion criteria. This novel method consisted of finding the level of the cricoid cartilage on an axial cut of the SPECT/CT and drawing a horizontal line bisecting the tracheoesophageal groove. The participants were then to identify whether the adenoma is anterior or posterior to that line. Data was recorded and participants were given immediate feedback as to their diagnostic accuracy. Participants were given 30 scans in one session to prevent fatigue.

The primary outcome was the accuracy of the novel technique of parathyroid adenoma localization based on SPECT/CT using intra-operative identification as the gold standard. The accuracy was compared to that of the original radiology report using cohen's kappa. Our secondary outcomes were inter-rater reliability of using this novel technique. A clinical diagnosis of PHPT included hypercalcemia and high PTH levels. Operative reports were used to identify the correct location of the adenoma causing hyperparathyroidism. Calcium, PTH, intraoperative identification of the adenoma location, radiology report identification, and the result of the performed task by participants were all recorded.

Statistical analysis was carried out using SPSS software (Statistical Package for the Social Sciences, Version 1.0.0.950). The percentages were calculated by adding the correct answers when compared to the operative report as gold standard. Percentage of each adenoma was recorded and the overall accuracy was the mean of all rater accuracies. Cohen's kappa was used to determine the inter-rater reliability between the original radiology report and the operative report. Fleiss kappa was used to calculate inter-rater

Table 1 Patient Demographics

Variable	$N = 130$
Age	59.3 (24–86)
Gender	
Males	26 (20%)
Females	104 (80%)
Preoperative PTH (Average)	20.2 pmol/L (6.1–81.5 pmol/L)
Postoperative PTH (Average)	3.06 pmol/L (.60–12.40 pmol/L)
Preoperative Calcium (Average)	2.77 mmol/L (2.37–2.77 mmol/L)
Parathyroid Location	
Left Inferior	37 (28%)
Left Superior	26 (20%)
Right Inferior	39 (30%)
Right Superior	28 (22%)

reliability between the raters and the operative report and the raters themselves.

Results

Three hundred ninety-eight patients were reviewed. 267 patients did not meet inclusion criteria and were excluded. 130 patients met inclusion and exclusion criteria and were included in the study. 104 were female, and 26 were male. The mean age of the patients was 59.3 years. The mean preoperative PTH was 20.2 pmol/L (6.1–81.5 pmol/L) and the mean postoperative PTH was 3.06 pmol/L (0.60–12.40 pmol/L). The mean calcium was calculated to be 2.77 mmol/L (2.37–2.77 mmol/L) (Table 1). 37 patients were identified to have left inferior parathyroid adenomas and 26 patients had left superior parathyroid adenomas. 39 patients had right inferior parathyroid adenomas and 28 patients had right superior parathyroid adenomas (Table 1).

Accuracy was calculated by total correct identified adenoma when compared to the original operative report. The combined accuracy for all raters using the novel method was 80.4% [76–84%]. The accuracy of the original radiology report compared to the operative report was 48.5% [4–78%] (Fig. 1). The accuracy of inferior and superior parathyroid adenomas was also calculated. The overall accuracy of inferior parathyroid adenomas was 83% (73–89%) compared to the original radiology report of 78% (Fig. 2). The overall accuracy for superior parathyroid adenomas was 78% (69–89%) compared to the original radiology report of 19% (Fig. 2).

Reliability was calculated using Cohen's Kappa and Fleiss Kappa. The original radiology report was compared to the operative report and Cohen's Kappa was calculated to be 0.468 [0.366–0.570] (Table 2). This is considered to be moderate agreement. When comparing raters to the operative report there was substantial agreement. The Fleiss Kappa was calculated to be 0.717 [0.691–0.743] (Table 3). Overall Fleiss Kappa between raters was calculated and inter-rater reliability was 0.706 [.674–.738] (Table 4). This is considered to be substantial agreement between raters.

Discussion

The gold standard of treatment for PHPTH caused by a parathyroid adenoma is surgical resection [10]. When compared to four gland exploration, a minimally invasive approach has been associated with reduced complications such as including injury to the recurrent laryngeal nerve, hypocalcemia and bleeding risks, as well as shorter hospital stay [11–13].

Technological advances have technology has improved accuracy of correct localization of parathyroid

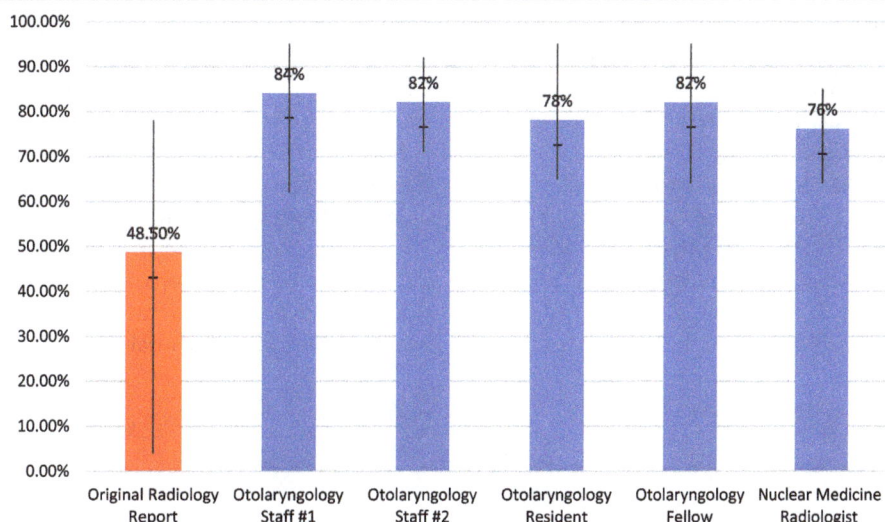

Fig. 1 Combined accuracy of correct localization of parathyroid adenomas

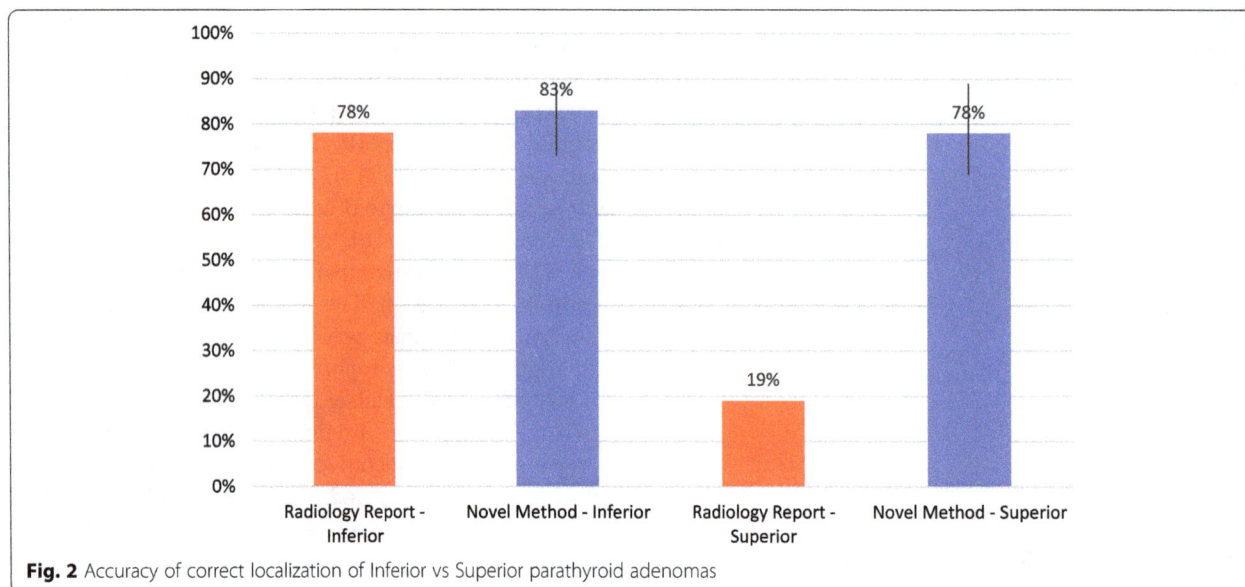

Fig. 2 Accuracy of correct localization of Inferior vs Superior parathyroid adenomas

adenomas. Preoperatively, it is important to localize these adenomas, as it dictates the surgical approach used to resect the enlarged gland. Of significant clinical importance is the ability to predict the location of the adenoma with respect to the recurrent laryngeal nerve. All superior adenomas (Fig. 3) that would be embryologically and anatomically deep to the recurrent laryngeal nerve require positive identification of the nerve prior to dissection, and resection of, the involved gland. Inferior adenomas are anterior to the recurrent laryngeal nerve and, therefore, dissection on the anterior surface of the gland is safely performed prior to identification of the nerve. Indeed, in some cases the inferior adenoma can be safely excised without identifying the nerve, though in our practice the nerve is identified prior to closure in virtually all cases. Multiple modalities have been used to help achieve localization, however, there is still ambiguity, especially with regards to identifying superior versus inferior gland enlargement.

In 2009, Perrier et al. have developed a nomenclature that provides a precise means of communicating the most frequently encountered parathyroid adenoma locations. Using the Perrier method, a uniform and reliable description of exact locations of parathyroid adenomas can aid in proper localization preoperatively [14]. The system essentially uses the letters A – G to describe exact gland locations. Keidar et al. found that using the

Perrier method, 80% of cases accurately localized parathyroid adenomas preoperatively using SPECT/CT [15]. This method however is not widely used in radiology reports due to its complexity.

Instead, radiologists often use the relationship between the parathyroid adenoma and the thyroid gland to decide on its location [16, 17] (Fig. 4). This can be misleading however, as the exact cranio-caudal location with respect to the thyroid gland can vary. Intra-operatively, surgeons more commonly use the relationship to the plane of the recurrent laryngeal nerve in order to localize parathyroid adenomas. Hauty et al., found using technetium-thallium scintiscanning for localizing parathyroid adenomas, a sensitivity in the detection of parathyroid adenomas of 82%, a diagnostic accuracy of 78% and a positive predictive value of 94% [18]. These accuracies are using the thyroid gland as standard of reference. It is important to note that the reason why we see these differences in accuracy is because there is a difference in the standard of reference. The method we have described uses a more embryologically and anatomically sound technique than standard radiological reporting and is thus shown to be more clinically relevant for the surgical approach.

It is important to take into account that the superior glands may never be separated from the thyroid gland during embryological migration [2]. If a superior gland is adenomatous, the potential course could result in the

Table 2 Cohen's Kappa comparing Operative Report and Original Radiology Report

Weighting	Kappa	Asymptotic Standard Error	Z	Lower 95% Asymptotic CI Bound	Upper 95% Asymptotic CI Bound
Linear	.468	.052	8.891	.366	.570

Table 3 Overall Fleiss Kappa for Inter-rater Reliability

Rating Category	Conditional Probability	Kappa	Asymptotic Sandard Error	Z	Lower 95% Asymptotic CI Bound	Upper 95% Asymptotic CI Bound
Inferior	.792	.706	.028	25.441	.651	.760
Superior	.769	.708	.028	25.536	.654	.763

Table 4 Fleiss Kappa for Overall Inter-rater Reliability and between Raters and Operative Report

	Kappa	Asymptotic Standard Error	Z	Lower 95% Asymptotic CI Bound	Upper 95% Asymptotic CI Bound
Overall Inter-rater	.706	.016	43.558	.674	.738
Overall Between Raters and Operative Report	.717	.013	54.203	.691	.743

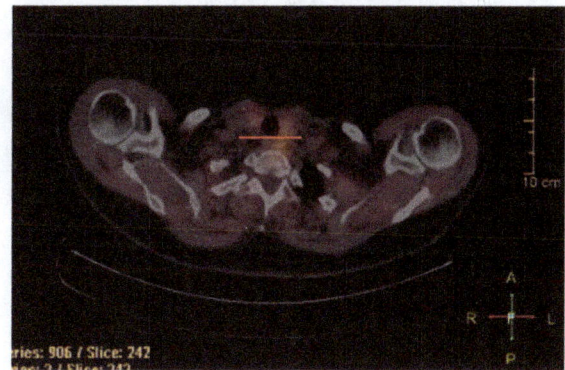

Fig. 4 Left superior parathyroid adenoma, as determined by the novel method. This adenoma was reported radiologically as inferior

gland in the inferior and posterior position. Dasgupta et al. reported that when radiology reports are duel reported by a surgeon and a nuclear medicine physician, there was a statistically significant improvement in localization [2, 3]. This finding may be attributed to the fact that surgeons may have a better understanding of the anatomy and embryology of the parathyroid glands than the nuclear medicine physician [3, 19]. The use of multiple imaging modalities, our newly described method, and dual reporting with nuclear medicine physicians and surgeons may improve the accuracy of preoperative localization.

The importance of preoperative localization by the operating surgeon cannot be underestimated. Increasing the localization accuracy allows an endocrine surgeon to further minimize the amount of dissection required during surgery which directly reduces the risk profile associated with minimally invasive parathyroid surgery.

There are a few limitations that can be identified in this present study. Using SPECT/CT in itself has limitations including patient motion during the study for accurate registration in SPECT/CT, attenuation and scatter correction, spatial registration, and radiation exposure considerations [20]. Another limitation is the size of the thyroid gland. Theoretically, if the thyroid gland size is larger, it would potentially push the parathyroid glands either more posterior or anterior with respect to the tracheoesophageal groove and could therefore alter

our findings or explain some of the incorrect localization results. A larger prospective study may help to address these limitations in the future.

Another limitation is that when the radiology reports were originally dictated, the radiologist did not have the benefit of knowing whether or not there indeed was an adenoma present before reading the study, as opposed to the subjects used for this research study. Thus, localization may have been more challenging for the original radiologist. We attempted to correct for this by eliminating patients that were originally described as non-localizing, regardless of the final operative findings.

We also did not perform intra-rater reliability testing, nor were we able to track a learning curve for our novel method. We plan to collect and analyze these metrics in a follow-up study.

Conclusion

The Harris method correctly identified the location of the parathyroid adenoma in terms of both side and superior/inferior position in 80.4% of patients, which considerably outperformed the original radiology reports accuracy of 48.5%. There was substantial agreement between our method and the operative report (Kappa = 0.717 [0.691–0.743]), as well as the inter-rater reliability (Kappa = 0.706 [0.674–0.738]). The Harris method is easily performed by the surgeon and radiologist and is less complex and time consuming than the previously reported Perrier method, with very similar localization success. By using this method, preoperative localization of parathyroid adenomas can be improved allowing the surgeon to plan for efficient, effective, and safe minimally invasive parathyroidectomy.

Authors' contributions
RL carried out the study design, collected and recorded the data, performed the data analysis, and drafted the manuscript. AI performed the novel method and participated in creating the study design, helped with statistical analysis, as well as edited the manuscript. JA, VB, MH all performed the novel

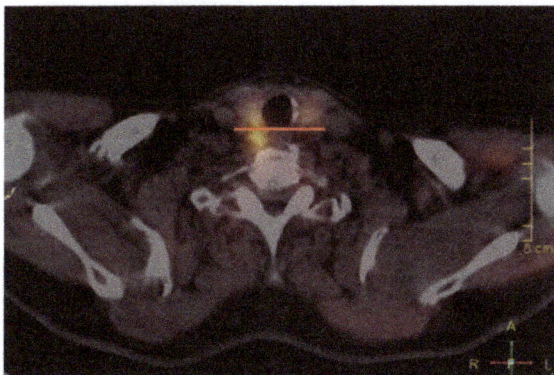

Fig. 3 Posterior to the horizontal line on the right deems this to be a right superior parathyroid adenoma

method and helped edit the manuscript. DC helped with statistical analysis and manuscript review. DOC participated in study design, data aquisition and manuscript review. HS participated in the study design and helped revise the manuscript. JH participated in study design, performed the novel method, and manuscript revision. All authors read and approved the final manuscript.

Competing interests
The authors declare that they have no competing interests.

Author details
[1]Division of Otolaryngology—Head and Neck Surgery, University of Alberta, 1E4 Walter Mackenzie Center, 8440 112 Street, Edmonton, AB T6G 2B7, Canada. [2]Department of Radiology & Diagnostic Imaging, Royal Alexandra Hospital, 1046 Royal Alexandra Hospital – Diagnostic Treatment Center, 2J2.00 WC Mackenzie Health Sciences Centre, 8440 112 Street, Edmonton, AB T6G 2R7, Canada.

References

1. Moreno MA, Callender GG, Woodburn K, Edeiken-Monroe BS, Grubbs EG, Evans DB, Lee JE, Perrier ND. Common locations of parathyroid adenomas. Ann Surg Oncol. 2011;18(4):1047–51. https://doi.org/10.1245/s10434-010-1429-x Epub 2010 Nov 20.
2. Dasgupta DJ, Navalkisoor S, Ganatra R, Buscome J. The role of single-photon emission computed tomography/ computed tomography in localizing parathyroid adenoma. Nucl Med Commun. 2013;34:621–6.
3. Judson BL, Shaha AR. Nuclear imaging and minimally invasive surgery in the management of hyperparathyroidism. J Nucl Med. 2008;49(11):1813–8.
4. Heffess CS. Embryology, anatomy, and histology. In: Wenig B, editor. Atlas of head and neck pathology. 2nd ed. China: Saunders Elsevier; 2008. p. 1012–28.
5. Carlson D. Parathyroid pathology: hyperparathyroidism and parathyroid tumors. Arch Pathol Lab Med. 2010;134(11):1639–44.
6. Gray SW, Skandalakis JE, Akin JT. Embryological considerations of thyroid surgery: developmental anatomy of the thyroid, parathyroids and the recurrent laryngeal nerve. Am Surg. 1976;42(9):621–8.
7. Ciappuccini R, Morera J, Pascal P, Rame JP, Heutte N, Aide N, et al. Dual-phase 99mTc sestamibi scintigraphy with neck and thorax SPECT/CT in primary hyperparathyroidism: a single institution experience. Clin Nucl Med. 2012;37:223–8.
8. Kluijfhout WP, Pasternak JD, Beninato T, Drake FT, Gosnell JE, Shen WT, Duh QY, Allen IE, Vriens MR, de Keizer B, Hope TA, Suh I. Diagnostic performance of computed tomography for parathyroid adenoma localization; a systemic review and meta-analysis. Eur J Radiol. 2017;88:117–28.
9. Hinson AM, Lee DR, Hobbs BA, Fitzgerald RT, Bodenner DL, Stack BC. Preoperative 4D CT localization of nonlocalizing parathyroid adenomas by ultrasound and SPECT-CT. Otolaryngol Head Neck Surg. 2015;153(5):775–8.
10. Fraser WD. Hyperparathyroidism. Lancet. 2009;374:145–58.
11. Ebner Y, Garti-Gross Y, Margulis A, et al. Parathyroid surgery: correlation between pre-operative localization studies and surgical outcomes. Clin Endocrinol. 2015. https://doi.org/10.1111/cen.12835.
12. Grant CS, Thompson G, Farley D, et al. Primary hyperparathyroidism surgical management since the introduction of minimally invasive parathyroidectomy: Mayo Clinic experience. Arch Surg. 2005;140:472–8.
13. Westerdahl J, Bergenfelz A. Unilateral versus bilateral neck exploration for primary hyperparathyroidism: five-year follow-up of a randomized controlled trial. Ann Surg. 2007;246:976–80.
14. Perrier ND, Edeiken B, Nunez R, et al. A novel nomenclature to classify parathyroid adenomas. World J Surg. 2009;33:412–6.
15. Keidar Z, Solomonov E, Karry R, Frenkel A, Israel O, Mekel M. Preoperative [99mTc] MIBI SPECT/CT interpretation criteria for localization of parathyroid adenomas—correlation with surgical findings. Mol Imaging Biol. 2017;19:265–70.
16. Smith JR, Oates ME. Radionuclide imaging of the parathyroid glands: patterns, pearls, and Ptifalls. Radiographics. 2004;24(4):1101–15.
17. Piciucchi S, Barone D, Gavelli G, Dubini A, Oboldi D, Matteuci F. Primary hyperparathyroidism: imaging to pathology. J Clin Imaging Sci. 2012;2:59.
18. Hauty M, Swartz K, McClung M, Lowe DK. Technetium-thallium scintiscanning for localization of parathyroid adenomas and hyperplasia. A reappraisal. Am J Surg. 1987;153:479–86.
19. Melton GB, Somervell H, Friedman KP, Zeiger MA, Civelek AC. Interpretation of 99mTc sestamibi parathyroid SPECT scan is improved when read by the surgeon and nuclear medicine physician together. Nucl Med Commun. 2005;26:633–8.
20. Livieratos L. Technical pitfalls and limitations of SPECT/CT. Semin Nucl Med. 2015;45:530–40.

26

When symptoms don't fit: a case series of conversion disorder in the pediatric otolaryngology practice

Lisa Caulley[1,2,3], Scott Kohlert[1,2,3], Hazen Gandy[1,4], Janet Olds[1,5] and Matthew Bromwich[1,2,3]*

Abstract

Background: Conversion disorder refers to functional bodily impairments that can be precipitated by high stress situations including trauma and surgery. Symptoms of conversion disorder may mimic or complicate otolaryngology diseases in the pediatric population.

Case presentation: In this report, the authors describe 3 cases of conversion disorder that presented to a pediatric otolaryngology-head and neck surgery practice. This report highlights a unique population of patients who have not previously been investigated. The clinical presentation and management of these cases are discussed in detail. Non-organic otolaryngology symptoms of conversion disorder in the pediatric population are reviewed. In addition, we discuss the challenges faced by clinicians in appropriately identifying and treating these patients and present an approach to management of their care.

Conclusion: In this report, the authors highlight the importance of considering psychogenic illnesses in patients with atypical clinical presentations of otolaryngology disorders.

Keywords: Pediatrics, Conversion disorders, Otolaryngology, Misdiagnosis

Background

The prevalence of mental illness is estimated to be 10–20% amongst children and adolescents worldwide, making it the leading cause of disability in young people [1]. Furthermore, treatments (both behavioral and pharmacological) of mental illness and the demand for them for children and adolescents has increased significantly in the past decade [2]. Untreated psychiatric disorders can impair a child's development and limit educational achievement [1].

Conversion disorders refer to body dysfunction characterized by neurological symptoms, either sensory or motor, that cannot be explained by a medical condition. Given their somatosensory nature, they typically require a medical assessment and the diagnosis of conversion disorder can only be established after organic diseases have been excluded or if they fail to account for the severity of a patient's impairment. In pediatric patients, the presentations of conversion disorder tend to be complex, and multiple conversion symptoms are the norm [3–5]. As it has been found to be associated with bodily stress, it is imperative that surgeons are aware of this disorder in the post-operative setting [5–9]. Developing an approach to this issue requires an appreciation for the multifactorial nature of its etiology.

It is prudent that clinicians be informed about the prevalence of mental illness in their patient population and its implications. Misdiagnosis or delayed diagnosis can have a significant impact on patients and creates a burden not only on the healthcare system, but also on the patient and their family members. In this article, the authors discuss 3 pediatric cases referred for otolaryngologic complaints that were complicated by conversion disorder. We discuss the implications of conversion disorder for the diagnosis and treatment for the otolaryngologist - head and neck surgeon and the need for an awareness of the impact of conversion disorders on presentation, treatment and recovery.

* Correspondence: mbromwich@cheo.on.ca
[1]Faculty of Medicine, University of Ottawa, Ottawa, ON, Canada
[2]Department of Otolaryngology-Head and Neck Surgery, The Ottawa Hospital, Ottawa, ON, Canada
Full list of author information is available at the end of the article

Case presentations

Patient 1 was a previously healthy 11-year-old girl who presented to hospital with a 2-week history of "dizziness". Her symptoms were described as disequilibrium precipitated by standing and sitting and relieved by lying flat. Her symptoms were unaffected by eye opening. Her symptoms were debilitating and she had difficulty ambulating. Her symptoms were unresponsive to antiemetics and she presented to the Children's Hospital of Eastern Ontario emergency room where she was diagnosed with vestibular neuronitis. When her symptoms persisted, she was admitted to hospital and assessed by the Otolaryngology-Head and Neck Surgery service. In addition to a history and focused head and neck examination, an oto-neurological examination was performed including evaluation of cranial nerves, voluntary saccades, spontaneous and gaze-evoked nystagmus, rapid head thrust and dix-hall pike maneuver. She did not demonstrate any clinical findings suggestive of vestibular neuronitis, migraine variant nor benign positional paroxysmal variant. Routine laboratory investigations were within normal limits. Magnetic resonance imaging of the brain was non-contributory. She was admitted to hospital for 4 days. She received instructions for daily strengthening exercises from the physiotherapy service. These interventions validated her experiences and offered a mechanism for symptom resolution that was psychologically and emotionally acceptable to the patient and her family, which resulted in a complete resolution of her symptoms. A previous diagnosis of social anxiety some 5 years ago may have been a relevant risk factor in the development of her symptoms.

Patient 2 was an 11-year-old girl who presented to hospital with a history of head trauma while somersaulting 3 weeks prior to her presentation. She described progressive headaches, disequilibrium, choreiform movements and ataxia following the mild traumatic head injury. Her symptoms were debilitating and she was unable to sit upright or ambulate. She had no significant past medical history. She was admitted to the medical service for 23 days, during which she was assessed by multiple subspecialties including the Otolaryngology – Head and Neck Surgery service. After a complete oto-neurological examination, she was found to have no evidence of a vestibular pathology to account for her symptoms, and a head computed tomography (CT) and magnetic resonance imaging (MRI) were normal. Routine laboratory investigations were within normal limits. Further assessment from Mental Health services identified the following contributing factors: post concussive symptomatology including high anxiety, high family expectations in the presence of limited communication and sibling rivalry, and the presence of a pre-existing significant traumatic event. A diagnosis of conversion disorder was made, and conceptualized

as an unconscious avoidant coping mechanism. While an inpatient, she was followed by a multidisciplinary team including Psychiatry, Psychology and Physiotherapy. The focus of mental health interventions was on communication and expression of emotion, while Physiotherapy provided exercises to improve her symptoms and validation of her psychological distress. She improved significantly over the course of hospitalization and was discharged to outpatient follow-up through Mental Health Services for continued intervention and support.

Patient 3 was a 13-year-old boy who underwent an adenoidectomy. He had a past medical history of significant nasal obstruction due to adenoid hypertrophy. His post-operative course was complicated by recurrent adenoid bleeds. One month post-operatively, the patient began to complain of daily headaches. Over the two weeks following, he reported daily nausea and disequilibrium. He returned to the emergency department when he developed complete paralysis of the lower limbs, essentially rendering him paraplegic and disabled. A complete head and neck examination including oto-neurologic examination was within normal limits. Routine laboratory investigations were within normal limits. An MRI and MR venogram of the brain failed to reveal evidence of any intracranial pathology. He remained in hospital for 17 days. His gait progressively improved with physiotherapy until he returned to baseline. The Mental Health service identified pre-existing significant traumatic events and psychosocial stressors for the entire family associated with multiple moves and living in a refugee camp for a year and a half prior to immigrating to Canada. In addition, the patient was found to have some evidence of anxiety and perfectionism that were exacerbated by his inability to participate in school, secondary to the surgery.

Discussion

To our knowledge, this is the first reported case series of pediatric psychiatric disorders that presented for consideration of otolaryngology-related pathology. Mental health disorders are misdiagnosed as organic diseases more frequently than clinicians expect due to several disease, patient and clinician factors. Furthermore, the ability to accurately diagnose patients with a psychiatric illness may often fall outside of the scope of practice for the average Otolaryngologist – Head and Neck Surgeon. However, as highlighted in the following section, it is crucial that clinicians keep psychiatric illnesses on the differential diagnosis, especially for patients who present with atypical or contradictory physical signs and symptoms. In addition, an approach to the management of these patients is provided as a resource for clinicians.

Functional disorders have been linked in the adult literature with a wide breadth of head and neck complaints, such as hearing loss, anosmia, stridor, dysphonia, and vision loss [10–14]. In children and adolescents, the most recent literature has reported symptoms arising from disorders such as pseudohypacusis and functional upper airway obstruction [15–17]. Paradoxical vocal cord motion, or psychogenic stridor, refers to the inappropriate adduction of the vocal cords during the respiratory cycle, and remains a common and frequently misdiagnosed functional disorder in the pediatric population. Over 50% of patients with paradoxical vocal cord motion are diagnosed with conversion disorder [12]. The differential diagnosis in the pediatric population is challenging, given the high base rates of pediatric mental health disorders including conversion disorder, adjustment disorder and autism spectrum disorder. This has the potential to be mistakenly diagnosed as primary otolaryngologic disease, as observed in this case series.

Conversion disorder (CD), or functional neurological symptom disorder, is characterized by disturbances in body function that are inconsistent with known anatomy or pathophysiology [18]. The Diagnostic and Statistical Manual of Mental Disorders V defines the conversion disorder as the presence of "one or more symptoms of altered voluntary motor or sensory function" in the absence of any identifiable neurological or medical cause. While the symptoms are psychogenic in origin, conversion disorder distinguishes itself from malingering and factitious disorder as the CD patient is not intentionally experiencing these symptoms [18, 19]. The patient population affected can be characterized as having perfectionist tendencies with high expectations regarding achievements and high levels of anxiety associated with illness [20–25]. There is no clear etiology of conversion disorder. However, in general, theories focus on the management of affect and stress [5, 18, 20–22, 24, 25].

There are no bedside tests or investigations to establish the diagnosis of conversion disorder. The diagnosis is made after organic disease has been ruled out [5, 18]. As such, diagnosing conversion disorder can put the clinician in the difficult position of having to communicate the presence of a non-organic illness as the source of the patient's severe disability, while validating the authenticity of their symptoms [20]. However, this communication combined with appropriate intervention assists in validating symptoms and provides a mechanism for their resolution.

Although it is rare for the practicing surgical specialist to encounter this disorder, its atypical sensory and motor manifestations make it a potential diagnosis in any specialist's practice. For instance, these patients may find themselves under the care of an Otolaryngologist-Head and Neck Surgeon to rule out organic hearing loss or peripheral vertigo as the etiology of their symptoms [26]. Objective tests of hearing and vestibular dysfunction, including audiometry, electronystagmography and rotational chair testing are essential to rule out organic pathology. Ancillary studies to detect non-organic pathology in children, including the Stenger Test, can be considered to identify pseudohypoacusis. The authors encourage consideration of psychological stressors as factors to be considered, which may be associated with conversion, or other, disorders encountered in severe disease and in the postoperative period as demonstrated in the presented cases. Early diagnosis and therapy can significantly improve health outcomes in these patients [19], and the prognosis is considered to be excellent (with roughly 95% of affected individuals experiencing spontaneous resolution of their symptoms within one month of diagnosis) [27].

A diagnostic challenge
Understanding the patient
With the support of online resources and media publicity, patients now present with a plethora of computer-generated differential diagnoses and planned diagnostic investigations independent of their physician's input [28]. However, the new age of knowledgeable and autonomous patients poses both benefits and challenges to clinicians.

Patients may find it challenging to accept a psychiatric diagnosis, which is based heavily on clinical judgment, when they have initially become invested in the concept of an organic disease as the etiology of their symptoms. The agnostic approach, where possible diagnoses and explanations are equally valid, is used by clinicians to manage relaying a lack of diagnosis to a family [29]. This approach may avoid questions about the authenticity of symptoms that can contribute to a hostile physician-patient relationship [20, 29]. Clinicians should be aware of the very sensitive and frank discussion that needs to take place with patients regarding the nature of their illness. Establishing a forum for discussion will also assist in providing guidance around patient-specific therapy for this disorder [20]. This discussion, validating both physical and mental symptoms, optimally could include an open invitation for the value of mental health professionals as part of the health care team.

Superfluous diagnostic testing
Diagnosis of mental illness continues to rely heavily on clinical judgment and judicious use of diagnostic testing. This means that clinicians must balance patient perspectives and values with clinical practice guidelines and professional expertise. This can be challenging in the context of unexplained symptoms and patients' conceptualizations about the symptoms, but optimally can be an opportunity to assist the patient in accessing evidence-based resources and care.

The patient-physician relationship is founded heavily in trust from both parties. This may invoke some restraint on the part of the clinician in opposing patient requests for non-beneficial investigations and procedures [28]. However, clinicians must be wary of the fact that both patients as well as physicians can introduce biases into clinical decision-making that can complicate care and increase health care costs [30]. Brett and McCullogh [28, 31] described an approach to clinical practice in the context of differing interests to facilitate patient-physician relationships. The authors recommend that a patient's preference for a diagnostic or therapeutic intervention dictate medical decision-making only when there is a modicum of potential clinical benefit. It is only if they meet this criterion that physicians proceed with patient-selected interventions [28, 31].

In addition to their patients, clinicians also have a fiscal responsibility to the health care system on a societal level to ensure its sustainability and judicious use of its resources [28, 32]. Although cost should not prevent patients from receiving optimal medical care, the fact remains that non-beneficial interventions have implications for individual patients and society as a whole and should be considered essential to professional integrity [28, 33–35]. Eliminating waste in diagnostic interventions, including duplicate and non-beneficial testing, can reduce a significant cost burden on the health care system [33]. At a certain threshold, challenging a patient's request when supported by clinical evidence should not be misconstrued as a denial of patient's perspective, but rather a professional responsibility to ensure cost-effective medical care [28]. This is best managed through transparent and collaborative dialogue, focused on the value of further investigations in improving the understanding of the evolving clinical picture and/or changing the clinical management.

Approach to the atypical otolaryngology-head and neck surgery patient

The appropriate management of pediatric patients with atypical symptoms can be a challenging task for Otolaryngologists. This report should stand as a resource for clinicians who encounter difficult cases in this context (Table 1). Open dialogue should be maintained with the patient and their family throughout the patient interaction. In challenging cases, such as those presented in this article, it is important for clinicians to broaden their differentials to include non-organic etiologies of otolaryngology disorders. Evaluation of these patients should be initiated with a thorough history and should note any potential risk factors for mental health and psychosocial factors which may impact the resiliency of the patient to cope with medical interventions, including surgery. Physical examination should include a complete

Table 1 Approach to the atypical ENT patient

Establish broad differential diagnoses[a]	
Organic diseases	
Non-organic diseases	Pseudohypacusis
	Functional upper airway obstruction
	Conversion disorder
	Adjustment disorder
	Autism spectrum disorders
Patient evaluation	Thorough history and physical examination including flexible nasolaryngoscopy
	Audiometry and vestibular testing should be performed to rule out organic pathology as indicated by the presenting complaint
	Consultation with relevant specialists including neurology and psychiatry
	Consider neuroimaging to rule out structural pathology
Treatment overview	Assessment of goals with staff, patient and family
	Confirm belief in presenting symptoms
	Avoid accusation
	Ensure patient and family is connected with appropriate community resources including physical or psychological rehabilitation
	Arrange follow-up visits

[a] This should be a resource utilized by clinicians in appropriate cases where an organic pathology has been ruled out

oto-neurologic examination and test of vestibular function. Rehabilitation should be prescribed based on results of screening and diagnostic testing. A consultation with Neurology and Mental Health services should be contemplated early, and where appropriate, an integrated team approach considered. The final care plan for these patients should commence with an understanding of the patient and family's goals, validation of the patient's symptomology and appropriate plan of care.

Conclusion

Delayed identification of mental illness can result in significant medical and psychological consequences for patients, increase the burden of care, and can impact their faith in the health care system. Furthermore, it creates a significant economic burden for the health-care system as a whole. In this case series, the authors present 3 patients in whom presentation and management of otolaryngology-related concerns were confounded by underlying conversion disorder.

While most patients referred to an Otolaryngology-Head and Neck Surgeon will have organic explanations for their symptoms, it is important for the clinician to keep psychogenic causes and contributors on the differential, especially in patients with atypical clinical presentations. The diagnostic approach to these patients requires a comprehensive assessment of the contributing factors, including the features of converson disorder associated with otolaryngology diseases, and impact the relationship between patients and clinicians. This article is intended to stimulate discussion between patients and clinicians regarding safe and efficient diagnosis of challenging clinical cases.

Abbreviations

CD: Conversion disorder; CT: Computed tomography; MRI: Magnetic resonance imaging

Authors' contributions

Conceptualization: MB. Methodology: LC, MB. Data curation: LC, SK, JO, HG, MB. Writing original draft preparation: LC, SK, JO, HG, MB. Writing review and editing: LC, SK, JO, HG, MB. All authors read and approved the final manuscript No authors have any financial or non-financial competing interests in regards to this manuscript.

Competing interests

The authors declare that they have no competing interests.

Author details

[1]Faculty of Medicine, University of Ottawa, Ottawa, ON, Canada. [2]Department of Otolaryngology-Head and Neck Surgery, The Ottawa Hospital, Ottawa, ON, Canada. [3]Division of Otolaryngology – Head and Neck Surgery, Children's Hospital of Eastern Ontario, 400 Smyth Road, Ottawa, ON K1H 8L1, Canada. [4]Department of Psychiatry, Children's Hospital of Eastern Ontario, University of Ottawa, Ottawa, ON, Canada. [5]Department of Psychology, Children's Hospital of Eastern Ontario, University of Ottawa, Ottawa, ON, Canada.

References

1. Organization WH: Child and adolescent mental health.. 2015.
2. Olfson M, Druss BG, Marcus SC. Trends in mental health care among children and adolescents. N Engl J Med. 2015;372(21):2029–38.
3. Ani C, Reading R, Lynn R, Forlee S, Garralda E. Incidence and 12-month outcome of non-transient childhood conversion disorder in the U.K. and Ireland. Br J Psychiatry. 2013;202:413–8.
4. Kozlowska K, Nunn KP, Rose D, Morris A, Ouvrier RA, Varghese J. Conversion disorder in Australian pediatric practice. J Am Acad Child Adolesc Psychiatry. 2007;46(1):68–75.
5. Kozlowska K, Palmer DM, Brown KJ, Scher S, Chudleigh C, Davies F, Williams LM. Conversion disorder in children and adolescents: a disorder of cognitive control. J Neuropsychol. 2014;9:87–108. https://doi.org/10.1111/jnp.12037.
6. van der Kruijs SJ, Bodde NM, Vaessen MJ, Lazeron RH, Vonck K, Boon P, Hofman PA, Backes WH, Aldenkamp AP, Jansen JF. Functional connectivity of dissociation in patients with psychogenic non-epileptic seizures. J Neurol Neurosurg Psychiatry. 2012;83(3):239–47.
7. Cojan Y, Waber L, Carruzzo A, Vuilleumier P. Motor inhibition in hysterical conversion paralysis. Neuroimage. 2009;47(3):1026–37.
8. de Lange FP, Toni I, Roelofs K. Altered connectivity between prefrontal and sensorimotor cortex in conversion paralysis. Neuropsychologia. 2010;48(6):1782–8.
9. Voon V, Brezing C, Gallea C, Ameli R, Roelofs K, LaFrance WC Jr, Hallett M. Emotional stimuli and motor conversion disorder. Brain. 2010;133(Pt 5):1526–36.
10. Rintelmann WF, Schwan SA, Blakley BW. Pseudohypacusis. Otolaryngol Clin N Am. 1991;24(2):381–90.
11. Kumpf W. Auscultatory detection of respiratory responses to olfactory stimuli. Approach to feigned anosmia (author's transl). Laryngol Rhinol Otol (Stuttg). 1978;57(9):830–3.
12. Lacy TJ, McManis SE. Psychogenic stridor. Gen Hosp Psychiatry. 1994;16(3):213–23.
13. Norton A, Roberton G. Functional upper airway obstruction. Anaesth Intensive Care. 1998;26(2):216–8.
14. Pula J. Functional vision loss. Curr Opin Ophthalmol. 2012;23(6):460–5.
15. Pracy JP, Walsh RM, Mepham GA, Bowdler DA. Childhood pseudohypacusis. Int J Pediatr Otorhinolaryngol. 1996;37(2):143–9.
16. Psarommatis I, Kontorinis G, Kontrogiannis A, Douniadakis D, Tsakanikos M. Pseudohypacusis: the most frequent etiology of sudden hearing loss in children. Eur Arch Otorhinolaryngol. 2009;266(12):1857–61.
17. Tomoda A, Kinoshita S, Korenaga Y, Mabe H. Pseudohypacusis in childhood and adolescence is associated with increased gray matter volume in the medial frontal gyrus and superior temporal gyrus. Cortex. 2012;48(4):492–503.
18. American Psychiatric Association. DSM-5 Task Force. Diagnostic and statistical manual of mental disorders : DSM-5. 5th ed. Arlington, VA: American Psychiatric Association; 2013.
19. Krasnik C, Grant C. Conversion disorder: not a malingering matter. Paediatr Child Health. 2012;17(5):246.
20. Kozlowska K. Good children with conversion disorder: breaking the silence. Clinical Child Psychology and Psychiatry. 2003;8(1):73–90.
21. Grattan-Smith P, Fairley M, Procopis P. Clinical features of conversion disorder. Arch Dis Child. 1988;63(4):408–14.
22. Leslie SA. Diagnosis and treatment of hysterical conversion reactions. Arch Dis Child. 1988;63(5):506–11.
23. Garralda ME. A selective review of child psychiatric syndromes with a somatic presentation. The British journal of psychiatry : the journal of mental science. 1992;161:759–73.
24. Bass C, Benjamin S. The management of chronic somatisation. The British journal of psychiatry : the journal of mental science. 1993;162:472–80.
25. Kozlowska K. Good children presenting with conversion disorder. Clinical Child Psychology and Psychiatry. 2001;6:575–91.
26. Nicholson TR, Stone J, Kanaan RA. Conversion disorder: a problematic diagnosis. J Neurol Neurosurg Psychiatry. 2011;82(11):1267–73.
27. Carlson ML, Archibald DJ, Gifford RH, Driscoll CL. Conversion disorder: a missed diagnosis leading to cochlear reimplantation. Otol Neurotol. 2011;32(1):36–8.
28. Brett AS, McCullough LB. Addressing requests by patients for nonbeneficial interventions. Jama. 2012;307(2):149–50.
29. Miller E. Defining hysterical symptoms. Psychol Med. 1988;18(2):275–7.
30. Crosskerry P, Nimmo GR. Better clinical decision making and reducing diagnostic error. Journal of the Royal College of Physicians and Edinburgh. 2011;41(2):155–62.
31. Brett A, McCullough LB. When patients request specific interventions: defining the limits of the physician's obligations. N Engl J Med. 1986;315(21):1347–51.
32. American College of Physicians. How Can Our Nation Conserve and Distribute Health Care Resources Effectively and Efficiently? Philadelphia: American College of Physicians; 2011: Policy Paper. (Available from American College of Physicians, 190 N. Independence Mall West, Philadelphia, PA 19106.). https://www.acponline.org/system/files/documents/advocacy/current_policy_papers/assets/health_care_resources.pdf.
33. Reuben DB, Cassel CK. Physician stewardship of health care in an era of finite resources. Jama. 2011;306(4):430–1.
34. Brody H. Medicine's ethical responsibility for health care reform–the top five list. N Engl J Med. 2010;362(4):283–5.
35. Newman-Toker DE, McDonald KM, Meltzer DO. How much diagnostic safety can we afford, and how should we decide? A health economics perspective. BMJ Qual Saf. 2013;22:ii11–20.

27

Endoscopic management of maxillary sinus inverted papilloma attachment sites to minimize disease recurrence

Vincent Wu[1], Jennifer Siu[2], Jonathan Yip[2] and John M. Lee[2,3*]

Abstract

Background: Inverted papillomas (IPs) are benign neoplasms, most commonly arising from the mucosal lining of the maxillary sinus. IPs can have single or multifocal sites of attachment. Although pedicle location is an important factor to consider in surgical planning, it is less clear whether the location or number of IP attachment sites hold any prognostic value. Herein, we aimed to determine the prognostic significance of the number and location of attachment sites of IPs originating from the maxillary sinus when managed by a pure endoscopic approach.

Methods: This was a single-center, single-surgeon retrospective chart review. Patients with maxillary sinus IPs who were managed by endoscopic approaches only, from January 1, 2010 to June 30, 2016, were identified. Demographic data, operative technique, number and location of IP attachment sites, follow-up duration, recurrence, and presence of malignant transformation were captured.

Results: Twenty-eight maxillary IP patients (61% males) were included, with a mean age of 54.9 (standard deviation (SD): 16.5) years. Approximately 36% of patients were referred from other institutions for management of recurrent IPs after failing previous surgical treatment. All patients were managed with an endoscopic approach, and all required an endoscopic medial maxillectomy to facilitate access to the maxillary sinus. At a mean follow-up of 31.1 (SD: 22.6) months, there were no recurrences identified. IPs with single (46%) and multifocal (54%) attachments were predominately to the medial and lateral walls. Maxillary IPs with multifocal attachments most frequently involved 2-3 walls of the sinus. Osteitis (36%) was commonly seen.

Conclusion: IPs originating from the maxillary sinus frequently had multifocal attachments, but this did not impact disease recurrence. Despite the surgical challenges of accessing all of the maxillary sinus walls, IPs originating from the maxillary sinus can be effectively managed via a pure endoscopic approach.

Keywords: Endoscopic, Sinus surgery, Maxillary sinus, Inverted papilloma, Prognosis, Recurrence, Attachment site, Multifocal, Medial maxillectomy

Background

Inverted papillomas (IPs) are benign neoplasms arising from the mucosal lining of the nasal cavity and paranasal sinuses [1]. IPs can have either single or multifocal sites of origin, with a recurrence rate ranging from 14 to 25% if surgical resection is not complete [2, 3]. This is of clinical significance as IPs are associated with a 5 – 15% malignant transformation rate to squamous cell carcinoma [4, 5].

The majority of IPs develop within the maxillary sinus, often originating from the medial wall [6–8]. Invasion into adjacent structures is the main complication of disease progression and can involve the orbit, lacrimal system, and skull base [9–12]. These tumors also have a tendency to erode and re-model bone, leading to devastating sequelae [13, 14].

Surgery is the mainstay of treatment for IPs and historically have included several approaches: 1) non-endoscopic

* Correspondence: leejo@smh.ca
[2]Division of Rhinology, Department of Otolaryngology – Head and Neck Surgery, St. Michael's Hospital, University of Toronto, Toronto, Ontario, Canada
[3]Li Ka Shing Knowledge Institute, St. Michael's Hospital, Toronto, Ontario, Canada
Full list of author information is available at the end of the article

endonasal, 2) limited external (i.e. Caldwell-Luc), 3) radical external (i.e. lateral rhinotomy or midfacial degloving with en bloc resection), and 4) endoscopic endonasal [5, 7, 12, 15]. A pedicle-oriented strategy is currently widely implemented in the resection of IPs with the surgical approach employed specific to the pedicle location. It has been reported that the endoscopic approach alone was insufficient in reaching all maxillary IPs pedicle sites, especially with IPs that originated from the lateral, anterior, and inferior sinus walls [7]. In these instances, external approaches such as the Caldwell-Luc were required for complete resection [7]. However, with advancements in endoscopic technologies and techniques, tumors originating from the maxillary sinus have increasingly been managed by a pure endoscopic approach alone.

Although the pedicle location is an important factor to consider in surgical planning, it is less clear whether the location or number of IP attachment sites hold any prognostic value. Herein, we aimed to determine the prognostic significance of the number and location of attachment sites of IPs originating from the maxillary sinus, when managed by a pure endoscopic approach. We hypothesize that IPs of multiple attachment sites are associated with increased recurrence.

Methods

Patient selection

We carried out a single surgeon (JML), single centre retrospective chart review. All patients who had resection for IPs originating only from the maxillary sinus, from January 1, 2010 to June 30, 2016, were included in the study. Patients who had expressed prior wishes not to be included in any clinical research at our academic centre were excluded. There were no other exclusion criteria.

Patient charts including pre-operative consults, operative notes, and post-operative follow-up reports were obtained and reviewed. All operative notes were dictated by the staff surgeon (JML). Demographic data, history of previous IP resection, surgical technique(s), presence of any perioperative complication(s), length of stay (LOS), and follow-up length were extracted.

Surgical approach

Once pathology of IP was confirmed via intraoperative frozen sections, the mass was resected systematically with a microdebrider initially to debulk the tumor that was free-floating in the sinonasal cavity. The goal of the surgery is to identify the site(s) of attachment(s) so that the mucosa can be removed and the underlying bone drilled down to decrease the chance of tumor recurrence. Angled endoscopes, along with curved instruments, microdebriders and burrs were used for tumor resection within the maxillary sinus. A medial maxillectomy was performed to facilitate removal of the tumor

origin (if it was attached to the medial maxillary sinus wall) or simply to allow increased access to all walls of the sinus cavity. For IPs originating from the anterior maxillary wall, a transseptal approach was used for increased angulation [16]. Frozen sections of resection margins were sent at the end of the operation to ensure complete removal of IP.

Outcome measures

The primary outcome measures were IP attachment site(s) and recurrence. The number and location(s) of the IP attachment site(s) were determined based on direct visualization by the surgeon, and were extracted from the operative note. A secondary measure was the presence of malignant transformation including dysplasia.

Statistical analysis

Descriptive statistics were used to summarize the frequency and percentage of categorical variables. Continuous variables are reported as mean and standard deviation (SD). Student's t-test was performed to determine the differences between single and multiple sites of IP attachment for age, follow-up time, LOS, and disease recurrence. Fisher's exact test was used to analyze differences in gender and previous recurrence. All statistical analyses were performed using Prism (v.7, GraphPad, USA), with significance set to $\alpha=0.05$.

Results

Twenty-eight maxillary IP patients (61% males) were identified and included for analysis, with a mean age of 54.9 (SD: 16.5) years. At a mean follow-up of 31.1 (SD: 22.6) months, no recurrences were identified. Ten patients (36%) were referred for IPs, which recurred after failing initial surgical treatment from another surgeon. Osteitis (36%) was commonly seen. Patient characteristics are shown in Table 1.

Comparisons of baseline characteristics between single and multiple attachment sites IPs are shown in Table 2. There was no statistically significant difference in the rate of recurrence between single and multiple attachment IPs

Table 1 Baseline Characteristics

Variables	Total Patient ($n = 28$)
Gender (male:female)	17:11
Age, years (mean, SD)	54.9 (16.5)
Prev. recurrence (n, %)	10 (36%)
Recurrence (n, %)	0 (0.0%)
Malignant transformation (n, %)	0 (0.0%)
Follow-up, months (mean, SD)	31.1 (22.6)
Length of stay, days (mean, SD)	0.68 (1.3)
Perioperative complications (n, %)	0 (0.0%)

Table 2 Comparison of Baseline Characteristics between Single and Multiple Attachment Sites

Variables	Single Attach. (n = 13)	Multiple Attach. (n = 15)	P-value
Gender (male:female)	7:6	10:5	0.700
Age, years (mean, SD)	55.8 (16.8)	54.2 (16.8)	0.807
Prev. recurrence (n, %)	3 (23%)	7 (47%)	0.254
Follow-up, months (mean, SD)	37.6 (23.7)	25.4 (20.7)	0.158
Length of stay, days (mean, SD)	0.31 (0.48)	1.0 (1.6)	0.145

group prior to revision surgery. Additionally, no statistically significant difference was noted in follow-up time between single attachment IP patients, with a length of 37.6 (SD: 23. 7) months, as compared to 25.4 (SD: 20.7) months in multifocal IP patients. LOS in hospital was short within both groups, and did not differ between groups.

Attachments of IP to the maxillary sinus walls were classified as either single (46%) or multiple (54%). IPs with single attachment predominately originated from the medial maxillary wall, while those with multiple pedicles involved primarily the medial, lateral, and anterior walls (Table 3). For maxillary IPs with multifocal sites of attachment, 67% of cases originated from 2 to 3 walls of the sinus cavity, but can also have multiple attachments to a single wall (Table 4).

All patients were managed with a pure endoscopic approach, with all requiring an endoscopic medial maxillectomy. No adjunctive external approaches were required and no perioperative complications were encountered.

Discusssion

The complete resection of maxillary sinus IPs is crucial due to the propensity for recurrence and its malignancy risk. During surgery, the tumor must be followed down to its origin to facilitate a wide local excision of the pedicle site [7, 17, 18]. In our series, IPs were followed to their attachments, with diseased mucosa resected and bone drilling performed at the pedicle sites. The number of attachment sites can theoretically be associated with tumor recurrence, since most IP recurrences occur at the pedicle and multifocal IPs may be more difficult to manage surgically [7, 19]. Previous reports have demonstrated successful surgical results stemming from a pure endoscopic approach for maxillary IPs originating from

the medial, superior, and posterior walls [4, 7, 20, 21]. However, endoscopic access to the anterior and inferior walls was noted to be more challenging, inadequate for reaching all of the tumor, which often necessitated adjunctive external approaches [7, 21–23].

Dean et al., (2014) reported that using a transseptal surgical approach in combination with medial maxillectomy facilitated full visualization of anterolateral maxillary IPs with multiple attachment sites, which allowed for the complete resection of the tumor pedicle [16]. During their study, with a mean follow-up of 29 months, no recurrences were noted for both the single and multiple IP attachment site groups [16]. Compared to results from our study, this is a similar findings as we noted no disease recurrence between single and multifocal sites at 31.1 months, while using a similar transseptal approach for accessing the anterior maxillary wall. However, contrasting our findings of no perioperative complications, Dean et al. reported infraorbital paresthesia in 9% of patients, secondary to tumor invasion of the nerve [16].

In a study by Hong et al. (2015), evaluating surgical approaches used in resecting maxillary IPs, only 16.1% of patients underwent a pure endoscopic approach [7]. External approaches, including Canine fossa puncture via Caldwell-Luc approach or Caldwell-Luc operation, were added gradually as required if endoscopy was insufficient in resecting all parts of the IP. External approaches were mainly added for lateral, anterior, and inferior wall involvement [7]. Hong et al. showed that 48.4% of maxillary IPs originated from the anterior and/or inferior walls, comparable to 42.9% in our study [7]. Similar to our results, no recurrences were reported in patients who underwent a pure endoscopic approach at a mean follow-up of 64.2 months [7]. Of interest, the recurrence rate

Table 3 Wall of Maxillary Sinus Involved in Cases with Single and Multiple Attachment Sites

Maxillary Sinus Wall	Single Attach.	Multiple Attach.
Posterior	1	7
Inferior	0	7
Lateral	2	9
Anterior	1	9
Medial	8	10
Superior	1	3

Table 4 Number of Maxillary Sinus Walls Involved in Cases of Multifocal Attachment

Number of Walls Involved	Cases
1	2
2	5
3	5
4	1
5	0
6	2

was found to be 9.7% in patients with IPs of multiple attachment sites, who underwent adjunctive external approaches [7]. In our experience, we found that an external approach is not necessary for access to all IP attachment sites. Instead, an endoscopic medial maxillectomy and use of angled scopes can facilitate visualization to the anterior and inferior maxillary walls.

The results of our study have several clinical implications. First, pure endoscopic management of sino-nasal disease decreases the need for prolonged LOS in hospital. A previous report by Sautter et al. (2007) demonstrated that patients who underwent endoscopic IP resection spent significantly fewer days in hospital as compared to patients who had open surgery [24]. Similarly, our study demonstrates low LOS of both our single and multifocal IPs. Other clinical implications of a pure endoscopic approach to maxillary sinus IPs have been well described in the literature and include avoidance of facial incision, minimizing scarring, decreased pain, swelling, and dysesthesia as compared to open surgery [20, 22]. Moreover, one of the largest single cohort studies on IP reported a reduction in recurrence with the implementation of endoscopic approaches [25]. These results were reiterated by a recent meta-analysis, which noted that endoscopic management of IPs reduced recurrence risk by 44% as compared to external approaches [26]. Additionally, endoscopic medial maxillectomy has been described as effective and reproducible for IP resection, with decreased operating time and morbidity as compared to open maxillectomy [27]. As we noted no perioperative complications within our series, our results may provide further evidence indicating the low morbidity stemming from the endoscopic approach.

This study has limitations. While we aimed to acquire long-term data on IP recurrence within our cohort, with a mean follow-up of 31.1 months, this still may not have adequately captured all cases of recurrence. It has been reported that up to 20% of recurrences may occur 5 years after resection for all IPs [28]. However, specific for maxillary IPs, recurrences have been noted to occur within a mean time of 20 months [7]. This study was also retrospective in nature, and has limitations inherent to such analysis. Our analysis focused on surgical outcomes by distinguishing single from multiple attachment sites IPs. With a larger sample size, analysis may be performed for surgical outcomes based on the exact number of attachments. Future studies should aim to assess longer-term outcomes.

Conclusion

No differences in recurrence were noted between single and multifocal attachment maxillary IPs. The majority of IPs originating from the maxillary sinus frequently had multi-focal attachments. Despite surgical challenges of reaching all sinus walls, maxillary IPs may be managed effectively via a pure endoscopic approach.

Abbreviations
IP: Inverted papilloma; LOS: Length of stay; SD: Standard deviation

Acknowledgements
This study was presented as a poster presentation at the Canadian Society of Otolaryngology – Head and Neck Surgery annual meeting in Saskatoon, Saskatchewan, 2017.

Funding
This study received no funding.

Authors' contributions
All authors were involved with the conception and design of the study, analysis and interpretation of data, revision of the manuscript, and have approved the final manuscript.

Competing interests
The authors declare that they have no competing interests.

Author details
[1]School of Medicine, Faculty of Health Sciences, Queen's University, Kingston, Ontario, Canada. [2]Division of Rhinology, Department of Otolaryngology – Head and Neck Surgery, St. Michael's Hospital, University of Toronto, Toronto, Ontario, Canada. [3]Li Ka Shing Knowledge Institute, St. Michael's Hospital, Toronto, Ontario, Canada.

References
1. Wood JW, Casiano RR. Inverted papillomas and benign nonneoplastic lesions of the nasal cavity. Am J Rhinol Allergy. 2012;26(2):157.
2. Shahrjerdi B, AngoYaroko A, Abdullah B. Co-existing of sinonasal inverted papilloma and angiofibroma: care report and review of the literature. Acta Inform Med. 2012;20(4):261–3.
3. Mirza S, Bradley PJ, Acharya A, Stacey M, Jones NS. Sinonasal inverted papillomas: recurrence, and synchronous and metachronous malignancy. J Laryngol Otol. 2007;121(9):857–64.
4. Krouse JH. Endoscopic treatment of inverted papilloma: safety and efficacy. Am J Otolaryngol. 2001;22(2):87–99.
5. Hyams VJ. Papillomas of the nasal cavity and the paranasal sinuses, a clinicopathologic study of 315 cases. Ann Otol Rhinol Laryngol. 1971; 80(2):192–6.
6. Buchwald C, Nielsen LH, Nielsen PL, Ahlgren P, Tos M. Inverted papilloma: a follow-up study including primarily unacknowledged cases. Am J Otolaryngol. 1989;10(4):273–81.
7. Hong SL, Mun SJ, Cho KS, Roh HJ. Inverted papilloma of the maxillary sinus: surgical approach and long-term results. Am J Rhinol Allergy. 2015;29(6):441–4.
8. Schneyer MS, Milam BM, Payne SC. Sites of attachment of Schneiderian papilloma: a retrospective analysis. Int Forum Allergy Rhinol. 2011;1(4):324–8.
9. Chaudhry IA, Taiba K, Al-Sadhan Y, Riley FC. Inverted papilloma invading the orbit through the nasolacrimal duct: a case report. Orbit. 2005;24(2):135–9.
10. Bajaj MS, Pushker N. Inverted papilloma invading the orbit. Orbit. 2002; 21(2):155–9.
11. Elner VM, Burnstine MA, Goodman ML, Dortzbach RK. Inverted papillomas that invade the orbit. Arch Ophthalmol. 1995;113(9):1178–83.
12. Pitak-Arnnop P, Bertolini J, Dhanuthai K, Hendricks J, Hemprich A, Pausch NC. Intracranial extension of Schneiderian inverted papilloma: a case report and literature review. Ger Med Sci. 2012;10:12.

13. Krouse JH. Development of a staging system for inverted papilloma. Laryngoscope. 2000;110(6):965–8.
14. Wolfe SG, Schlosser RJ, Bolger WE, Lanza DC, Kennedy DW. Endoscopic and endoscope-assisted resections of inverted sinonasal papillomas. Otolaryngol Head Neck Surg. 2004;131:174–9.
15. Sham CL, Woo JK, van Hasselt CA. Endoscopic resection of inverted papilloma of the nose and paranasal sinuses. J Laryngol Otol. 1998; 112(8):758–64.
16. Dean NR, Illing EA, Woodworth BA. Endoscopic resection of anterolateral maxillary sinus inverted papillomas. Laryngoscope. 2015;125(4):807–12.
17. Xiao-Ting W, Peng L, Xiu-Qing W, Hai-Bo W, Wen-Hui P, Bing L, Er-Peng Z, Guang-Gang S. Factors affecting recurrence of sinonasal inverted papilloma. Eur Arch Otorhinolaryngol. 2013:1–5.
18. Kamel RH, Abdel FA, Awad AG. Origin oriented management of inverted papilloma of the frontal sinus. Rhinology. 2012;50(3):262–8.
19. Dubin MG, Kuhn FA. Unilateral multifocal inverted papilloma of the maxillary and frontal sinus. Am J Otolaryngol. 2006;27(4):263–5.
20. Lund V, Stammberger H, Nicolai P, Castelnuovo P. European position paper on endoscopic Management of Tumours of the nose, paranasal sinuses and Skull Base introduction. Rhinology. 2011:1–43.
21. Dragonetti A, Gera R, Sciuto A, Scotti A, Bigoni A, Barbaro E, Minni A. Sinonasal inverted papilloma: 84 patients treated by endoscopy and proposal for a new classification. Rhinology. 2011;49(2):207–13.
22. Busquets JM, Hwang PH. Endoscopic resection of sinonasal inverted papilloma: a meta-analysis. Otolaryngol Head Neck Surg. 2006;134(3):476–82.
23. McCollister KB, Hopper BD, Ginsberg LE, Michel MA. Inverted papilloma: a review and What's new. Neurographics. 2015;5(3):96–103.
24. Sautter NB, Cannady SB, Citardi MJ, Roh HJ, Batra PS. Comparison of open versus endoscopic resection of inverted papilloma. Am J Rhinol. 2007;21(3):320–3.
25. Bugter O, Monserez DA, van Zijl FVWJ, Baatenburg de Jong RJ, Hardillo JA. Surgical management of inverted papilloma; a single-center analysis of 247 patients with long follow-up. J Otolaryngol Head Neck Surg. 2017 Dec 20;46(1):67.
26. Amedee RG. Recurrence of Sinonasal inverted papilloma following surgical approach: a meta-analysis. Am J Rhinol. 2017;31(3):207.
27. Sadeghi N, Al-Dhahri S, Manoukian JJ. Transnasal endoscopic medial maxillectomy for inverting papilloma. Laryngoscope. 2003;113(4):749–53.
28. Jiang XD, Dong QZ, Li SL, Huang TQ, Zhang NK. Endoscopic surgery of a sinonasal inverted papilloma: surgical strategy, follow-up, and recurrence rate. Am J Rhinol Allergy. 2017;31(1):51–5.

28

The role of induction chemotherapy followed by surgery in unresectable stage IVb laryngeal and hypopharyngeal cancers: a case series

Pichit Sittitrai*[iD], Donyarat Reunmarkkaew and Saisaward Chaiyasate

Abstract

Background: The purpose of this study was to evaluate the benefit of induction chemotherapy followed by surgery in locally advanced unresectable stage IVb laryngeal and hypopharyngeal squamous cell carcinoma (LHSCC).

Methods: Data of patients with stage IVb LHSCC who received induction chemotherapy for the purpose of tumor resection between January 2007 and January 2016 were retrospectively collected. Definitive surgery with postoperative adjuvant therapy was performed in patients whose tumors became resectable (resectable group). Chemoradiotherapy, radiotherapy, or supportive care was considered in patients whose tumors remained unresectable (unresectable group).

Results: Thirty-two patients were identified; the tumor resectability rate after induction chemotherapy was approximately 56%. The median overall survival (OS) rates of the resectable and unresectable groups were 20.0 months (range, 16.0–35.5 months) and 9.5 months (range, 6.0–15.0 months), respectively ($p = 0.008$). The estimated 2-year OS rates of the resectable and unresectable groups were 59.5% (95% confidence interval [CI], 33.2–78.3%) and 10.7% (95% CI, 1.1–35.4%), respectively ($p = 0.008$). The estimated 2-year disease-free survival (DFS) rates of the resectable and unresectable groups were 53.5% (95% CI, 27.9–73.6%), and 14.3% (95% CI, 2.3–36.6%), respectively ($p = 0.009$). On multivariate analysis, factors positively impacting OS and DFS in all patients were surgical resection, a laryngeal primary site, and induction chemotherapy with docetaxel, cisplatin, and fluorouracil.

Conclusions: In advanced unresectable stage IVb LHSCC patients, surgical resection following induction chemotherapy appears to improve survival outcomes.

Keywords: Larynx, Hypopharynx, Chemotherapy, Unresectable tumor

Background

Head and neck squamous cell carcinoma (HNSCC) accounts for approximately 6% of all cancers worldwide; most patients present with locally advanced diseases [1–3]. The standard treatment for advanced resectable HNSCC is surgery followed by radiotherapy or a combination of chemotherapy and radiotherapy [1, 3, 4]. In more advanced unresectable tumors, radiotherapy was considered the conventional treatment [5]. However, with these modalities' limited responses and low survival rates, alternative approaches including altered fractionation radiotherapy, combined radiotherapy and chemotherapy, and combined radiotherapy and targeted therapy were devised [5–7]. Meta-analyses and clinical trials have previously demonstrated the superiority of combined radiotherapy and chemotherapy over radiation therapy alone in advanced unresectable head and neck cancer patients; however, the survival advantage remained inadequate [6–9]. For advanced unresectable laryngeal and hypopharyngeal squamous cell carcinoma (LHSCC), multimodality treatment has also been introduced, with induction chemotherapy

* Correspondence: psittitrai@yahoo.com
Department of Otolaryngology, Chiang Mai University, Chiang Mai 50200, Thailand

administered before definitive local therapy as the most promising option [1, 4, 10]. The use of induction chemotherapy to reduce tumor size and improve surgical resectability has been investigated in previous studies; however, almost all patients had oral cavity cancers, and the criteria for unresectability remain very heterogeneous [11–13].

Although the criteria for unresectability are widely debated, stage IVb HNSCC, as defined by the American Joint Committee on Cancer (AJCC) Staging Manual (7th edition), is the clearest and most accepted cutoff for resectability [14]. The purpose of this study was to evaluate the benefit of induction chemotherapy that achieved adequate tumor shrinkage followed by surgery in patients with locally advanced unresectable stage IVb laryngeal and hypopharyngeal squamous cell carcinoma.

Methods

We conducted a retrospective study of patients with unresectable LHSCC who underwent induction chemotherapy to render tumors resectable at the Department of Otolaryngology, Faculty of Medicine, Chiang Mai University between January 2007 and January 2016. The patients were evaluated with clinical examination and imaging studies (computed tomography and/or magnetic resonance imaging); primary tumors and/or cervical lymph nodes were initially considered unresectable if they had 1) prevertebral fascia invasion, 2) carotid artery encasement of more than 270 degrees, or 3) mediastinal structure involvement. Patients who had distant metastasis, Eastern Cooperative Oncology Group performance status ≥2, or had not completed all 3 cycles of induction chemotherapy were excluded.

The induction chemotherapy regimen was as follows: 1) cisplatin 100 mg/m^2 on day 1, and 5-fluorouracil (5-FU) 1000 mg/m^2/d from days 1–4 (PF regimen), 2) carboplatin at an area under the curve of 5 on day 1 and paclitaxel 175 mg/m^2 on day 1 (CP regimen), and 3) docetaxel 75 mg/m^2 on day 1, cisplatin 75 mg/m^2 on day 1, and 5-FU 750 mg/m^2/d from day 1 to 4 (TPF regimen). The choice of the regimen was decided based on the patient's performance status, creatinine clearance, and financial constraints. Induction chemotherapy was administered in 3 cycles every 3 weeks; 2–3 weeks after completing the third cycle, the patients were re-evaluated for tumor response by clinical examination and imaging studies according to the RECIST version 1.1 [15]. If the tumor had shrunk and was considered resectable, the patient was scheduled for surgery 3–4 weeks after completing induction chemotherapy. Surgical treatment consisted of either total laryngectomy with partial laryngectomy or total laryngectomy with total pharyngectomy and flap reconstruction (pectoralis major myocutaneous or radial forearm free flaps). The types of performed neck dissections were modified

radical, radical, or extended radical. Chemoradiotherapy with weekly cisplatin (30 mg/m^2) or carboplatin at an area under the curve of 1.5 combined with radiotherapy at the total dose of 60–70 Gy or radiotherapy alone at the dose of 66–70 Gy were recommended postoperatively.

Patients with unresectable tumors after induction chemotherapy were managed with concurrent chemoradiotherapy, radiotherapy, or supportive care according to their medical conditions. All patients were followed for a minimum of 12 months after treatment completion or until death. The institutional review board approved this study.

SPSS version 18.0 for Windows (IBM Corporation, Armonk, NY, USA) was used to analyze the patients' characteristics. Variables were compared using Pearson's chi-square or independent samples t-test, as appropriate. The Stata statistical software version 12.0 (Stata Corporation, Texas, USA) was used for survival analysis. Estimated survival function was calculated by using the Kaplan-Meier method and compared using the log-rank test. Logistic regression was used for univariate and multivariate analyses of factors affecting resectability. The Cox proportional hazards model was used for univariate and multivariate analyses of factors affecting survival function.

Results

Thirty-two patients were included in the study; all had stage IVb diseases (T4bN3 = 12 patients, T4bN2 = 9 patients, and T3 N3 = 11 patients). The median follow-up time was 18 months (range, 6–35.5 months). According to our unresectability criteria, there were 9 patients with prevertebral fascia invasion, 17 with carotid artery encasement, 5 with both prevertebral fascia invasion and carotid artery encasement, and 1 with mediastinal structure involvement. The patient's clinical characteristics are presented in Table 1. After 3 cycles of induction chemotherapy, none of the patients achieved complete tumor response. However, 21 patients had partial tumor response, 7 had stable disease, and 4 had progressive disease.

Pathological examination of the surgical specimens revealed free, close, and positive margins in 1, 7, and 10 cases, respectively. Pathological extracapsular extension of the resected lymph node was observed in 9 cases.

Postoperative chemoradiotherapy was recommended in all surgical cases. Thirteen patients were able to complete the 6 cycles of chemotherapy, while 3 complete 1–3 cycles. Two patients had radiotherapy alone owing to a tumor-free surgical margin and no extracapsular extension of the dissected lymph node. Five patients with unresectable diseases were treated with concurrent chemoradiotherapy, 3 with radiotherapy, and 6 with supportive care. Pulmonary metastasis was noted in 3 patients during the follow-up period

Table 1 Baseline Patient Characteristics

Characteristics	Resectable group N = 18 (%)	Unresectable group N = 14 (%)	p-value
Age, year			
Mean (SD)	59.5 (3.13)	62.3 (3.29)	0.053
Sex			
Male	14 (77.8)	10 (71.4)	0.681
Female	4 (22.2)	4 (28.6)	
Performance status			
0	12 (66.7)	7 (50)	0.341
1	6 (33.3)	7 (50)	
Smoking			
Yes	12 (66.7)	10 (71.4)	0.773
No	6 (33.3)	4 (28.6)	
Alcohol			
Yes	8 (44.4)	8 (57.1)	0.476
No	10 (55.6)	6 (42.9)	
Primary site			
Larynx	9 (50)	3 (21.4)	0.098
Hypopharynx	9 (50)	11 (78.6)	
TN stage			
T3 N3	6 (33.3)	5 (35.7)	0.888
T4bN2	5 (27.8)	4 (28.6)	
T4bN3	7 (38.9)	5 (35.7)	
Causes of unresectability			
Preveterbral fascia invasion	4 (22.2)	5 (35.7)	0.960
Carotid artery encasement	12 (66.7.)	5 (35.7)	
Preveterbral fascia invasion and carotid artery encasement	2 (11.1)	3 (21.4)	
Mediastinal structure involvement	0	1 (7.1)	
Regimen			
TPF	11 (61.1)	3 (21.4)	0.080
CP	3 (16.7)	5 (35.7)	
PF	4 (22.2)	6 (42.9)	
Differentiation			
Poor	7 (38.9)	7 (50)	0.641
Moderate	6 (33.3)	5 (35.7)	
Well	5 (27.8)	2 (14.3)	

TPF = docetaxel, cisplatin, and 5-fluorouracil, CP = carboplatin and paclitaxel, PF = cisplatin and 5-fluorouracil

(12 months after surgery and adjuvant chemoradiotherapy in 1 patient, and 5 and 10 months after initiating supportive care in the other 2 patients, respectively).

Resectability rate

Following induction chemotherapy, 18 patients with a partial response had sufficient tumor reduction and were considered resectable (i.e., the resectable group). The remaining 14 patients still had unresectable diseases (and comprised the unresectable group). The resectability rate was 56.3%.

Factors predicting tumor resectability

Clinical variables including primary site, T stage, N stage, the cause of unresectability, chemotherapy regimen, and tumor differentiation were analyzed to determine tumor resectability after induction chemotherapy. On univariate analysis, laryngeal cancer and

TPF regimen were the factors associated with tumor resectability ($p = 0.048$, and $p = 0.006$, respectively). Multivariate analysis showed that receiving a TPF regimen was the only predictive factor associated with producing sufficient tumor reduction; patients who underwent TPF had a tumor resectability rate of 78.6%, while those who underwent PF and CP regimens had resectability rates of 40% and 37.5%, respectively ($p = 0.044$). (Table 2)When considering the characteristics of resectable tumors, those with carotid artery encasement had the highest chance of undergoing surgical resection, with a rate of 70.6%. However, tumors with prevertebral fascia invasion alone, prevertebral fascia invasion plus carotid artery encasement, and mediastinal structure involvement had resection rates of 44.4%, 40%, and 0%, respectively; the differences were not significant ($p = 0.088$).

Overall survival (OS)

The median OS of all patients was 16 months (range, 9.5–35.5 months). The median OS rates of the resectable and unresectable groups were 20.0 months (range, 16.0–35.5 months), and 9.5 months (range, 6.0–15.0 months), respectively ($p = 0.008$).

The estimated 2-year OS of all patients was 39.1% (95% confidence interval [CI], 22.1–55.7%). The estimated 2-year OS rates of the resectable and unresectable groups were 59.5% (95% CI, 33.2–78.3%), and 10.7% (95% CI, 1.1–35.4%), respectively ($p = 0.0008$) (Fig. 1).

Disease-free survival (DFS)

The median DFS of all patients was 13.5 (range, 7.5–21.5 months). The median DFS of the resectable and unresectable groups were 20.0 months (range, 12.5–25.0 months), and 6.0 months (range, 5.0–11.0 months), respectively ($p = 0.009$).

The estimated 2-year DFS of all patients was 36% (95% CI, 19.6–52.7%). The estimated 2-year DFS of the resectable and unresectable groups were 53.5% (95% CI, 27.9–73.6%), and 14.3% (95% CI, 2.3–36.6%), respectively ($p = 0.0009$) (Fig. 2).

Locoregional recurrence occurred in 20 patients; 8 (44.4%) were in the resectable group and 12 (85.7%) in the unresectable group.

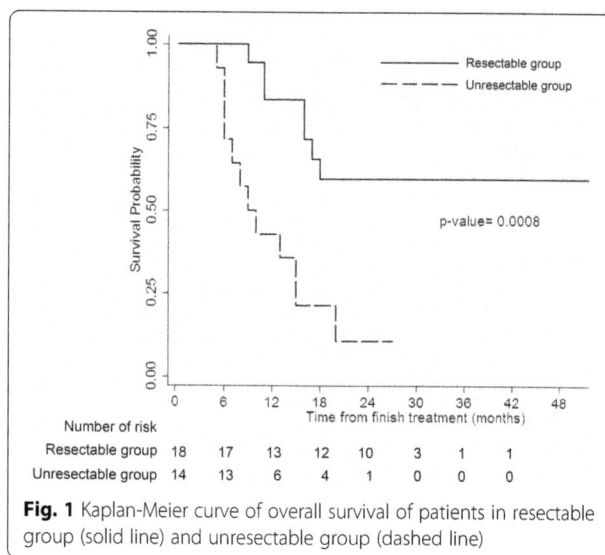

Fig. 1 Kaplan-Meier curve of overall survival of patients in resectable group (solid line) and unresectable group (dashed line)

Factors influencing OS and DFS

Clinical variables including age, sex, performance status, smoking, alcohol usage, primary site, T stage, N stage, the cause of unresectability, chemotherapy regimen, surgical resection, and tumor differentiation were analyzed to determine factors influencing OS and DFS rates in all patients. Univariate analysis revealed factors positively affecting OS and DFS rates were patients with performance status = 0 ($p = 0.041$, and $p = 0.038$, respectively), laryngeal cancer ($p = 0.009$, and $p = 0.012$, respectively), receiving the TPF regimen ($p = 0.006$, and p = 0.009, respectively), and surgical resection ($p = 0.010$, and $p = 0.008$, respectively).

However, on multivariate analysis, factors positively affecting the OS and DFS rates in all patients were surgical resection ($p = 0.007$ and 0.007, respectively), laryngeal

Table 2 Multivariate analysis of factors predicting tumor resectability after induction chemotherapy

Variable	Odds ratio	95% confidence interval	p-value
Chemotherapy regimen			
TPF vs. CP/PF	9.76	1.20–79.69	0.044

TPF = docetaxel, cisplatin, and 5-fluorouracil, CP = carboplatin and paclitaxel, PF = cisplatin and 5-fluorouracil

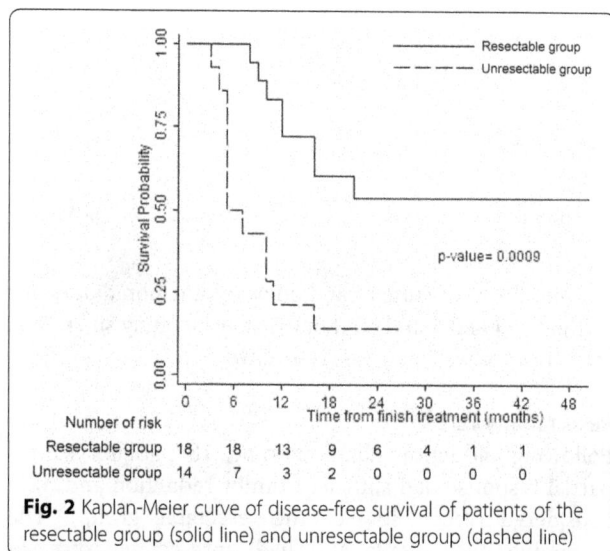

Fig. 2 Kaplan-Meier curve of disease-free survival of patients of the resectable group (solid line) and unresectable group (dashed line)

primary (p = 0.009 and 0.005, respectively), and receiving the TPF regimen (p < 0.001 and = 0.006, respectively). (Table 3 and Table 4) No factor influencing OS and DFS were identified in the resectable group, while definitive chemoradiotherapy extended DFS in the unresectable group (p = 0.001).

Discussion

For locally advanced resectable LHSCC, organ-preservation strategies using combined chemotherapy and radiotherapy as induction, concurrent, sequential, or alternating therapies have been studied in recent decades [16–18]. In more advanced LHSCC with cartilage invasion, extralaryngeal soft tissue invasion, or high-volume tumor, primary surgery with postoperative adjuvant therapy has remained the recommended therapy [16–19].

Induction chemotherapy in HNSCC has been aimed at reducing distant metastasis, inducing tumor shrinkage, and allowing for the assessment of tumor responsiveness in order to plan subsequent therapies [4]. Although induction chemotherapy followed by radiotherapy or chemoradiotherapy in locally advanced unresectable HNSCC (including LHSCC) showed an advantage for OS, the patients' prognoses remained unsatisfactory [1, 10, 20]. Separately, induction chemotherapy has also been used to achieve surgical resection and improve prognosis in unresectable HNSCC [11, 12]. Patil et al. [11] investigated oral cavity cancer patients who had "technically unresectable tumors" because 1) the disease extended to the zygoma, 2) there was soft tissue involvement that reached the hyoid bone, 3) there was infratemporal fossa involvement, 4) oral tongue cancer extending to the vallecula was present, or 5) extensive soft tissue invasion impacting the achievement of a negative surgical margin was present. Approximately 43% of their patients experienced sufficient tumor shrinkage to allow surgery after induction chemotherapy. Schmaltz et al. [12] performed a

Table 3 Multivariate analysis of factors positively affecting the overall survival rate

Variables	Hazard ratio	95% confidence interval	p-value
Primary site			
Larynx vs. Hypopharynx	0.14	0.03–0.60	0.009
Chemotherapy regimen			
TPF vs. CP/PF	0.08	0.01–0.45	< 0.001
Treatment			
Surgery vs. Non-surgery	0.26	0.09–0.69	0.007

TPF = docetaxel, cisplatin, and 5-fluorouracil, CP = carboplatin and paclitaxel, PF = cisplatin and 5-fluorouracil

Table 4 Multivariate analysis of factors positively affecting the disease-free survival rate

Variables	Hazard ratio	95% confidence interval	p-value
Primary site			
Larynx vs. Hypopharynx	0.12	0.03–0.53	0.005
Chemotherapy regimen			
TPF vs. CP/PF	0.09	0.02–0.51	0.006
Treatment			
Surgery vs. Non-surgery	0.27	0.10–0.69	0.007

TPF = docetaxel, cisplatin, and 5-fluorouracil, CP = carboplatin and paclitaxel, PF = cisplatin and 5-fluorouracil

study of patients with oral cavity cancer, oropharyngeal cancer, metastatic lymphadenopathy of unknown primary, and hypopharyngeal cancer; their criteria for unresectability were a high risk of incomplete surgical resection, advanced nodal status of N2b or more, thrombosis of the internal jugular vein, and major scalability. They achieved a resectability rate of 87.8% in their patients after induction chemotherapy.

The term 'unresectable' is difficult to define, as resectability has improved over time owing to advances in surgical and reconstruction techniques [11, 21]. The criteria for unresectability of the primary site or of the adenopathy generally include fixation to the spine or prevertebral muscles; or involvement of the skin, dura, base of skull, or brachial plexus [21]. We included patients with advanced unresectable laryngeal and hypopharyngeal cancers in our study. The criteria for unresectability were prevertebral fascia invasion, carotid artery encasement, and mediastinal structure involvement, which are classified as very advanced stage IVb (T4b and /or N3) by the AJCC Cancer Staging Manual, 7th edition. It revealed that hypopharyngeal cancers were detected more frequently to be unresectable in our patients because they are characterized by the extensive submucosal spread and high risk of nodal involvement which are usually more aggressive than laryngeal cancers [22]. To the best of our knowledge, there has been no study of the management of unresectable stage IVb LHSCC exclusively.

None of our patients achieved complete tumor response after 3 cycles of induction chemotherapy, but 18 patients with partial responses had sufficient tumor reduction for resection; their resectability rate was 56.3%. The only significant predictive factor for tumor response was receiving a TPF regimen. Among tumors that met our unresectability criteria, those with carotid artery encasement had the highest rate of resectability (70.6%) post-induction chemotherapy, but with no statistical significance.

Induction chemotherapy with the addition of docetaxel to cisplatin and 5-FU was previously shown to significantly improve OS and DFS in patients with unresectable HNSCC [1, 3, 11, 17]; this was also confirmed in our study. We also demonstrated that surgical resection had a positive impact on both OS and DFS, which is consistent with data from Patil et al. [11] and from Schmaltz et al. [12]. In primary site-specific analysis, patients with laryngeal cancer had longer survival than those with hypopharyngeal cancer.

In patients undergoing surgical resection, postoperative adjuvant therapy and favorable pathological response had previously been identified as factors that improved survival [11, 13]. However, none of these factors (including tumor stage, tumor differentiation, pathological surgical margin, pathological extracapsular extension of lymph node, or postoperative treatment) affected patient outcomes in our study. However, definitive chemoradiotherapy had a positive impact on DFS in the unresectable group.

The survival rates in our study appear to be lower than in patients who received sequential therapy for locally advanced larynx and hypopharynx cancer in the TAX 324 study [17]. However, this was expected since patients in our study had far more advanced disease stages. Therefore, the concept of surgical resection following induction chemotherapy, even in patients who initially had stage IVb disease, appears to be viable.

The limitations of our study include its retrospective nature, single-arm study, and small sample size. The chemotherapy regimen was decided based on the patient's performance status, creatinine clearance and financial constraints. The TPF regimen was more likely to be administered in the resectable group, although there was no significant difference between the groups. However, this may cause selection bias and may affect the outcomes.

Conclusion

In advanced unresectable stage IVb LHSCC, induction chemotherapy converted 56% of tumors to resectable status. Surgical resection following induction chemotherapy with TPF regimen appears to improve survival outcomes, especially in patients with laryngeal primary tumor sites. Concurrent chemoradiotherapy results in better DFS than either radiotherapy alone or supportive care in patients whose tumors remain unresectable after induction chemotherapy.

Abbreviations

C: Carboplatin; CI: Confidence interval; DFS: Disease-free survival; F: 5-Fluorouracil; HNSCC: Head and neck squamous cell carcinoma; LHSCC: Laryngeal and hypopharyngeal squamous cell carcinoma; OS: Overall survival; P: Cisplatin; P: Paclitaxel; T: Docetaxel; TNM: Tumor/node/metastasis

Authors' contributions

PS, DR, and SC conceptualized the study. PS wrote the final manuscript. PS and DR was responsible for maintenance of the database, data analysis and manuscript preparation including revision and editing. SC performed the statistical analyses along with revision and editing of the manuscript. All authors read, provided revisions and approved the final manuscript.

Competing interests

The authors declare that they have no competing interests.

References

1. Vermorken JB, Remenar E, van Herpen C, et al. Cisplatin, fluorouracil, and docetaxel in unresectable head and neck cancer. N Engl J Med. 2007; 357(17):1695–704.
2. Parkin DM, Bray F, Ferlay J, et al. Global cancer statistics, 2002. CA Cancer J Clin. 2005;55(2):74–108.
3. Posner MR, Hershock DM, Blajman CR, et al. Cisplatin and fluorouracil alone or with docetaxel in head and neck cancer. N Engl J Med. 2007; 357(17):1705–15.
4. Nwizu T, Ghi MG, Cohen EE, et al. The role of chemotherapy in locally advanced head and neck squamous cell carcinoma. Semin Radiat Oncol. 2012;22(3):198–206.
5. Jeremic B, Shibamoto Y, Stanisavljevic B, et al. Radiation therapy alone or with concurrent low-dose daily either cisplatin or carboplatin in locally advanced unresectable squamous cell carcinoma of the head and neck: a prospective randomized trial. Radiother Oncol. 1997;43(1):29–37.
6. Ruo Redda MG, Ragona R, Ricardi U, et al. Radiotherapy alone or with concomitant daily low-dose carboplatin in locally advanced, unresectable head and neck cancer: definitive results of a phase III study with a follow-up period of up to ten years. Tumori. 2010;96(2):246–51.
7. Adelstein DJ, Li Y, Adams GL, et al. An intergroup phase III comparison of standard radiation therapy and two schedules of concurrent chemoradiotherapy in patients with unresectable squamous cell head and neck cancer. J Clin Oncol. 2003;21(1):92–8.
8. Budach W, Hehr T, Budach V, et al. A meta-analysis of hyperfractionated and accelerated radiotherapy and combined chemotherapy and radiotherapy regimens in unresected locally advanced squamous cell carcinoma of the head and neck. BMC Cancer. 2006;6:28.
9. Pignon JP, le Maître A, Maillard E, Bourhis J, MACH-NC Collaborative Group. Meta-analysis of chemotherapy in head and neck cancer (MACH-NC): an update on 93 randomised trials and 17,346 patients. Radiother Oncol. 2009; 92(1):4–14.
10. Paccagnella A, Orlando A, Marchiori C, et al. Phase III trial of initial chemotherapy in stage III or IV head and neck cancers: a study by the Gruppo di studio sui Tumori della Testa e del Collo. J Natl Cancer Inst. 1994; 86(4):265–72.
11. Patil VM, Prabhash K, Noronha V, et al. Neoadjuvant chemotherapy followed by surgery in very locally advanced technically unresectable oral cavity cancers. Oral Oncol. 2014;50(10):1000–4.
12. Schmaltz H, Borel C, Ciftci S, et al. Induction chemotherapy before surgery for unresectable head and neck cancer. B-ENT. 2016;12(1):29–32.
13. Zhong LP, Zhang CP, Ren GX, et al. Randomized phase III trial of induction chemotherapy with docetaxel, cisplatin, and fluorouracil followed by surgery versus up-front surgery in locally advanced resectable oral squamous cell carcinoma. J Clin Oncol. 2013;31(6):744–51.
14. Edge SB, Byrd DR, Compton CC, Fritz AG, Greene FL, Trotti A III, editors. Larynx AJCC Cancer staging manual. 7th ed. New York: Springer; 2010. p. 57–62.
15. Eisenhauer EA, Therasse P, Bogaerts J, et al. New response evaluation criteria in solid tumours: revised RECIST guideline (version 1.1). Eur J Cancer. 2009; 45(2):228–47.
16. Lefebvre LJ, Rolland F, Tesselaar M, et al. Phase 3 randomized trial on larynx preservation comparing sequential vs alternating chemotherapy and radiotherapy. J Natl Cancer Inst. 2009;101(3):142–52.
17. Posner MR, Norris CM, Wirth LJ, et al. Sequential therapy for the locally advanced larynx and hypopharynx cancer subgroup in TAX 324: survival, surgery, and organ preservation. Ann Oncol. 2009;20(5):921–7.

18. Forastiere AA, Zhang Q, Weber RS, et al. Long-term results of RTOG 91–11: a comparison of three nonsurgical treatment strategies to preserve the larynx in patients with locally advanced larynx cancer. J Clin Oncol. 2013;31(7):845–52.

19. Scherl C, Mantsopoulos K, Semrau S, et al. Management of advanced hypopharyngeal and laryngeal cancer with and without cartilage invasion. Auris Nasus Larynx. 2017;44(3):333–9.

20. Zorat PL, Paccagnella A, Cavaniglia G, et al. Randomized phase III trial of neoadjuvant chemotherapy in head and neck cancer: 10-year follow-up. J Natl Cancer Inst. 2004;96(22):1714–7.

21. Culliney B, Birhan A, Young AV, Choi W, Shulimovich M, Blum RH. Management of locally advanced or unresectable head and neck cancer. Oncology (Williston Park). 2008;22(10):1152–61.

22. Wei WI. The dilemma of treating hypopharyngeal carcinoma: more or less: Hayes Martin lecture. Arch Otolaryngol Head Neck Surg. 2002;128(3):229–32.

29

The 678 Hz acoustic immittance probe tone: a more definitive indicator of PET than the traditional 226 Hz method

Justin M. Pyne[1,2], Tarek Ibrahim Lawen[1,2], Duncan D. Floyd[2] and Manohar Bance[1,2,3*]

Abstract

Background: The accurate diagnosis of Eustachian tube (ET) dysfunction can be very difficult. Our aim is to determine whether a 678 Hz probe tone is a more accurate indicator of Patulous ET (PET) than the 226 Hz probe tone when used in compliance over time (COT) testing.

Methods: Twenty subjects (11 normal ET ears and 7 PET ears) were individually seated in an examination room and connected to a GSI TympStar Middle Ear Analyzer. The order of probe tone frequency (678 or 226 Hz) was randomized. Baseline "testing" COT recordings for each ear undergoing testing were completed. Subjects were instructed to occlude their contralateral nostril and to breathe forcefully in and out through their ipsilateral nostril until the test had run to completion. This process was repeated with the probe tone that had not been previously run. For the control group, each subject had one random ear tested. For the experimental group, only the affected ear(s) was tested. Wilcoxon rank rum tests were performed to determine statistical significance.

Results: The baseline COT measurements for the control group and PET group were similar, 0.86 mL (SD = 0.34) and 0.74 (SD = 0.33) respectively. Comparing the 226 Hz tone between groups revealed that PET patients had a median COT difference 0.19 mL higher than healthy ET patients, and for the 678 Hz tone, PET patients had a median COT difference of 0.57 mL higher than healthy ET patients. Both were deemed to be statistically significant ($p = 0.002$, $p = 0.004$ respectively). The was a statistically significant median COT difference between the 678 Hz and 226 Hz of 0.61 mL ($p = 0.034$) for the PET group, while the same comparison for the control group of 0.05 mL was not significant ($p = 0.262$), suggesting that the 678 Hz tone yields a larger response for PET than the 226 Hz tone, and no difference for the control group, thus making it less prone to artifact noise interference.

Conclusion: The 678 Hz probe tone is a more reliable indicator of ET patency, and should be preferably used over the 226 Hz tone for future COT testing.

Background

The Eustachian tube (ET) is a narrow, epithelial-lined osseocartilaginous tube that connects the middle ear cavity to the nasopharynx [1, 2]. It functions to maintain middle ear health and to facilitate sound transmission from the tympanic membrane (TM) to the inner ear [3]. The ET accomplishes this by fulfilling three major physiologic roles, which include drainage of middle ear secretions, prevention of nasopharyngeal reflux and,

most importantly, pressure equalization across the TM [4, 5]. The proper functioning of the ET greatly depends on the regular intermittent opening and closing of the tube. At rest, the ET is passively collapsed; however, the ET can be actively opened under the control of paratubal muscles during such activities as swallowing, yawning and chewing [2, 6]. Any aberration in opening and closing is considered ET dysfunction (ETD) and can be further classified as either obstructive or patulous dysfunction [3, 4, 7].

Obstructive ETD is inadequate tubal opening caused by either paratubal muscular failure or obstruction of the ET by intrinsic changes. Failure of the ET to open typically results in patients complaining of aural fullness,

* Correspondence: m.bance@dal.ca

[1]Faculty of Medicine, Dalhousie University, Halifax, NS, Canada

[2]Department of Surgery, Division of Otolaryngology – Head and Neck Surgery, Dalhousie University, Faculty of Medicine, Halifax, NS, Canada

Full list of author information is available at the end of the article

periodic 'popping' sounds, muffled hearing and tinnitus [8]. Left untreated, patients with obstructive ETD can develop cholesteatoma, perforation, middle ear effusions and conductive hearing loss [4, 9].

A patulous Eustachian tube (PET) is a far less common type of ETD where the ET remains abnormally open intermittently or permanently, allowing for excessive communication between the middle ear and nasopharynx [10]. Reported potential risk factors for PET include sudden and severe weight loss, pregnancy, radiation therapy and congenital ET defects; nonetheless, many patients do not have any predisposing factors [10–16].

The most typical symptoms of PET include autophony (hearing one's own voice) and aerophony (hearing one's own breathing), and often aural fullness [17]. Vertigo, tinnitus and conductive hearing loss have been described, but in our experience, are less common [18]. In severe cases, symptoms are so distressing that patients progress to develop psychiatric sequelae, such as suicidal ideation and major depressive episodes [15]. Some symptoms, such as autophony can overlap with other disorders, such as superior canal dehiscence. Classically, autophony and aerophony are made worse with standing and exercise, and are improved by lying down [19]. However, symptoms can be intermittent and not present when the patient is seen in clinic. The definitive diagnosis of PET is made on direct otoscopic observation of the tympanic membrane moving synchronously with respiration: this is the result of transmission of nasopharyngeal air pressures directly to the middle ear cavity (MEC) through the patent ET. The movement of the tympanic membrane can be exacerbated by having the subject sit upright and take deep breaths while occluding one nostril, to accentuate nasopharyngeal pressure changes [19].

Despite several different methods being employed over the years, there is no universally accepted protocol for the evaluation of a patent ET [10]. Nasal endoscopy is frequently used to examine the pharyngeal opening of the ET; however, due to a narrow tubular lumen, the opening being eccentric to the line of visualization, the valve area being mostly hidden, and the presence of secretions, diagnostic visualization of the ET is usually very difficult [20].

Various researchers have suggested the use of acoustic immittance and standard tympanometry to indirectly observe the respiratory-synchronous movements of the tympanic membrane in the presence of PET [4, 21, 22].

During an acoustic immitance measurement, the tympanometer generates a pure tone of a specific frequency that is delivered into the ear canal via its probe component., and the reflected sound measured. This is a measure of the acoustic impedance and admittance. The typical, tympanometric probe tone is 226 Hz. Acoustic admittance (the reciprocal of acoustic impedance) is a reliable surrogate for compliance when the tone is of a relatively low frequency.

A tympanometer can graph the compliance over time (COT) of the tympanic membrane (sometimes called long time-base tympanometry, and often found on the reflex decay testing function in commercial tympanometers), and this is helpful in the evaluation ET function. During the test, the patient is asked to perform various breathing exercises (e.g. ipsilateral nostril breathing or sniffing) to see the effect on the tympanic membrane's COT. Exaggerated changes in tympanic membrane compliance synchronous with inhalation and exhalation are indicative of a PET [10].

Compliance over time using 226 Hz pure tones has been shown to identify PET via respiratory-synchronous middle ear compliance with occlusion of the contralateral nostril and forced ipsilateral nostril breathing [10, 22–24]. Nonetheless, we have found in our ET practice that alterations in COT measurements using a 678 Hz pure tone is more powerfully predictive of PET than any other tone used before. This was observed when using COT testing with the 226 Hz frequency in the Eustachian Tube clinic; anecdotally, the false-positive rate was too high and the signals too small to reliably interpret with the 226 Hz tone.

The aim of this study was to evaluate results of COT testing in presumed closed and patulous Eustachian tubes, and to compare the 226 Hz and 678 Hz probe tones to determine if the latter provides a clearer distinction between patulous ET and closed ET, which has not been previously described. We hypothesize, based on our observations, that the PET group will produce stronger, clearer, and more identifiable patterns of COT using a 678 Hz pure tone when compared with the 226 Hz frequency, while the closed ET group will yield similar results for each respective tone.

Methods

Subject selection

Ethics approval was obtained from our institutional research ethics board. Through the Eustachian Tube Clinic at our institution, subjects were identified as having suspected PET and asked to participate in this study. These subjects experienced one or more of the symptoms of autophony, aerophony, and/or aural fullness. All PET subjects were examined with otoscopy and microscopy to confirm that there was no obstruction in the ear canal, no current visible ear disease, and that the TM was moving with respiration prior to testing. Any subjects not meeting these criteria were excluded from the PET group (experimental group). These were our confirmed PET subjects.

To obtain our healthy ET group (control group), subjects with no prior history of ear disease, no previous ear surgery, and no current ET dysfunction were recruited. All healthy subjects were examined with otoscopy to confirm that there was no obstruction in the ear canal, no current visible ear disease, and that the TM was not moving with respiration prior to testing. Any ears not meeting these criteria were excluded from the control group.

Data collection

Data was collected prospectively. Subjects were seated upright in an examination room and connected to a GSI TympStar Middle Ear Analyzer (Grason-Stadler, MN, USA). A typical tympanogram was completed on each subject. The machine was then set to the acoustic reflex decay test protocol (allowing for a 15-s recording/10 s analysis window) and either the 226 Hz probe tone or the 678 Hz probe tone was selected. The acoustic reflex stimulus setting was set to the CONTRA option, but the contralateral earphone was not placed in the subject's opposite ear; the stimulus level was also set to 35 dB, i.e. there was no acoustic stimulus applied that could cause a stapedial reflex. The order of probe tone frequency (678 or 226 Hz) was randomized. Baseline "testing" COT recordings for each ear undergoing testing were completed. This measured the middle ear admittance over the 15 s window in the absence of any acoustic stimuli or subject maneuvering. As such, this was the admittance over time with the middle ear "at rest." COT testing for PET was then completed. Just prior to initiating the test, each subject was instructed to occlude their contralateral nostril. The testing protocol was initiated, and each subject was instructed breathe forcefully in and out through their ipsilateral nostril until the test had run to completion, which increases nasopharyngeal pressure changes, and therefore emphasize the effects of a PET. This process was repeated with the probe tone that had not been previously run. For the control group, each subject had one random ear tested. For the experimental group, only the affected ear(s) was tested. All results were retrieved from the TympStar printer upon completion of each test run.

Statistical analysis

A descriptive analysis was performed on patient demographics. These are represented by averages, range, and standard deviation. For statistical analysis, COT values at both 226 Hz and 678 Hz were compared between healthy and PET subjects, as well as within each subject group. A case control design was implemented. With PET patients representing cases and healthy ET patients representing controls. Wilcoxon rank sum tests were performed to determine statistical significance. All

analysis was performed with R version 3.3.1 ("Bug in Your Hair"). Effect sizes are presented as medians and approximate 95% confidence intervals. Non-parametric testing was utilized as sample sizes in our study were insufficient to rely on assumptions of asymptomatic normality for the purposes of hypothesis testing. A p value < 0.05 was considered statistically significant (95% confidence interval.)

Study population

The control group consisted of eight males and three females with a mean age of 28.7 years (range: 24 years to 46 years; SD = 5.8 years). Of this group, three members described having symptoms of tinnitus intermittently. None had hearing loss or experienced autophony.

The experimental group consisted of four males and three females with a mean age of 35.7 years (range: 23 years to 50 years; SD = 12.3 years). Of these patients, two had a sensorineural hearing loss and one had a hearing loss that was conductive in nature. Three patients from the experimental group could volitionally open their ET, and tests were performed when they were sure their ETs were open, which was confirmed by observation of movement of the TM with respiration. Four patients reported symptoms of autophony. None reported tinnitus. Data are reported as means and standard deviations (SD).

Results

The study included a total of 18 patients (18 ears) who underwent COT testing, demographics are in Table 1. Both the average and range of magnitude of MEC were recorded for each group.

In the control group (11 ears), the resting tympanogram compliance average was 0.86 mL (SD = 0.34 mL), which is comparable to that of the experimental group (0.74 mL, SD = 0.33 mL), however two PET ears were missed for this stage of testing. The average change in middle ear compliance (COT) was 0.07 mL (SD = 0.05 mL) for the 226 Hz frequency, and 0.12 mL (SD = 0.12 mL) for the 678 Hz frequency (Table 2). Figure 1 shows COT tracings for a healthy ET subject at the 226 Hz and 678 Hz frequencies. For the PET group (7 ears), the average middle ear compliance change was 0.26 mL (SD = 0.08 mL) and 0.69 mL (SD = 0.35 mL) for the 226 Hz and 678 Hz frequencies, respectively (Table 2). Figure 2 shows COT tracings for a PET subject at the 226 Hz and 678 Hz frequencies.

Table 1 Demographics of study population

	Mean Age, yrs (range)	Male	Female
Healthy ET	28.63 (24–46)	8	3
PET	35.71 (22–50)	4	3

Table 2 Comparison of healthy ET and PET COT following testing of 226 Hz and 678 Hz probe tones

	226 Hz		678 Hz	
	Average COT (mL)	SD (mL)	Average COT (mL)	SD (mL)
Healthy ET	0.07	0.05	0.12	0.12
PET	0.26	0.08	0.69	0.35

For comparison of results between groups, the difference between median COT at each frequency was evaluated (Table 3). It was found that for the 226 Hz frequency, the experimental group had an average COT of 0.19 mL more than the control group (0.26 mL vs 0.07 mL) and this was statistically significant ($p = 0.002$, Fig. 3). The median COT difference between groups at the 678 Hz frequency the difference was found to be 0.57 mL (0.69 mL vs. 0.12 mL) and this statistically significant ($p = 0.004$, Fig. 4). The difference between COT at 678 Hz and 226 Hz for the control group was 0.05 mL, while for the experimental group, this difference was 0.61 mL. The later was found to be statistically significant ($p = 0.034$) while there was no significant relationship seen in the former ($p = 0.262$).

Discussion

Evaluation of ET function via tympanometry has been used for many years, but it certainly has its challenges. Primarily, the 226 Hz tone provides only limited reliability for distinguishing between healthy and diseased ET

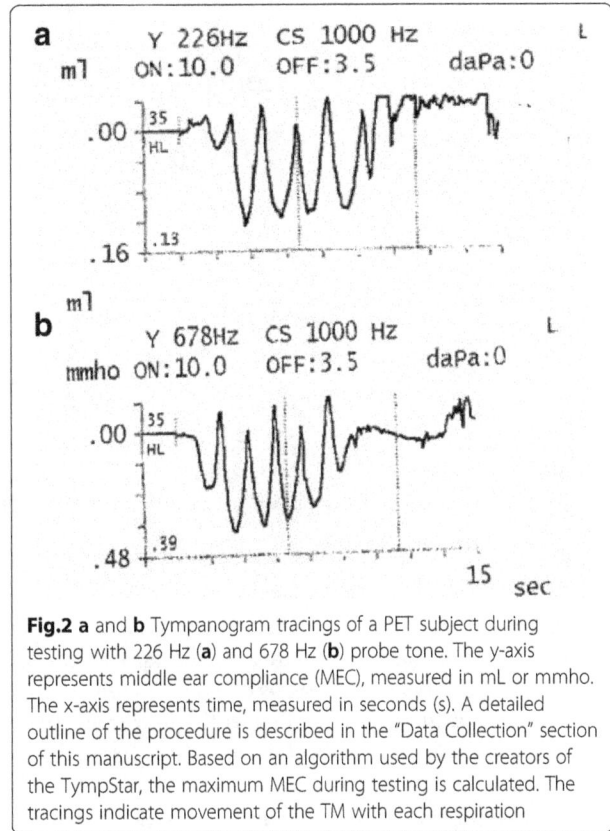

Fig. 1 **a** and **b** Tympanogram tracings of a healthy ET subject during testing with 226 Hz (**a**) and 678 Hz (**b**) probe tone. The y-axis represents middle ear compliance (MEC), measured in mL or mmho. The x-axis represents time, measured in seconds (s). A detailed outline of the procedure is described in the "Data Collection" section of this manuscript. Based on an algorithm used by the creators of the TympStar, the maximum MEC during testing is calculated. The tracings indicate movement of the TM with each respiration

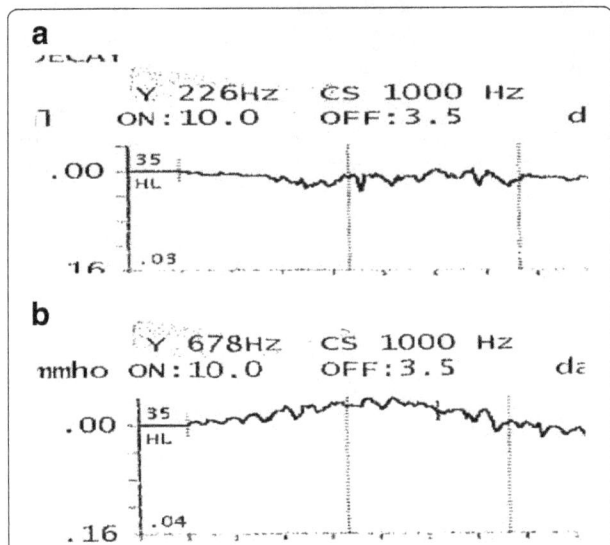

Fig.2 **a** and **b** Tympanogram tracings of a PET subject during testing with 226 Hz (**a**) and 678 Hz (**b**) probe tone. The y-axis represents middle ear compliance (MEC), measured in mL or mmho. The x-axis represents time, measured in seconds (s). A detailed outline of the procedure is described in the "Data Collection" section of this manuscript. Based on an algorithm used by the creators of the TympStar, the maximum MEC during testing is calculated. The tracings indicate movement of the TM with each respiration

states. This study investigated the compliance over time (COT) of patulous ET and healthy ET patients when subjected to 226 Hz and 678 Hz tones, with the goal of determining if the latter yielded a clearer distinction between the healthy and disease ET states. Although based on our statistical analysis, both the 226 Hz and 678 Hz frequencies yielded results that indicate they can distinguish between healthy ET and PET states, in comparison with the former, the latter method shows a very strong response for PET subjects, and in some cases, the response was higher than the limits of the TympStar instrument. This limitation is due to the fact the we have independently adapted this machine to run the tests we have set up. As such, the TympStar as commercially

Table 3 Wilcoxon Rank-Sum test for COT difference between healthy ET and PET at 226 Hz and 678 Hz probe tones

	Median Difference	95 CI	p
PET 226 Hz vs. healthy ET 226 Hz	0.19	(0.09 to 0.28)	0.002
PET 678 Hz vs. healthy ET 678 Hz	0.57	(0.25 to 0.93)	0.004
Healthy 678 Hz vs Healthy 226 Hz	0.05	(−0.02 to 0.09)	0.262
PET 678 Hz vs PET 226 Hz	0.61	(0.01 to 0.79)	0.034

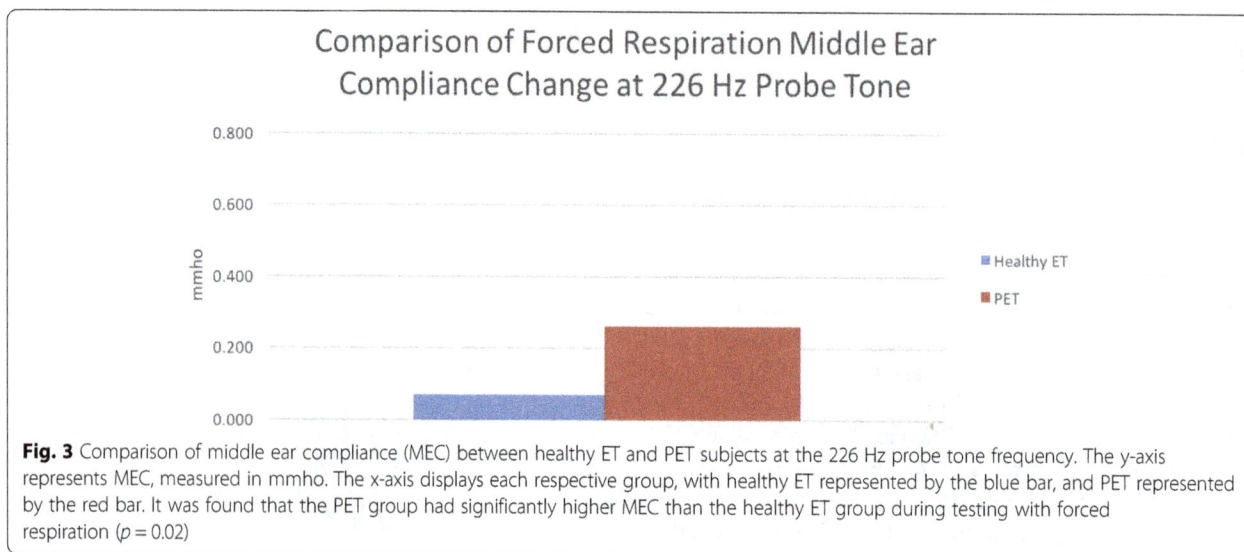

Fig. 3 Comparison of middle ear compliance (MEC) between healthy ET and PET subjects at the 226 Hz probe tone frequency. The y-axis represents MEC, measured in mmho. The x-axis displays each respective group, with healthy ET represented by the blue bar, and PET represented by the red bar. It was found that the PET group had significantly higher MEC than the healthy ET group during testing with forced respiration ($p = 0.02$)

configured is not the ideal instrument for measuring positive PET responses. Nonetheless, the upper limit of recording was 0.99 mmho and any response that exceeded this value were recorded as the maximum (0.99 mmho). If an instrument with the capability of reading up to 2.0 mmho or even 3.0 mmho was available, a more exact measurement of MEC would be possible. While the 226 Hz frequency does appear to show a distinction between healthy ET and PET states, the response is much lower than the 678 Hz probe tone, suggesting that the former could yield false positive results due to random noise.

One interesting aspect of our analysis was the comparison of probe tones within each subject group. There was no statistically significant difference between the 226 Hz and 678 Hz frequencies COT responses for the control group, which would support the notion that both are equally as effective at avoiding a false positive non-healthy ET state. However, comparing the same two tones for the experimental group, we found that the 678 Hz frequency had a significantly higher response than the 226 Hz frequency, offering further support that the former is the ideal frequency for this methodology of testing.

When evaluating the readouts from the instrument, it appeared that there was an apparent discrepancy between the displayed reading and the paper tracing produced. According to the manufacturer of the TympStar machine, a complicated and proprietary algorithm – which is beyond the scope of this paper – is used to produce the peak value reading, and little weight should be given to the tracings per se, rather

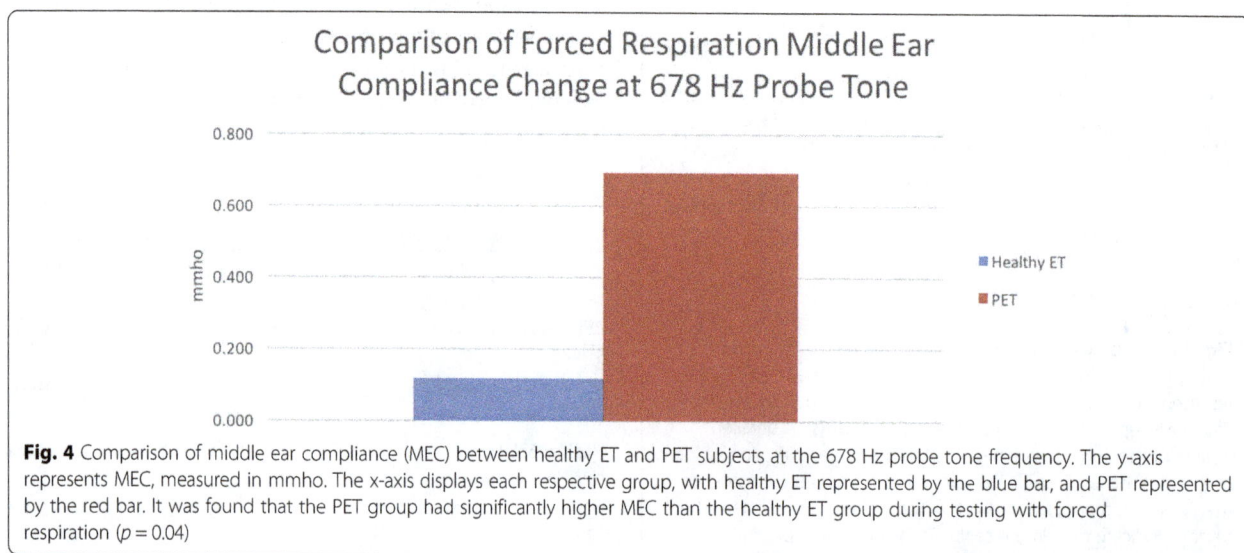

Fig. 4 Comparison of middle ear compliance (MEC) between healthy ET and PET subjects at the 678 Hz probe tone frequency. The y-axis represents MEC, measured in mmho. The x-axis displays each respective group, with healthy ET represented by the blue bar, and PET represented by the red bar. It was found that the PET group had significantly higher MEC than the healthy ET group during testing with forced respiration ($p = 0.04$)

the actual numbers reported on screen are more accurate.

It is important to acknowledge one of the limitations to our study: the sample size. However, given that many subjects with intermittent PET displayed no eardrum movements at the time of testing, or they stopped between microscopic examination and going to the testing area, it is difficult to obtain a large population of gold standard subjects. Thus, a longer study period may afford the necessary amount of time to discover a larger group of subjects.

Conclusion

To our knowledge, this is the first study to describe the 678 Hz probe tone in evaluation of middle ear immitance and compliance over time. Based on the evidence presented here, this suggests that this tone is a more reliable distinguisher between healthy ET and PET states than the previously accepted frequency. A study aimed at a larger population would be ideal for further evaluation. Additionally, using an instrument with the ability to record larger amplitude responses would allow more precise and accurate measurements of PET responses.

Abbreviations
ET: Eustachian Tube; ETD: Eustachian Tube dysfunction; MEC: Middle ear cavity; PET: Patulous Eustachian tube; TM: Tympanic membrane

Acknowledgements
The authors would like to thank members of the Sensory Encoding and Neuro-Sensory Engineering (SENSE) Lab for their assistance with the experimental setup.

Authors' contributions
JMP, TIL, DDF, and MB all assisted in the preparation of this manuscript. Study design by JMP, TIL, DDF, and MB. Data collection by JMP, TIL and DDF. Data analysis by JMP and DDF. Statistical analysis by JMP. All authors read and approved the final manuscript.

Authors' information
Justin Pyne is a third-year medical student at Dalhousie Medical School in Halifax, Nova Scotia, Canada.

Competing interests
The authors declare that they have no competing interests.

Author details
[1]Faculty of Medicine, Dalhousie University, Halifax, NS, Canada. [2]Department of Surgery, Division of Otolaryngology – Head and Neck Surgery, Dalhousie University, Faculty of Medicine, Halifax, NS, Canada. [3]Department of Clinical Neurosciences, University of Cambridge, Cambridge, UK.

References
1. Bartlett C, Pennings R, Ho A, Kirkpatrick D, Van Wijhe R, Bance M. Simple mass loading of the tympanic membrane to alleviate symptoms of patulous Eustachian tube. J Otolaryngol Head Neck Surg. 2010;39:259–68.
2. Alper CM, Swarts JD, Singla A, Banks J, Doyle WJ. Relationship between the electromyographic activity of the paratubal muscles and eustachian tube opening assessed by sonotubometry and videoendoscopy. Arch Otolaryngol Head Neck Surg. 2012;138:741–6.
3. Smith ME, Scoffings DJ, Tysome JR. Imaging of the Eustachian tube and its function: a systematic review. Neuroradiology. 2016;58(6):543–56.
4. Bluestone CD. Eustachian Tube. Structure, Function, Role in Otitis Media. Raleigh: BC Decker Inc.; 2005.
5. Poe, DS, Gopen, Q. Eustachian Tube Dysfunction. In: Ballenger's Textbook of Otolaryngology, Wackym, PA (Eds), BC Decker, Toronto 2008.
6. Sadé J, Ar A. Middle ear and auditory tube: middle ear clearance, gas exchange, and pressure regulation. Otolaryngol Neck Surg. 1997;116:499–524.
7. Bluestone CD, Klein JO. Otitis media and Eustachian tube dysfunction. In: Bluestone CD, Sylven SE, Alper CM, et al, editors. Pediatric Otolaryngology, 4. Philadelphia: W.B. Saunders; 2003. p. 474.
8. McCoul ED, Anand VK, Christos PJ. Validating the clinical assessment of eustachian tube dysfunction: the Eustachian tube dysfunction questionnaire (ETDQ-7). Laryngoscope. 2012;122:1137–41.
9. Schilder AGM, Bhutta MF, Butler CC, Holy C, Levine LH, Kvaerner KJ, et al. Eustachian tube dysfunction: consensus statement on definition, types, clinical presentation and diagnosis. Clin Otolaryngol. 2015;40:407–11.
10. McGrath AP, Michaelides EM. Use of middle ear immittance testing in the evaluation of patulous eustachian tube. J Am Acad Audiol. 2011;22(4):201–7.
11. Munoz D, Aedo C, Der C. Patulous eustachian tube in bariatric surgery patients. Otolaryngol Head Neck Surg. 2010;143:521–4.
12. Kuo C-Y, Wang C-H. Patulous Eustachian tube causing hypermobile eardrums. N Engl J Med. 2014;371:e37.
13. Poe DS. Diagnosis and management of the patulous eustachian tube. Otol Neurotol. 2007;28:668–77.
14. Karwautz A, Hafferl A, Ungar D, Sailer H. Patulous eustachian tube in a case of adolescent anorexia nervosa. Int J Eat Disord. 1999;25:353–5.
15. Doherty JK, Slattery WH 3rd. Autologous fat grafting for the refractory patulous eustachian tube. Otolaryngol Head Neck Surg. 2003;128:88–91.
16. O'Connor AF, Shea JJ. Autophony and the patulous eustachian tube. 1981.
17. Patel AA. Patulous Eustachian Tube: Background, Epidemiology, Etiology: Medscape. New York; 2017.
18. Robinson PJ, Hazell JWP. Patulous eustachian tube syndrome: the relationship with sensorineural hearing loss; treatment by eustachian tube diathermy. JLaryngol Otol. 1989;103:739–41.
19. Spear SA, Arriaga MA. In: Lalwani AK, Pfister MHF, editors. Recent advances in otolaryngology head and neck surgery, Vol. 2. New Delhi: Jaypee Brothers Medical Publishers (P) Ltd; 2013. Otol Neurotol 2013;34. p. 105–106.
20. Mathew GA, Kuruvilla G, Job A. Dynamic slow motion video endoscopy in Eustachian tube assessment. Am J Otolaryngol. 2007;28(2):91–7.
21. Northern JL. Clinical measurement procedures. In: Jerger J, editor. Handbook of Clinical Impedance Audiometry. Dobbs Ferry: American Electromedics Corp; 1975. p. 21–46.
22. Henry DF, DiBartolomeo JR. Patulous Eustachian tube identification using tympanometry. J Am Acad Audiol. 1993;4(1):53–7.
23. Kitajima N, Sugita-Kitajima A, Kitajima S. A case of patulous Eustachian tube associated with dizziness induced by nasal respiration. Auris Nasus Larynx. 2016;43:702–5.
24. Amoako-Tuffour Y, Jufas N, Quach J, Le L, Earle G, Kotiya AA, et al. Acoustic transmission characteristics of a Eustachian tube volitionally opened in two living subjects. Otol Neurotol. 2016;37:1055–8. https://doi.org/10.1097/MAO. 0000000000001130.

Improved symptomatic, functional, and fluoroscopic outcomes following serial "series of three" double-balloon dilation for cricopharyngeus muscle dysfunction

Derrick R. Randall[1,2*], Lisa M. Evangelista[1], Maggie A. Kuhn[1] and Peter C. Belafsky[1]

Abstract

Background: Cricopharyngeus muscle dysfunction (CPMD) is a common cause of dysphagia. We employ a progressive series of three double-balloon dilations separated by 4–6 weeks between procedures as a primary treatment option. The purpose of this study was to evaluate subjective, functional and objective improvement in swallowing after three serial dilations for CPMD.

Methods: We retrospectively evaluated patients between June 1, 2014, and June 30, 2016, who underwent a series of three double-balloon dilations for CPMD. Pre- and post-dilation Eating Assessment Tool-10 (EAT-10), Functional Oral Intake Scale (FOIS), pharyngeal constriction ratio, pharyngeal area, and pharyngoesophageal segment (PES) opening were compared.

Results: Seventeen patients with CPMD underwent serial double-balloon dilation procedures separated by one month. Mean age of the cohort was 73.5 (SD ± 13.3) years, and 53% were female. The mean EAT-10 improved from 24.7 (SD ± 7.8) to 15.9 (SD ± 10.2) [$p = 0.0021$]. Mean FOIS improved from 5.4 (SD ± 1.4) pre- to 6.3 (SD ± 0.9) post-treatment ($p = 0.017$). Mean UES opening increased from 1.05 (SD ± 0.34) cm to 1.48 (SD ± 0.41) cm ($p = 0.0003$) in the anteroposterior fluoroscopic view and from 0.58 (SD ± 0.18) to 0.76 (SD ± 0.30) cm ($p = 0.018$) in the lateral view. Pharyngeal constriction ratio (PCR), a surrogate measure of pharyngeal strength, improved from 0.49 (SD ± 0.37) to 0.24 (SD ± 0.15) ($p = 0.015$), however pharyngeal area (PA) was unchanged.

Conclusions: A progressive series of three double-balloon dilations for cricopharyngeus muscle dysfunction resulted in improved patient reported dysphagia symptom scores and objective fluoroscopic swallowing parameters.

Keywords: Dysphagia, Cricopharyngeus muscle dysfunction, Otolaryngology, Laryngology, Swallowing, Transnasal esophagoscopy

Background

Oropharyngeal swallowing dysfunction is common and costly. Complications include malnutrition, dehydration, depression, social isolation, pneumonia, hospital admission, increased length of stay, and death [1–3]. Early recognition allows implementation of appropriate rehabilitation, diet allocation or surgical management to prevent sequelae of impairment [4–6]. The pharyngoesophageal segment (PES) is a manometric high-pressure zone extending 3–5 cm from the hypopharynx to the cervical esophagus. Dysphagia resulting from PES dysfunction is a result of obstruction, poor compliance, impaired laryngeal elevation or ineffective pharyngeal propulsive forces [7]. Persons with PES dysfunction may present with solid food dysphagia, choking with deglutition, throat clearing, and globus.

One of the most common causes of solid food oropharyngeal dysphagia is cricopharyngeus muscle dysfunction (CPMD) [8]. The cricopharyngeus muscle is an essential

* Correspondence: d.randall@ucalgary.ca
This manuscript was presented at the Canadian Society of Otolaryngology Annual Meeting, Charlottetown, PEI, June 11 – 14, 2016.
[1]Center for Voice and Swallowing, Department of Otolaryngology – Head & Neck Surgery, University of California Davis, Sacramento, CA, USA
[2]Section of Otolaryngology – Head & Neck Surgery, Department of Surgery, University of Calgary, Calgary, AB T2W 3K2, Canada

component of the PES and is responsible for preventing the ingestion of air during respiration and reflux of esophageal contents into the pharynx. CPMD manifests as a spectrum of videofluoroscopic swallowing study (VFSS) findings ranging from non-obstructing bars found in up to 30% of the asymptomatic population to severely obstructing bars that limit oral intake to solids and liquids (Fig. 1) [9]. Pharyngeal constriction against an obstructed PES can lead to the development of a dilated, weak pharynx and Zenker's diverticulum [10, 11]. Treatment options include diet modification, botulinum toxin injection, dilation and endoscopic or open myotomy [7]. A variety of procedural interventions have been demonstrated to improve both symptoms and radiographic evidence of CPMD [7, 12, 13]. The optimal treatment requires an individualized strategy that takes into account disease severity, patient comorbidities and functional status, prognosis and required duration of effect.

A recent systematic review of dilation for CPMD found a variable response rate, ranging from 64 to 100% [12]. The variability in treatment efficacy may be related to dilator size, number of procedures, and the underlying disease process [14–17]. Furthermore, measures of swallowing function can be assessed by one of the numerous dysphagia symptom indices, if at all, or objective outcomes from fluoroscopic investigations. In our center, we use a series

of progressively enlarging balloon dilations, utilizing two balloons simultaneously to achieve a greater dilation profile and better approximate the natural, kidney shape of the PES [18, 19]. Patients are asked to complete Eating Assessment Tool (EAT-10) and Functional Oral Intake Scale (FOIS) instruments at all patient encounters in order to measure their progress and assess the severity of their symptoms. The EAT-10 has been validated for impact on quality of life due to dysphagia for several different etiologies, while the FOIS evaluates the degree of oral diet capacity by considering variety of consistencies a patient can manage and the amount of enteral tube feeding required [20, 21]. The purpose of this investigation was to determine the short term subjective and objective outcomes of serial PES double-balloon dilation for CPMD.

Methods

Patient population and outcome measures

This investigation was approved by the University of California, Davis Institutional Review Board (protocol #905351–1). All patients with complete data who underwent a series of three progressively increased balloon dilations for CPMD between June 1, 2014, and June 30, 2016 were included. The diagnosis of CPMD was made on VFSS. Patients who had undergone intervention for CPMD prior to the VFSS and those with either Zenker

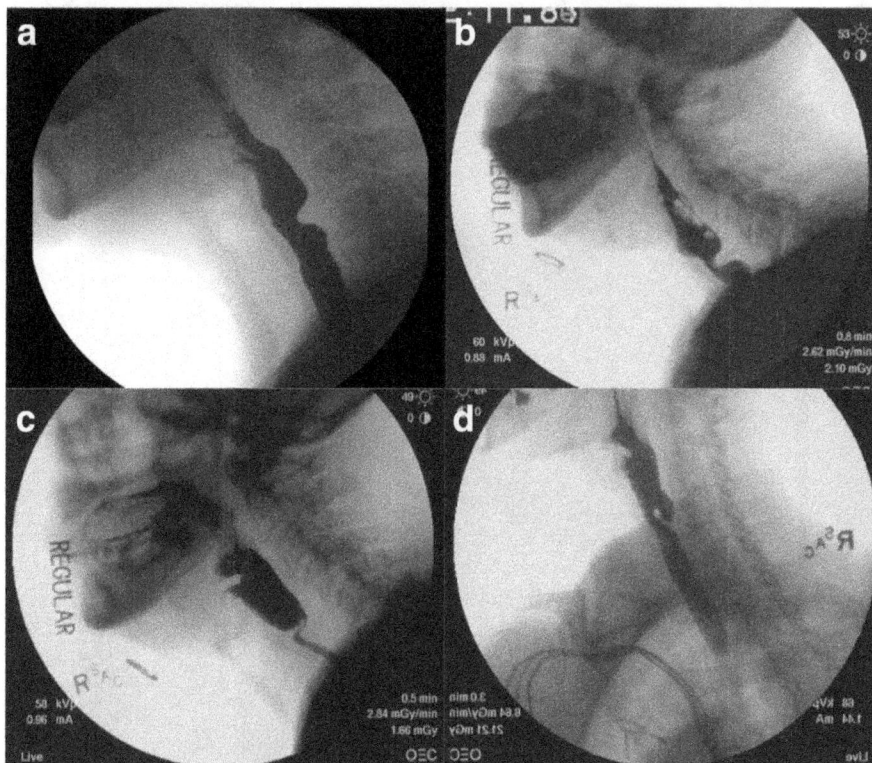

Fig. 1 Spectrum of cricopharyngeus muscle dysfunction showing asymptomatic narrowing of pharyngoesophageal segment to severe narrowing and diverticulum formation. **a** Non-obstructing bar. **b** Moderately obstructing bar. **c** Severely obstructing bar. **d** Zenker's diverticulum

diverticulum or prior radiation therapy of the head and neck were excluded. Pre- and post-dilation validated EAT-10, FOIS, PES opening (cm) in the anteroposterior (PESAP) and lateral (PESL) fluoroscopic view (Fig. 2), pharyngeal constriction ratio (PCR), and pharyngeal area (PA) were retrospectively collected.

Videofluoroscopic analysis

Fluoroscopic studies were performed according to our center's standard protocol [22, 23]. Each subject was administered a bolus of liquid barium (EZ-PAQUE barium sulfate suspension, 60% w/v; 41% w/w, E-Z-EM, Inc., Westbury, NY) in the following order: 1, 3, and 20 mL. Each subject was also given a 3-cm^3 bolus of barium paste (EZpaste, E-Z-Em, Inc). Patients undergoing esophagram did not receive a 3 mL bolus of liquid or paste barium but did additionally receive a 13 mm barium tablet and large volume (> 60 mL) liquid barium trial via straw drinking. The fluoroscopic studies were recorded digitally with Olympus Image Stream Medical nStream G3 HD/SD Video Recording (Image Stream Medical, Littleton, MA) and were played back with WinDVD7 for Windows (Intervideo, Corel Corp., Ottawa, Canada).

Objective fluoroscopic displacement measures were obtained according to established protocols [9, 24–26]. In brief, pharyngeal area is measured in the lateral view on the 1 mL liquid barium 'hold' position. The posterior landmark starts superiorly at the posterior pharyngeal wall anterior to the tubercle of the atlas and follows inferiorly to the floor of the hypopharynx. The anterior boundary is traced from the posterior arytenoids to the surface of the arytenoid cartilages, proceeds to the laryngeal surface of the epiglottis, curves into the valleculae,

then follows along the base of tongue. The anterior/superior landmark ends at the velum. All measures requiring lateral views utilize these landmarks. PCR is the ratio of PA at maximal compression divided by the PA at rest and is a validated measure of pharyngeal contractility. An elevated PCR suggests diminished pharyngeal strength [23]. Standardized measures of the PESL and PESAP were obtained during the trial of 20 mL liquid barium bolus. Anteroposterior (AP) measures for the UES opening are obtained in the AP view with the same superior and inferior landmarks; lateral boundaries are defined as the maximal distention.

Surgical technique

All dilation procedures were performed under monitored anesthesia care with sedation administered per anesthesiologist preference. Typical sedation is achieved with a combination of midazolam and fentanyl. Our technique of dilation begins with the administration of a combination xylocaine (4%) and neosynephrine (0.25%) nasal spray administered 2–3 min prior to the procedure. Flexible esophagoscopy is performed through the more patent naris (Pentax VE-1530 transnasal esophagoscope, Pentax Precision Medical Company, KayPentax, Lincoln Park, NJ, USA). A diagnostic esophagoscopy is performed and a guidewire(s) from a Hercules® 3 Stage Wire Guided Balloon (Cook Medical, Bloomington, IN) is inserted through the side channel of the endoscope. The esophagoscope is then removed over the guidewire(s), replaced through the contralateral naris, and positioned in the hypopharynx to visualize the postcricoid region. The dilation balloon(s) are then advanced over the guidewire(s). Our protocol involves sequential

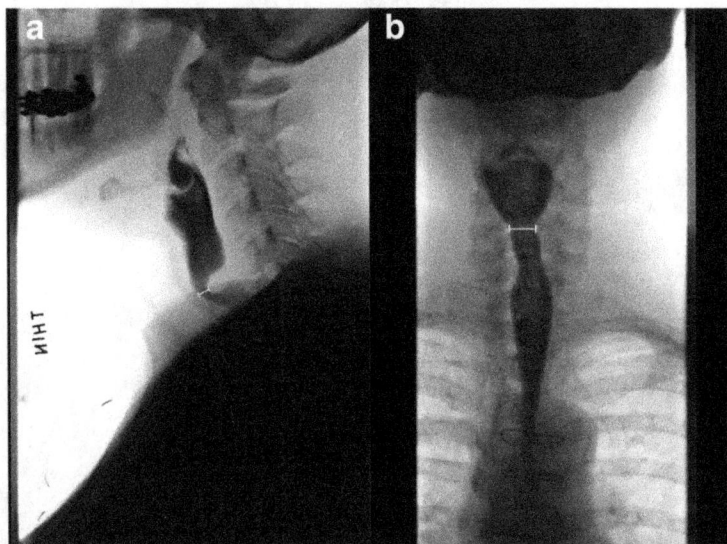

Fig. 2 Demonstration of pharyngoesophageal segment (PES) parameters in videofluoroscopy studies. **a** PES lateral view (PESL). **b** PES anteroposterior view (PESAP). Measurement bars indicate narrowest opening dimension during 20 mL barium volume test

dilation personalized for each patient but typically begins with one 18–20 mm balloon in the first procedure, followed by two 13–15 mm balloons in the second dilation and two 15–18 mm balloons for the third dilation (Fig. 3). Balloons were sequentially inflated through each diameter and then held at final dilation for 60 s. After deflation and removal, the PES was examined for signs of injury to the mucosa. The mucosa is examined at every stage of dilation and the procedure is terminated if any blood is seen on the balloon or evidence of mucosal laceration is visualized. The interval between dilations was 4–8 weeks, dependent on patient and OR availability, in accordance with use in prior studies [27, 28].

Statistical analysis

Statistical analysis was carried out using Stata 12.0 (StataCorp, College Way, TX), with descriptive statistics determined for baseline and demographic data. Comparison between pre- and post-dilation outcomes was performed using paired t-tests for continuous variables and Wilcoxon matched pairs–signed rank test for ordinal data. A Bonferroni correction was utilized to adjust for multiple comparisons.

Results

Seventeen patients with CPMD who underwent three serial balloon dilations with complete pre- and post-treatment fluoroscopy data were enrolled. The mean age of the cohort was 73 (SD ± 11.5) years, 59% female. Fifty-one dilations were done in total. The mean duration between pre- and post-treatment VFSS was 206 (SD ± 83) days and the mean time between final dilation and post-treatment fluoroscopy was 37 (SD ± 33) days. Median balloon dilator diameters for the first, second, and third stages of the "series of three" dilations were 20 mm, 15 + 15 mm, and 18 + 18 mm, respectively, situated in the PES as shown in Fig. 3.

Changes in symptom and functional scores are displayed in Table 1. The mean EAT-10 improved from 24.7 (SD ± 7.8) pre- to 15.9 (SD ± 10.2) post-treatment (p = 0.0021). The mean FOIS improved from a mean of 5.4 (SD ± 1.4) pre- to 6.3 (SD ± 0.9) post-treatment (p = 0.017). In our series, individual patient EAT-10 and FOIS scores either improved or were unchanged in 14/17 patients (82%) following the third dilation, compared to pre-treatment values.

Changes in radiographic outcome are displayed in Table 2. PESAP increased from 1.05 cm (SD ± 0.34 cm) to 1.48 cm (SD ± 0.41 cm) (p = 0.0003). PESL increased from 0.58 cm (SD ± 1.8 cm) to 0.76 cm (SD ± 0.30 cm) (p = 0.018). These values represent increases in PES opening width and anteroposterior space of 41 and 31%, respectively (Fig. 4). Among patients with severely obstructed CPMD (PESL opening less than 0.5 cm, n = 7) the anteroposterior opening increased by 72% from 0.39 cm (SD ± 0.07 cm) to 0.67 cm (SD ± 0.27 cm) (p = 0.047). Patients who underwent serial balloon dilation also showed improvement in PCR from 0.49 (SD ± 0.37) to 0.23 (SD ± 0.15) (p = 0.015), indicating improved ability to constrict the pharynx and propel a food bolus through the PES. Despite improved constriction, PA showed no difference between pre- and post-treatment values (p = 0.91). There were no perforations of the upper esophagus or PES identified in this study cohort, and no patients developed delayed infections in the neck.

To evaluate the durability of our treatment approach, we reviewed patient records to determine whether members of our cohort underwent additional treatments. We identified ten patients (59%) who underwent additional upper esophageal procedures, nine of whom had repeat dilations and one who opted for a cricopharyngeus myotomy. The mean duration of time between the third dilation and a repeat procedure was 416 days (SD ± 246, range = 124–849 days). Five patients who underwent subsequent treatments also had fluoroscopic studies repeated, however there were no statistically significant differences between the measures obtained after the third dilation and the later dilation. Similarly, there were

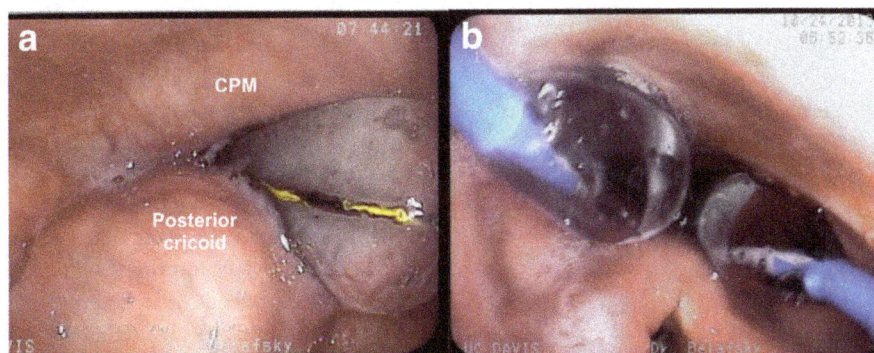

Fig. 3 Transnasal esophagoscope view of pharynx during sequential balloon dilation using **a**) one and **b**) two balloon dilators. CPM = cricopharyngeus muscle

Table 1 Pre-and post-treatment symptom scale and functional outcome measures

Parameter	n	Pre-treatment (+/− SD)	Post-treatment (+/− SD)	p value
EAT-10	17	24.7 (7.8)	15.9 (10.2)	0.0021*
FOIS	17	5.4 (1.5)	6.3 (0.9)	0.017**

EAT-10 eating assessment tool, *FOIS* functional oral intake scale
*Paired t-test
**Wilcoxon matched pairs–signed rank test

no differences between EAT-10 or FOIS scores ($n = 9$) following additional treatments.

Discussion

In this study, we investigated the effect of serial PES dilation for CPMD and report improved patient-reported symptoms, functional, and fluoroscopic short-term outcomes. We observed marked improvements in PES opening and EAT-10 scores, confirming existing data that PES dilation is an effective method to address CPMD [12]. Though symptom scores do not return to normal after intervention, they suggest significant improvement, which is compatible with measured fluoroscopic outcomes.

Our study provides several interesting findings related to the efficacy of serial double-balloon dilation to a size larger than what can be achieved with a single balloon. As expected, both PESAP and PESL opening increase in these patients but the increase is more pronounced in the anterior posterior projection (PESAP). The fluoroscopic finding of a hypertrophic cricopharyngeus muscle used to diagnose CPMD is typically identified on the lateral VFSS projection. We did not expect the greatest therapeutic benefit to be appreciated in the anteriorposterior fluoroscopic view (PESAP). Previous fluoroscopic data report improvement in the lateral fluoroscopic view only (PESL) [10, 16]. Fig. 3 illustrates that the increased dilation obtained by using two balloons occurs in a vector that should increase the lateral dimension of the PES, a consequence that would result in improved opening on the AP VFSS. This degree of lateral expansion cannot be effectively achieved with a single, circular balloon or bougie.

Table 2 Pre-and post-treatment VFSS outcome measures. All tests performed with paired t-tests

Parameter	n	Pre-treatment (+/− SD)	Post-treatment (+/− SD)	p value
PESAP opening (cm)	15	1.05 (0.34)	1.48 (0.41)	0.0003
PESL opening (cm)	17	0.58 (0.18)	0.76 (0.30)	0.018
Pharyngeal constriction ratio	13	0.49 (0.37)	0.24 (0.15)	0.015
Pharyngeal area (cm²)	12	9.45 (3.62)	9.52 (3.96)	0.91

PESAP upper esophageal sphincter in anterior-posterior view, *PESL* upper esophageal opening in lateral view

Anecdotal experience and case reports indicate reflux symptoms can worsen following cricopharyngeus myotomy in select populations [29–31], leading some authors to consider reflux or ineffective esophageal motility a contraindication [32]. However, manometric studies of PES pressures before and after cricopharyngeus muscle myotomy demonstrate reduction of resting pressure to normal values with no increase in pharyngeal acid regurgitation [33–35]. The cricopharyngeus muscle is not ablated or resected with dilation, and it has been reported that single balloon dilation reduces the size of an obstructing cricopharyngeus muscle less than myotomy [10]. We observed persistent fluoroscopic indentation of the PES in most patients post serial dilations. This suggests that serial dilation may cause less diminution to the protective function of the PES than myotomy.

Another interesting observation was the disparate change in PCR and PA following serial PES dilation. While pharyngeal contraction improved (PCR), the pharynx remained dilated (PA). These data are consistent with other reports after both dilation and myotomy [10], which suggests that some of the pharyngeal dilation caused by prolonged PES obstruction may be permanent. A dilated pharynx is associated with decreased pharyngeal contractility and resting tone and is a major risk factor for aspiration. The finding that some of the pharyngeal insult caused by the CPMD is permanent may support earlier intervention before end stage pharyngeal dilation occurs. This is similar to findings in esophageal achalasia, which support LES intervention before the development of an atonic, dilated, sigmoid esophagus [36, 37].

This investigation is not without limitations. Definitive conclusions cannot be drawn from this retrospective case series. As with all musculotendinous injuries, return to function and rehabilitation is generally measured in months rather than days or weeks [38], which exceeds the mean duration between the final dilation and fluoroscopic assessment of 37 days. Thus, it is possible that the maximum amount of improvement was not captured. In addition, we were not able to determine improvements between dilation procedures, so it is not known at what point patients experienced the greatest improvement. Our clinical experience suggests that a series of three double-balloon dilations with a gradual increase in balloon diameter provides the safest most effective treatment strategy. Previous investigation has reported lateral fluoroscopic PES opening improvement to 0.62 cm after single balloon dilation and 0.82 cm after myotomy [10]. While the improvement to 0.76 cm reported in this investigation suggests that a series of three sequential dilations provides improved outcomes over a traditional single balloon procedure, a randomized prospective comparison is required before definitive improvement can be confirmed. This may prove difficult, as dilation is often reserved for elderly persons with significant medical comorbidity and myotomy recommended for younger, healthier

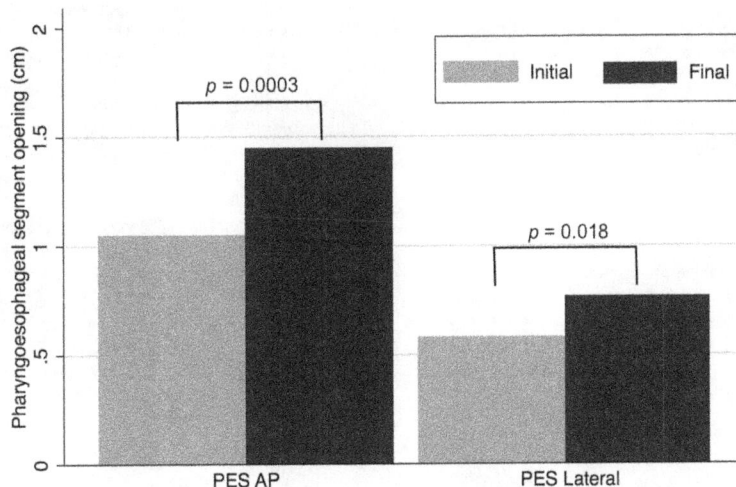

Fig. 4 Mean values of pre- and post-dilation opening dimensions of the pharyngoesphageal segment (PES). AP = anteroposterior view

individuals. This study was limited to persons with complete survey (EAT-10) and fluoroscopic data after three procedures. Individuals who experienced significant improvement after one or two dilations were excluded, as were individuals who were lost to follow-up or declined a postoperative fluoroscopic swallow study. The influence of this follow-up bias has an uncertain effect on the improvement reported in this investigation.

This investigation was designed to determine the short-term symptomatic and objective outcomes of a series of three PES dilations. Previous investigations suggest there is inadequate long-term response following dilation to 20 mm, particularly among persons with CPMD secondary to neurodegenerative disease such as oculopharyngeal muscular dystrophy [7, 39]. Ideally serial dilation would provide longer duration of benefit. We do not have patients routinely return for reassessment unless their symptoms recur, but our clinical experience with this technique suggests some patients develop symptomatic recurrence with less severe degree of cricopharyngeus muscle obstruction that responds to a single repeat treatment. We reviewed our cohort and found there was a subset of patients who returned for additional treatments. In this relatively small series, 59% of patients needed treatment again at a later date, on average 416 days after the third dilation. This is congruent with reported rates and timing of recurrence of swallowing dysfunction following dilation of the cricopharyngeus, but the heterogeneity of the data included in these studies makes direct comparison of any individual techniques difficult [7, 12, 39]. Indeed, recurrence and durability are important considerations in the management of CPMD and appropriate patient counseling, so rigorous future prospective investigation to properly address this question are needed. Defining recurrence based on either symptoms or objective data is challenging and

varies between patients, so our study advances understanding in what outcomes can be expected.

Though serial double-balloon dilation is performed at numerous centers, there is little literature on its safety. The key complication or side effect of concern in these procedures is upper esophageal perforation. During the study period we did not have any perforations of the upper aerodigestive tract. Presumably the risk of perforation is increased with greater dilation diameter. Mucosal lacerations occurred in some instances, but this was not discretely recorded and could not be measured. In our experience, a simple mucosal laceration did not lead to any instances of deep neck space infections or other complications. Although we believe progressive dilation over three serial encounters with appropriate recovery intervals reduces the likelihood of this complication, further investigation is required to confirm this assertion. Optimal interval between dilations is debatable, with repeat dilations for benign mucosal strictures of the esophagus often done in weekly intervals, but we believe CPMD treatment allows longer intervals between treatments without losing efficacy, given the apparent average duration of effect [12, 27, 28, 40]. Even with the inherent limitations of this retrospective case series, the data suggest that a "series of three" dilation approach is a safe and effective treatment of cricopharyngeus muscle dysfunction and support the need for further study.

Conclusion

Our data suggest a "series of three" serial balloon dilation is a safe and effective treatment for CPMD. The treatment results in a significant improvement in symptomatic dysphagia (EAT-10), functional oral intake (FOIS), and objective fluoroscopic parameters. Further investigation is required to evaluate the durability and compare outcomes of this approach to traditional techniques of single balloon PES dilation.

Abbreviations

CPMD: Cricopharyngeus muscle dysfunction; EAT-10: Eating Assessment Tool-10; FOIS: Functional Oral Intake Scale; PA: Pharyngeal area; PCR: Pharyngeal constriction ratio; PES: Pharyngoesophageal segment; PESAP: Pharyngoesophageal segment anteroposterior view; PESL: Pharyngoesophageal segment lateral view; SD: Standard deviation; VFSS: Videofluoroscopic swallowing study

Acknowledgments

The authors thank Sharon Clifford, Radiation Technologist, for image acquisition; Erik Steele, Anne Amador, Michelle Payne, Speech Language Pathologists, for fluoroscopy data collection analysis; Shannon Whitney, Barb Taylor, Mary Margaret Henson, Parul Puri, Registered Nurses, for data collection and operating room nursing; and Rebecca Anson, Surgical Scrub Technician, for operating room assistance.

Authors' contributions

DRR developed study concept and protocol, obtained clinical data, analyzed and interpreted patient data, and was a major contributor in writing the manuscript. LME provided study design details, interpreted patient data, and performed fluoroscopic swallowing studies. MAK obtained clinical data, and was a major contributor in writing the manuscript. PCB obtained clinical data, analyzed and interpreted patient data, and was a major contributor in writing the manuscript. All authors read and approved the final manuscript.

Competing interests

The authors declare that they have no competing interests.

References

1. McHorney CA, Robbins J, Lomax K, Rosenbek JC, Chignell K, Kramer AE, et al. The SWAL-QOL and SWAL-CARE outcomes tool for oropharyngeal dysphagia in adults: III. Documentation of Reliability and Validity Dysphagia. 2002;17:97–114. https://doi.org/10.1007/s00455-001-0109-1.

2. Guyomard V, Fulcher RA, Redmayne O, Metcalf AK, Potter JF, Myint PK. Effect of dysphasia and dysphagia on inpatient mortality and hospital length of stay: a database study. J Am Geriatr Soc. 2009;57:2101–6. https://doi.org/10.1111/j.1532-5415.2009.02526.x.

3. Altman KW, Yu G-P, Schaefer SD. Consequence of dysphagia in the hospitalized patient. Arch Otolaryngol Neck Surg. 2010;136:784. https://doi.org/10.1001/archoto.2010.129.

4. Perry L, Love CP. Screening for dysphagia and aspiration in acute stroke: a systematic review. Dysphagia. 2001;16:7–18. https://doi.org/10.1007/PL00021290.

5. White GN, O'Rourke F, Ong BS, Cordato DJ, Chan DKY. Dysphagia: causes, assessment, treatment, and management. Geriatrics 2008;63:15–20. http://www.ncbi.nlm.nih.gov/pubmed/18447407. Accessed 25 May 2017.

6. Altman K. Dysphagia evaluation and care in the hospital setting: the need for protocolization. Otolaryngol Head Neck Surg. 2011;145:895–8. https://doi.org/10.1177/0194599811415803.

7. Kuhn M, Belafsky P. Management of cricopharyngeus muscle dysfunction. Otolaryngol Clin N Am.2013;Dec;46:1087–99.

8. Hoy M, Domer A, Plowman EK, Loch R, Belafsky P. Causes of dysphagia in a tertiary-care swallowing center. Ann Otol Rhinol Laryngol. 2013;122:335–8. https://doi.org/10.1177/000348941312200508.

9. Leonard R, Kendall K, McKenzie S. UES opening and Cricopharyngeal bar in Nondysphagic elderly and nonelderly adults. Dysphagia. 2004;19:182–91. https://doi.org/10.1007/s00455-004-0005-6.

10. Allen J, White CJ, Leonard R, Belafsky PC. Effect of cricopharyngeus muscle surgery on the pharynx. Laryngoscope. 2010;120:1498–503. https://doi.org/10.1002/lary.21002.

11. Belafsky PC, Rees CJ, Allen J, Leonard RJ. Pharyngeal dilation in

cricopharyngeus muscle dysfunction and Zenker diverticulum. Laryngoscope. 2010;;NA-NA. doi:https://doi.org/10.1002/lary.20874.

12. Ashman A, Dale OT, Baldwin DL. Management of isolated cricopharyngeal dysfunction: systematic review. J Laryngol Otol. 2017;130:611–5. https://doi.org/10.1017/S0022215116007994.

13. Kocdor P, Siegel ER, Tulunay-Ugur OE. Cricopharyngeal dysfunction: a systematic review comparing outcomes of dilatation, botulinum toxin injection, and myotomy. Laryngoscope. 2016;126:135–41. https://doi.org/10.1002/lary.25447.

14. Wang AY, Kadkade R, Kahrilas PJ, Hirano I. Effectiveness of esophageal dilation for symptomatic cricopharyngeal bar. Gastrointest Endosc. 2005;61:148–52. https://doi.org/10.1016/S0016-5107(04)02447-2.

15. Clary MS, Daniero JJ, Keith SW, Boon MS, Spiegel JR. Efficacy of large-diameter dilatation in cricopharyngeal dysfunction. Laryngoscope. 2011;121:2521–5. https://doi.org/10.1002/lary.22365.

16. Dou Z, Zu Y, Wen H, Guifang W, Jiang L, Hu Y. The Effect of Different Catheter Balloon Dilatation Modes on Cricopharyngeal Dysfunction in Patients with Dysphagia. doi:https://doi.org/10.1007/s00455-012-9402-4.

17. Patel BJ, Mathur AK, Dehom S, Jackson CS. Savary dilation is a safe and effective long-term means of treatment of symptomatic Cricopharyngeal bar. J Clin Gastroenterol. 2013:1. https://doi.org/10.1097/MCG.0000000000000026.

18. Cates D, Plowman EK, Mehdizadeh O, Yen K, Domer A, Gilden M, et al. Geometric morphometric shape analysis in an ovine model confirms that the upper esophageal sphincter is not round. Laryngoscope. 2013;123:721–6. https://doi.org/10.1002/lary.23634.

19. Belafsky PC, Plowman EK, Mehdizadeh O, Cates D, Domer A, Yen K. The upper esophageal sphincter is not round: a pilot study evaluating a novel, physiology-based approach to upper esophageal sphincter dilation. Ann Otol Rhinol Laryngol. 2013;122:217–21. https://doi.org/10.1177/000348941312200401.

20. Crary MA, Mann GDC, Groher ME. Initial psychometric assessment of a functional oral intake scale for dysphagia in stroke patients. Arch Phys Med Rehabil. 2005;86:1516–20. https://doi.org/10.1016/J.APMR.2004.11.049.

21. Belafsky PC, Mouadeb DA, Rees CJ, Pryor JC, Postma GN, Allen J, et al. Validity and reliability of the eating assessment tool (EAT-10). Ann Otol Rhinol Laryngol. 2008;117:919–24. https://doi.org/10.1177/000348940811701210.

22. Leonard R, Belafsky P. Dysphagia following cervical spine surgery with anterior instrumentation: evidence from fluoroscopic swallow studies. Spine (Phila Pa 1976). 2011;36:2217–23. https://doi.org/10.1097/BRS.0b013e318205a1a7.

23. Randall DR, Strong EB, Belafsky PC. Altered pharyngeal structure and dynamics among patients with cervical kyphosis. Laryngoscope. 2016; https://doi.org/10.1002/lary.26417.

24. Kendall KA, McKenzie S, Leonard RJ, Gonçalves MI, Walker A. Timing of events in normal swallowing: a videofluoroscopic study. Dysphagia. 2000;15:74–83. https://doi.org/10.1007/s004550010004.

25. Kendall KA, Leonard RJ. Pharyngeal constriction in elderly dysphagic patients compared with young and elderly nondysphagic controls. Dysphagia. 2001;16:272–8. https://doi.org/10.1007/s00455-001-0086-4.

26. Leonard R, Kendall KA, McKenzie S. Structural displacements affecting pharyngeal constriction in nondysphagic elderly and nonelderly adults. Dysphagia 2004;19:133–141. http://www.ncbi.nlm.nih.gov/pubmed/15382802. Accessed 25 May 2017.

27. Francis DO, Hall E, Dang JH, Vlacich GR, Netterville JL, Vaezi MF. Outcomes of serial dilation for high-grade radiation-related esophageal strictures in head and neck cancer patients. Laryngoscope. 2015;125:856–62. https://doi.org/10.1002/lary.24987.

28. Piotet E, Escher A, Monnier P. Esophageal and pharyngeal strictures: report on 1,862 endoscopic dilatations using the Savary-Gilliard technique. Eur Arch Oto-Rhino-Laryngology. 2008;265:357–64. https://doi.org/10.1007/s00405-007-0456-0.

29. van Overbeek JJ, Betlem HC. Cricopharyngeal myotomy in pharyngeal paralysis. Cineradiographic and manometric indications. Ann Otol Rhinol Laryngol. 1979;88(5 Pt 1):596–602. https://doi.org/10.1177/000348947908800503.

30. Bonavina L, Khan NA, DeMeester TR. Pharyngoesophageal dysfunctions. The role of cricopharyngeal myotomy. Arch Surg 1985;120:541–549. http://www.ncbi.nlm.nih.gov/pubmed/3921004. Accessed 25 May 2017.

31. Sanei-Moghaddam A, Kumar S, Jani P, Brierley C. Cricopharyngeal myotomy for cricopharyngeus stricture in an inclusion body myositis patient with

Improved symptomatic, functional, and fluoroscopic outcomes following serial "series of three" double-balloon...

203

hiatus hernia: a learning experience. BMJ Case Rep. 2013;2013 https://doi.org/10.1136/bcr-2012-008058.

32. Kelly JH. Management of upper esophageal sphincter disorders: indications and complications of myotomy. Am J Med. 2000;:43S–46S. http://www.ncbi.nlm.nih.gov/pubmed/10718451. Accessed 25 May 2017.

33. Taillefer R, Duranceau AC. Manometric and radionuclide assessment of pharyngeal emptying before and after cricopharyngeal myotomy in patients with oculopharyngeal muscular dystrophy. J Thorac Cardiovasc Surg 1988;95:868–875. http://www.ncbi.nlm.nih.gov/pubmed/3361934. Accessed 25 May 2017.

34. Pera M, Yamada A, Hiebert CA, Duranceau A. Sleeve recording of upper esophageal sphincter resting pressures during Cricopharyngeal Myotomy. Ann Surg. 1997;225:229–34. https://doi.org/10.1097/00000658-199702000-00012.

35. Williams RBH, Ali GN, Hunt DR, Wallace KL, Cook IJ. Cricopharyngeal myotomy does not increase the risk of esophagopharyngeal acid regurgitation. Am J Gastroenterol. 1999;94:3448–54. https://doi.org/10.1111/j.1572-0241.1999.01507.x.

36. Gyawali CP. Achalasia: new perspectives on an old disease. Neurogastroenterol Motil. 2016;28:4–11. https://doi.org/10.1111/nmo.12750.

37. Roman S, Kahrilas PJ, Mion F, Nealis TB, Soper NJ, Poncet G, et al. Partial recovery of peristalsis after myotomy for achalasia: more the rule than the exception. JAMA Surg. 2013;148:157–64. https://doi.org/10.1001/2013.jamasurg.38.

38. Kuhn JE. Exercise in the treatment of rotator cuff impingement: a systematic review and a synthesized evidence-based rehabilitation protocol. J Shoulder Elb Surg. 2009;18:138–60. https://doi.org/10.1016/j.jse.2008.06.004.

39. Manjaly JG, Vaughan-Shaw PG, Dale OT, Tyler S, Corlett JCR, Frost RA. Cricopharyngeal dilatation for the long-term treatment of dysphagia in Oculopharyngeal muscular dystrophy. Dysphagia. 2012;27:216–20. https://doi.org/10.1007/s00455-011-9356-y.

40. Bilgin Buyukkarabacak Y, Taslak Sengul A, Pirzirenli MG, Basoglu A. Recurrent dilatation in resistant benign esophageal strictures: timing is significant. Turkish J Med Sci. 2016;46:79–83. https://doi.org/10.3906/sag-1412-72.

31

Hemorrhage within the tympanic membrane without perforation

Chang-Hee Kim and Jung Eun Shin*

Abstract

Background: Hemotympanum refers to both the presence of blood in the middle ear cavity and to ecchymosis of the tympanic membrane (TM), and a systematic study of intra-TM (iTM) hemorrhage without bleeding in the middle ear cavity has not been conducted. The goals of our study were to analyze the causes of iTM hemorrhage without TM perforation or bleeding in the middle ear cavity, and to demonstrate the clinical characteristics of the disease.

Methods: This Case series study included five patients with iTM hemorrhage between August 2014 and August 2017. An iTM hemorrhage was diagnosed when otoendoscopic examination demonstrated minor bleeding behind the intact TM, a hemorrhage was observed between the TM annulus and the epidermal layer, and temporal bone computed tomography revealed thickening of the TM without soft tissue density within the tympanic cavity or temporal bone fracture. Initial symptoms, and serial findings of otoendoscopy and pure tone audiometry (PTA) were investigated.

Results: iTM hemorrhage developed due to blunt head trauma in two patients, descent barotrauma during scuba diving in two patients, and spontaneous epistaxis in one patient. Otalgia and ear fullness were the most common symptoms, but PTA showed no or minimal conductive hearing loss in all patients.

Conclusions: An iTM hemorrhage may develop after blunt head trauma, barotrauma due to scuba diving, or spontaneous epistaxis; otological symptoms included otalgia, tinnitus, and aural fullness. An iTM hemorrhage resolved spontaneously without specific treatment, usually within 1 month.

Keywords: Tympanic membrane, Hemorrhage, Hemotympanum, Head trauma, Barotrauma, Epistaxis

Background

Hemotympanum refers to both the presence of blood in the middle ear cavity and to ecchymosis of the tympanic membrane (TM). A temporal bone fracture due to blunt head trauma, therapeutic nasal packing, epistaxis, blood disorders, anticoagulant therapy, barotrauma, and otitis media are common causes of hemotympanum [1–5]. Previous studies of hemotympanum have focused on hemorrhages within the middle ear cavity. To our knowledge, a systematic study of intra-TM (iTM) hemorrhage without bleeding in the middle ear cavity has not been conducted, even though there have been reports of two cases [6, 7]. Although the thickness of TM is only about

0.1 mm, the TM has capillaries between outer epidermal layer and inner mucous layer. So it is reasonable that hemorrhage within the TM may be resulted from various causes such as head trauma and barotrauma. The purpose of the present study was to analyze the causes of iTM hemorrhage and demonstrate the clinical course of the disease.

Methods

We conducted a retrospective case series study of patients who showed iTM hemorrhage without perforation. Between August 2014 and August 2017, medical records of the patients who were diagnosed with hemotympanum or whose TM showed abnormal findings were retrospectively reviewed, and five patients of iTM hemorrhage without perforation were enrolled in this study. The presence of iTM hemorrhage was determined

* Correspondence: 20050055@kuh.ac.kr
Department of Otorhinolaryngology-Head and Neck Surgery, Konkuk University School of Medicine, Konkuk University Medical Center, 120-1 Neungdong-ro (Hwayang-dong), Gwangjin-gu, Seoul 143-729, Republic of Korea

by otoendoscopy findings and temporal bone computed tomography (TBCT). On otoendoscopic examination, minor bleeding of a bright or dark red color was seen behind the intact TM; a hemorrhage was also observed between the tympanic annulus and the epidermis of the TM (Figs. 1, 2, 3, 4 and 5), as the tympanic annular ligament is embedded between the epidermal layer and the mucosal layer of the TM [8]. TBCT demonstrated thickening of the TM suggestive of an iTM hemorrhage without soft tissue density within the tympanic cavity, indicating a hemorrhage. Patients with TM perforation, middle ear effusion, or a hemorrhage in the tympanic cavity were excluded from the study. Patients who underwent intratympanic steroid injections were also excluded. Patients' symptoms were reviewed, otoendoscopic and TBCT findings were evaluated, and audiometric results were serially compared in these patients with iTM hemorrhage. This study was approved by the Institutional Review Board (KUH1110068).

Results

Clinical characteristics of five patients with iTM hemorrhage are summarized in Table 1. Among the five patients, iTM hemorrhage was associated with head trauma in two patients, barotrauma during scuba diving in two patients, and epistaxis in one patient. Otalgia and ear fullness were the most common symptoms, but pure

tone audiometry (PTA) showed no or minimal conductive hearing loss in all patients. Follow-up duration was 1 week to 1 month in these patients.

Patient 1 (Table 1) was a previously healthy 19-year-old man who presented with otalgia, tinnitus, and ear fullness in the left ear associated with vertigo; symptoms developed after head trauma to the occipital area due to a fall from the horizontal bar. Otoendoscopic examination revealed a red hemorrhage behind the intact left TM and along the tympanic annulus between the annular ligament and epidermal layer of the TM (Fig. 1a-e), suggesting iTM hemorrhage. The right TM was normal. PTA demonstrated a minimum air-bone gap on the left side (Fig. 1g). TBCT was conducted at the day of first visit, and axial views of TBCT showed a very small soft tissue density in the Prussak's space (Figures I, J) consistent with iTM hemorrhage observed on otoendoscopic examination without other abnormal findings. Neurologic examination revealed no focal neurologic deficit, but video nystagmography showed a peripheral, right-beating spontaneous nystagmus. The patient was hospitalized with a diagnosis of labyrinthine concussion and left iTM hemorrhage. He initially complained of severe vertigo accompanied by nausea and vomiting, but the symptoms improved greatly on the second day. A bithermal caloric test revealed 33% canal paresis on the left side. Over time, the ear fullness

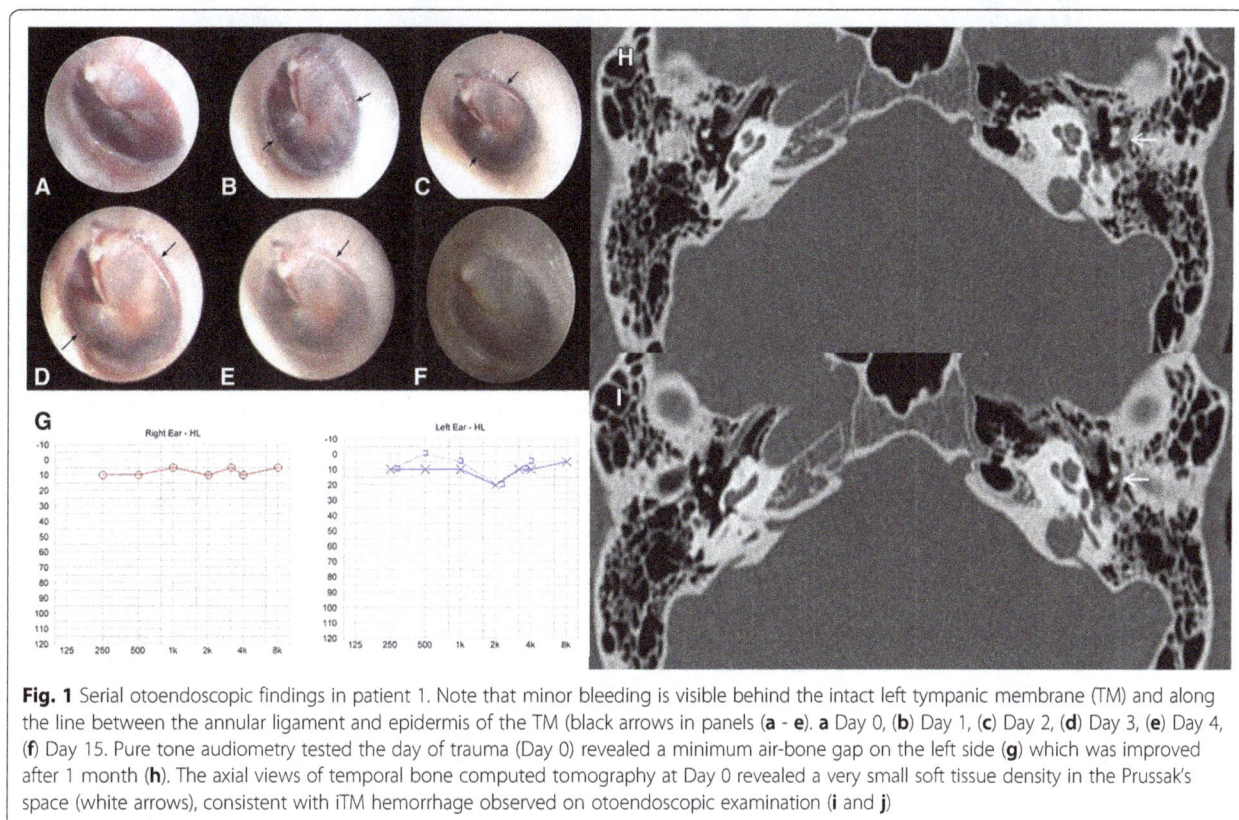

Fig. 1 Serial otoendoscopic findings in patient 1. Note that minor bleeding is visible behind the intact left tympanic membrane (TM) and along the line between the annular ligament and epidermis of the TM (black arrows in panels (**a** - **e**). **a** Day 0, (**b**) Day 1, (**c**) Day 2, (**d**) Day 3, (**e**) Day 4, (**f**) Day 15. Pure tone audiometry tested the day of trauma (Day 0) revealed a minimum air-bone gap on the left side (**g**) which was improved after 1 month (**h**). The axial views of temporal bone computed tomography at Day 0 revealed a very small soft tissue density in the Prussak's space (white arrows), consistent with iTM hemorrhage observed on otoendoscopic examination (**i** and **j**)

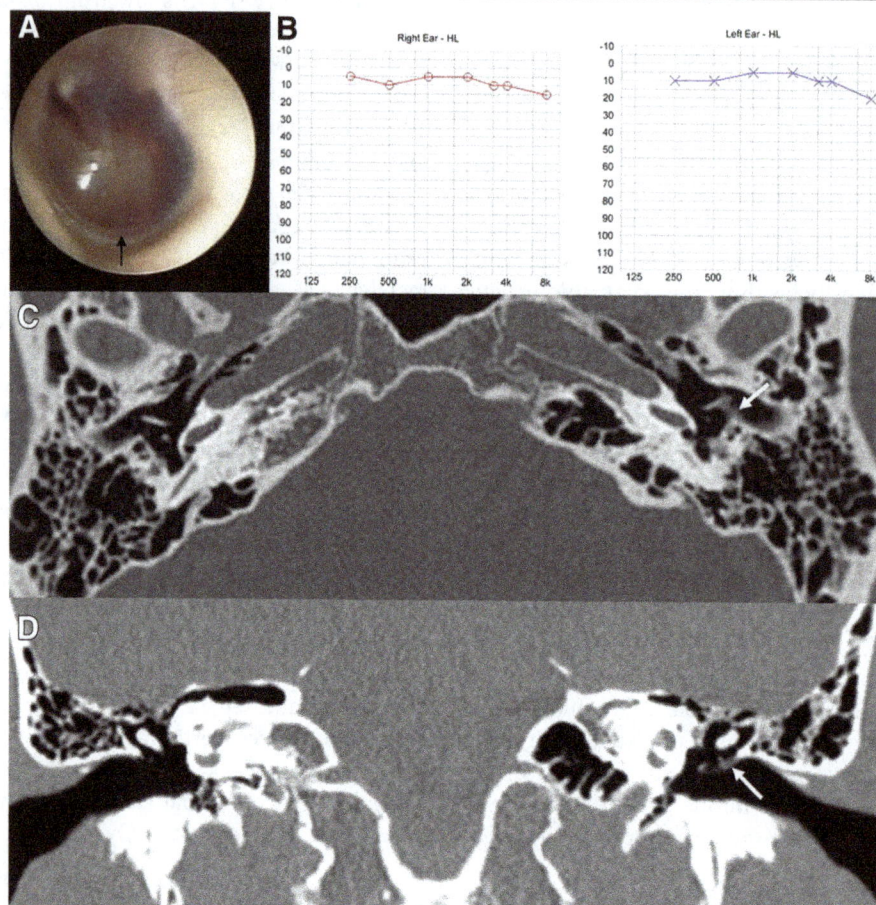

Fig. 2 Otoendoscopic examination (**a**) of patient 2 revealed a small hemorrhage behind the intact left tympanic membrane (TM) and along the line between the tympanic annulus and epidermal layer of the TM (black arrow). Initial pure tone audiometry showed normal hearing on the left side (**b**), and follow-up pure tone audiometry after 1 week revealed no change (**c**). Temporal bone computed tomography demonstrated mild thickening of the left TM (white arrows) on axial (**d**) and coronal views (**e**), suggesting iTM hemorrhage

gradually resolved. The amount of hemorrhagic fluid in the TM decreased (Fig. 1a-f) and resolved within 1 month, and air conduction threshold was improved in PTA (Fig. 1h).

Patient 2 (Table 1) was a previously healthy 33-year-old man who visited our clinic with symptoms of left facial tenderness, otalgia, tinnitus, and a sensation of ear fullness in the left ear that had developed after left facial trauma 1 day previously. He did not complain of vertigo, and a neurologic examination revealed no abnormality. Dark red bleeding was observed through the intact TM on the left side on otoendoscopic examination (Fig. 2a). The thin line of a hemorrhage was seen between the tympanic annular ligament and epidermal layer, which was suggestive of an iTM hemorrhage. PTA showed normal hearing on both sides (Fig. 2b) despite symptoms of ear fullness and tinnitus. TBCT was conducted at the day of first visit, and it demonstrated mild thickening of the left TM on axial (Fig. 2d) and coronal views (Fig. 2e) without other abnormal findings, which was consistent with otoendoscopic

findings indicating an iTM hemorrhage. One week later, the iTM hemorrhage had resolved without any complications and follow-up PTA showed no change (Fig. 2c).

Patient 3 (Table 1) was a previously healthy 51-year-old man who presented with ear fullness and severe otalgia of the left ear that developed during scuba diving 2 days previously. The diver had performed more than 30 dives. He felt that the descent during the most recent dive was faster than usual and experienced difficulty equalizing the pressure in his left ear with the surrounding water pressure. During descent, despite repeated middle ear autoinflation using the Valsalva maneuver, he experienced abrupt onset of severe otalgia on the left side. On otoendoscopic examination, bluish bulging of the anterior part of the left TM was observed, but TM perforation or bleeding was not noted (Fig. 3a). PTA revealed mild conductive hearing loss on the left side (Fig. 3b). TBCT was conducted at the day of first visit, which demonstrated thickening of the left TM on axial (Fig. 3d) and coronal views (Fig. 3e) without other abnormal findings, suggesting an iTM hemorrhage.

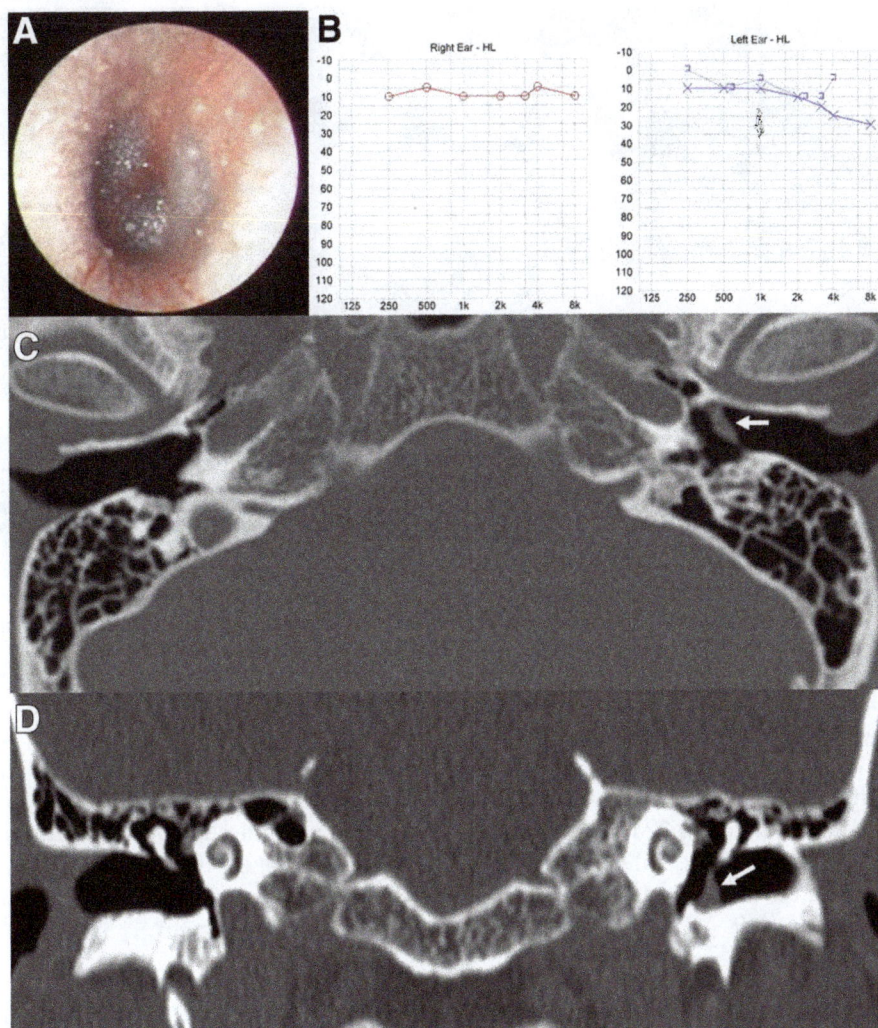

Fig. 3 Otoendoscopic examination (**a**) of patient 3 showed bluish thickening of the anterior part of the intact left tympanic membrane (TM). Pure tone audiometry revealed mild conductive hearing loss on the left side (**b**), which was improved after 2 weeks (**c**). Temporal bone computed tomography revealed thickening of the left TM (white arrows) on axial (**d**) and coronal views (**e**), suggesting iTM hemorrhage

Two weeks after the injury, the hematoma within the left TM resolved and the patient became asymptomatic, and PTA showed slight improvement (Fig. 3c).

Patient 4 (Table 1) had undergone aortic valve replacement due to aortic regurgitation 7 years previously and had been on anticoagulant medication since that procedure. He visited our clinic with a symptom of left ear fullness. He had gone scuba diving 10 days previously, and reported that he had felt otalgia and ear fullness on both sides during descent. Otoendoscopic examination showed minor bleeding along the manubrium of the malleus in the right TM (Fig. 4a) and minor hemorrhage behind the intact TM and along the annular ligament in the left ear (Fig. 4b). PTA revealed mild conductive hearing loss on the left side only (Fig. 4c). TBCT was conducted at the day of first visit, which revealed mild thickening of the left TM on axial (Fig. 4d) and

coronal views (Fig. 4e) without other abnormal findings, suggesting an iTM hemorrhage. After 1 week, his ear discomfort resolved without treatment.

Patient 5 (Table 1) was a 35-year-old woman referred to our clinic with a complaint of epistaxis. Epistaxis began spontaneously on both sides without trauma while the patient was preparing breakfast. Though the bleeding was not massive, she immediately visited the emergency department. Her vital signs were stable and her past medical history was unremarkable. She was not on anticoagulant or NSAID medication, but took alprazolam occasionally when she suffered from sleep disturbance. A nasal endoscopic examination revealed mild bleeding in the Kiesselbach's area of the bilateral nasal septa. Bleeding was easily controlled by electrocauterization, and antibiotic ointment was applied to the electrocauterized mucosa without nasal packing. After control

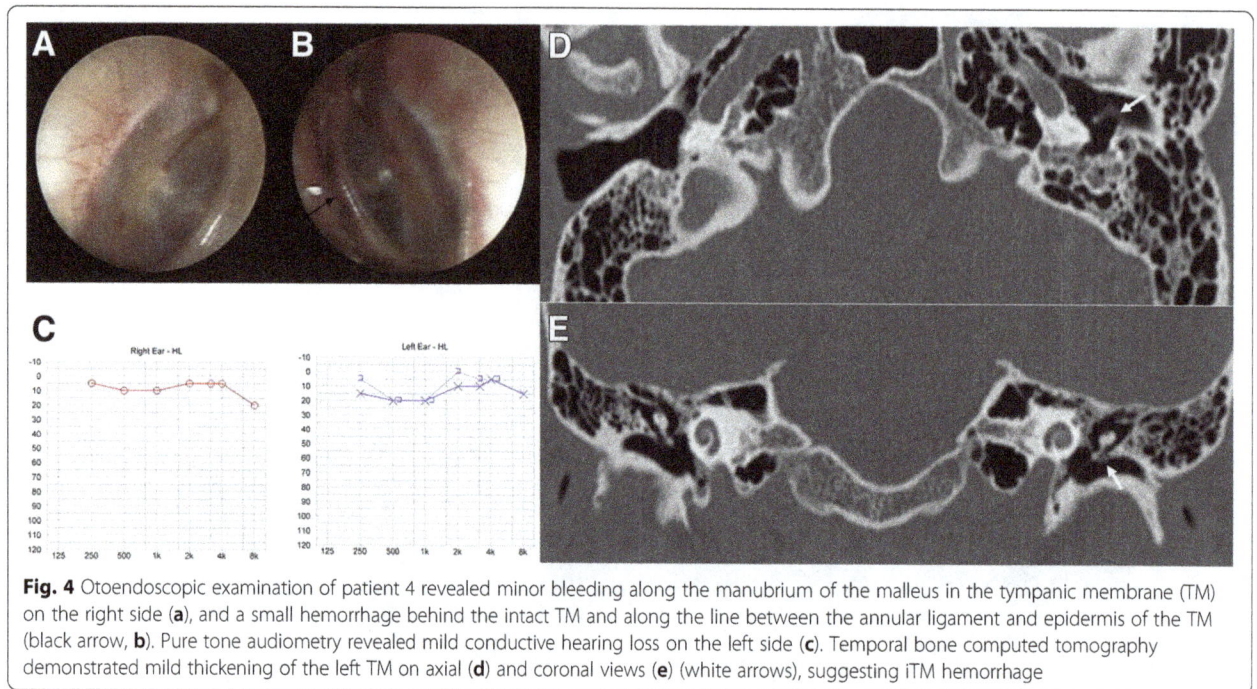

Fig. 4 Otoendoscopic examination of patient 4 revealed minor bleeding along the manubrium of the malleus in the tympanic membrane (TM) on the right side (**a**), and a small hemorrhage behind the intact TM and along the line between the annular ligament and epidermis of the TM (black arrow, **b**). Pure tone audiometry revealed mild conductive hearing loss on the left side (**c**). Temporal bone computed tomography demonstrated mild thickening of the left TM on axial (**d**) and coronal views (**e**) (white arrows), suggesting iTM hemorrhage

of the epistaxis, the patient reported mild aural fullness in both ears, and otoendoscopic examination revealed a hemorrhage along the manubrium of the malleus and a small hemorrhage behind the intact TM and along the annular ligament of the right (Fig. 5a) and left TMs (Fig. 5b). The volume of the hemorrhage was greater in the right ear than in the left. PTA revealed normal hearing on both sides (Fig. 5c). TBCT was conducted at the day of first visit, which revealed mild thickening of the right TM on axial (Fig. 5d) and coronal views (Fig. 5e) without other abnormal findings, suggesting an iTM hemorrhage. After 10 days, the iTM hematoma was resolved, and the patient's ear discomfort disappeared without treatment.

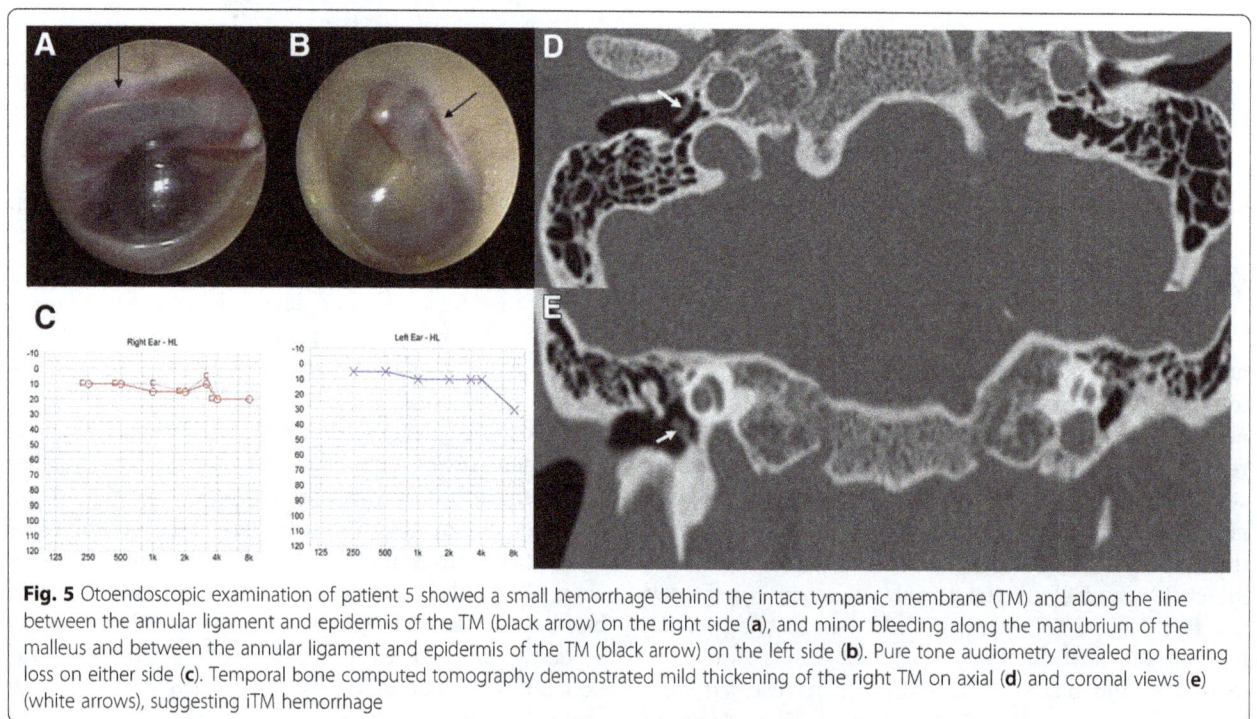

Fig. 5 Otoendoscopic examination of patient 5 showed a small hemorrhage behind the intact tympanic membrane (TM) and along the line between the annular ligament and epidermis of the TM (black arrow) on the right side (**a**), and minor bleeding along the manubrium of the malleus and between the annular ligament and epidermis of the TM (black arrow) on the left side (**b**). Pure tone audiometry revealed no hearing loss on either side (**c**). Temporal bone computed tomography demonstrated mild thickening of the right TM on axial (**d**) and coronal views (**e**) (white arrows), suggesting iTM hemorrhage

Table 1 Clinical characteristics of the patients with intra-tympanic membrane hemorrhage

No.	Sex/Age	Side	Cause	Ear symptoms	Underlying diseases
1	M/19	Left	Head trauma (occipital area)	Left tinnitus, ear fullness, otalgia, vertigo	None
2	M/33	Left	Head trauma (left zygomaticomaxillary area)	Left otalgia, tinnitus, ear fullness	None
3	M/51	Left	Barotrauma (SCUBA diving)	Left severe otalgia, ear fullness	None
4	M/30	Both	Barotrauma (SCUBA diving)	Both otalgia, ear fullness	Warfarin medication due to previous aortic valve replacement surgery
5	F/35	Both	Epistaxis	Both mild ear fullness	None

Discussion

An iTM hemorrhage without TM perforation or bleeding in the tympanic cavity is so rarely observed that only five patients were enrolled in this study in 3 years. The causes of iTM hemorrhage included blunt head trauma in two patients, barotrauma due to scuba diving in two patients, and spontaneous epistaxis in one patient. Although all patients complained of ear fullness in the affected ear, PTA revealed no or minimal conductive hearing loss. Moreover, iTM hemorrhage spontaneously resolved without complication in all of the five patients.

The TM serves essential roles in sound transmission and middle ear protection. Its shape is irregularly round and slightly conical. The TM varies in thickness; it is thicker in the center and periphery than in the intermediate area, and thicker in the pars flaccida than in the pars tensa [9]. Three layers are clearly distinguished in both the pars tensa and pars flaccida: the outer epidermal layer, middle lamina propria, and inner mucous layer. The middle lamina propria is composed of outer radial fibers, inner circular fibers with parabolic fibers between the radial and circular fibers in the pars tensa, and loose connective tissue with abundant elastic and collagen fibers in the pars flaccida [9]. Although the structural organization of the middle lamina propria layer is distinct between the pars tensa and pars flaccida, the capillaries supplying the TM are located within the loose connective tissue of the middle lamina propria in both the pars tensa and pars flaccida [9–11].

Studies of the vascular distribution of the TM have been performed in humans [12–15] and other animals [16–19]. They described a dual arterial source supplying the TM; one from the tympanic annulus (peripheral ring plexus) and the other along the malleus handle (manubrial plexus). The vascular supply is derived from three major arteries: the anterior tympanic artery, deep auricular artery, and stylomastoid artery. The posterior half of the TM is more richly perfused than the anterior half. The outer epidermal layer of the TM is continuous with the epidermis of the external auditory canal skin, and the inner mucous layer is connected to the mucosa of the middle ear at the peripheral margin of the TM [8]. The TM annulus is a horseshoe-like, fibrocartilaginous

structure that maintains attachment of the TM into the tympanic sulcus [8, 20]. As the TM annulus lies beneath the outer epidermal layer, slight bleeding between the TM annulus and the epidermal layer may indicate an iTM hemorrhage. In the present study, we determined the existence of iTM hemorrhage by otoendoscopic examination; minor bleeding of a bright or dark red color was seen behind the intact TM and between the TM annulus and the epidermal layer, in addition to TBCT findings that showed thickening of the TM with soft tissue density.

Most cases of hemotympanum caused by head trauma are also associated with temporal bone fracture [1]. In this case, bleeding within the tympanic cavity of the middle ear was observed on TBCT, and conductive or mixed hearing loss was revealed on audiometry. However, iTM hemorrhage without bleeding in the middle ear cavity caused by head trauma has not been reported. In the present study, two patients had iTM hemorrhage after head trauma; the region of trauma was the occipital area in one patient and the zygomaticomaxillary area in the other. It can be assumed that capillaries within the TM were injured due to head trauma.

Although scuba diving is popular as a recreational activity, it may expose participants to risks of injury, and more than 50% of all diving complications are associated with otologic pathology [21, 22]. Among them, middle ear barotrauma is the most common; it is associated with Eustachian tube dysfunction [23]. Two patients in this study who were experienced scuba divers developed iTM hemorrhage during descent despite their efforts at middle ear autoinflation. When the equilibration between middle ear and environmental pressures fails during descent, the pressure external to the TM exceeds that in the middle ear cavity and the TM bulges inward. An iTM hemorrhage may have developed due to injuries to the capillaries within the TM by acute retraction of the TM during descent.

Hemotympanum that occurred secondary to spontaneous epistaxis has been reported [2–4]. It developed after epistaxis without nasal packing in five patients. When posterior nasal packing was performed to control the epistaxis, Eustachian tube dysfunction due to peritubal lymphatic stasis was postulated as the cause [24]. However, in patients in previous studies, hemotympanum might have been caused by retrograde blood reflux via the Eustachian tube rather than by peritubal lymphatic stasis because nasal packing was not used [2–4]. The cause of iTM hemorrhage in our patient was unclear; we speculate that a sudden significant increase in blood pressure or attempting a Valsalva maneuver might have caused iTM hemorrhage in this patient.

The limitation of this study is that, owing to the nature of the case series study, there is no control group, intervention or outcome measured, and the authors suggested supposed causes of iTM hemorrhage without providing real pathophysiologic mechanisms.

Conclusions

Although very rare, iTM hemorrhage may develop due to blunt head trauma, barotrauma, or spontaneous epistaxis. The patients with iTM hemorrhage complained of ear symptoms such as otalgia, tinnitus, and aural fullness. However, audiometry revealed no or very mild conductive hearing loss. An iTM hemorrhage resolved spontaneously without complications within 2 weeks in all patients.

Abbreviations
iTM: Intra-tympanic membrane; PTA: Pure tone audiometry; TBCT: Temporal bone computed tomography; TM: Tympanic membrane

Acknowledgments
This paper was written as part of Konkuk University's research support program for its faculty on sabbatical leave in 2014.

Authors' contributions
CHK: design & perform research, data analysis & interpretation, and manuscript writing & review. JES: design & perform research, data analysis & interpretation, and manuscript writing & review. Both authors read and approved the final manuscript.

Competing interests
The authors report no conflicts of interest. The authors alone are responsible for the content and writing of the paper.

References
1. Cannon CR, Jahrsdoerfer RA. Temporal bone fractures. Review of 90 cases. Arch Otolaryngol. 1983;109(5):285–8.
2. Evans TC, Hecker J, Zaiser DK. Hemotympanums secondary to spontaneous epistaxis. J Emerg Med. 1988;6(5):387–9.
3. Fidan V, Ozcan K, Karaca F. Bilateral hemotympanum as a result of spontaneous epistaxis. Int J Emerg Med. 2011;4:3.
4. Hurtado TR, Zeger WG. Hemotympanums secondary to spontaneous epistaxis in a 7-year-old. J Emerg Med. 2004;26(1):61–3.
5. Lalwani AK, Jackler RK. Spontaneous hemotympanum associated with chronic middle ear effusion. Am J Otol. 1991;12(6):455–8.
6. Waninger KN, Gloyeske BM, Hauth JM, Vanic KA, Yen DM. Intratympanic hemorrhage and concussion in a football offensive lineman. J Emerg Med. 2014;46(3):371–2.
7. Rasmussen ER, Larsen PL, Andersen K, et al. Petechial hemorrhages of the tympanic membrane in attempted suicide by hanging: a case report. J Forensic Legal Med. 2013;20(2):119–21.
8. Merchant SN, Nadol JB. Schuknecht's pathology of the ear, 3rd ed. Shelton: People's medical publishing house; 2010.
9. Lim DJ. Human tympanic membrane. An ultrastructural observation. Acta Otolaryngol. 1970;70(3):176–86.
10. Lim DJ. Tympanic membrane. Electron microscopic observation. I: pars tensa. Acta Otolaryngol. 1968;66(3):181–98.
11. Lim DJ. Tympanic membrane. II. Pars flaccida. Acta Otolaryngol. 1968;66(6):515–32.
12. Applebaum EL, Deutsch EC. Fluorescein angiography of the tympanic membrane. Laryngoscope. 1985;95(9 Pt 1):1054–8.
13. Applebaum EL, Deutsch EC. An endoscopic method of tympanic membrane fluorescein angiography. Ann Otol Rhinol Laryngol. 1986;95(5 Pt 1):439–43.
14. Saini VK. Vascular Pattern Of Human Tympanic Membrane. Arch Otolaryngol. 1964;79:193–6.
15. Hamberger CA, Wersaell J. Vascular supply of the tympanic membrane and the OSSICULAR chain. Acta Otolaryngol Suppl. 1964;188(Suppl 188):308.
16. Uno Y, Ohtani O, Masuda Y. Vascular pattern of the Guinea pig tympanic membrane. Acta Anat (Basel). 1990;139(4):380–5.
17. Hellstrom S, Spratley J, Eriksson PO, Pais-Clemente M. Tympanic membrane vessel revisited: a study in an animal model. Otol Neurotol. 2003;24(3):494–9.
18. Albiin N, Hellstrom S, Salen B, Stenfors LE, Wirell S. The vascular supply of the rat tympanic membrane. Anat Rec. 1985;212(1):17–22.
19. Maher WP. Microvascular networks in tympanic membrane, malleus periosteum, and annulus perichondrium of neonatal mongrel dog: a vasculoanatomic model for surgical considerations. Am J Anat. 1988;183(4):294–302.
20. Kassem F, Ophir D, Bernheim J, Berger G. Morphology of the human tympanic membrane annulus. Otolaryngol Head Neck Surg. 2010;142(5):682–7.
21. Klingmann C, Praetorius M, Baumann I, Plinkert PK. Otorhinolaryngologic disorders and diving accidents: an analysis of 306 divers. Eur Arch Otorhinolaryngol. 2007;264(10):1243–51.
22. Klingmann C, Praetorius M, Baumann I, Plinkert PK. Barotrauma and decompression illness of the inner ear: 46 cases during treatment and follow-up. Otol Neurotol. 2007;28(4):447–54.
23. Edmonds C, Bennett M, Lippmann J, Mitchell S. Diving and Subaquatic Medicine, 5th ed. Boca Raton: CRC Press; 2015.
24. McCurdy JA Jr. Effects of nasal packing on eustachian tube function. Arch Otolaryngol. 1977;103(9):521–3.

32

A stepped approach for the management of symptomatic internal derangement of the temporomandibular joint

Candan Efeoglu[1*] (iD), Aylin Sipahi Calis[1], Huseyin Koca[1] and Esra Yuksel[2]

Abstract

Background: Internal derangement is the clinical and pathological condition of disc displacement of the temporomandibular joint. Management of these cases involve conservative and surgical treatment options. Minimally invasive surgical procedures namely arthrocentesis and arthroscopy are promising techniques in the management of internal derangement. However patient selection algorithms, indications for minimally invasive procedures and details of the techniques should be further studied for safe and cost effective management of these cases.

This manuscript aims to retrospectively analyze the significance of a stepped surgical treatment approach (arthrocentesis under local anaesthesia as the first line of treatment, followed by arthroscopic lysis and lavage under general anaesthesia in unresolving cases) of internal derangement with or without osteoarthritis.

Methods: This is a retrospective cohort study. Case notes of 1414 patients that were managed with a standard protocol were reviewed. Appropriate inclusion and exclusion criteria were set. Thirty-three patients were eligible for inclusion. Parameters recorded were pain-free inter-incisal opening, spontaneous pain, pain on function, difficulty on chewing, and perceived disability on jaw movements. Pre-operative and post-operative (at the end of the follow up period) pain free maximum interincisal opening values were compared with paired t test and the subjective parameters were evaluated with Chisquare analysis. Treatment outcome and success rate according to American Association of Oral and Maxillofacial Surgeons were descriptively shown.

Results: Interincisal opening values increased, and the number of patients with severe or medium rated subjective parameters were reduced at discharge. These improvements were found to be statistically significant. Clinical (Wilkes) staging of internal derangement pre-operatively and at discharge remained either unchanged or was lower. Treatment outcome and success according to American Association of Oral and Maxillofacial Surgeons criteria was 94%.

Conclusion: The stepped approach for the management of symptomatic internal derangement with or without osteoarthritis is a successful treatment strategy with favourable therapeutic outcomes.

Background

Internal derangement (ID) is the clinical and pathological condition of disc displacement of the temporomandibular joint (TMJ), and the usual coexisting osteoarthritis (OA). OA is also known as osteoarthrosis or degenerative joint disease (DJD) [1].

Although a small fraction of patients with ID experience symptoms that require treatment, it is considered to be the most common cause of serious TMJ pain and dysfunction. These symptoms lead to deterioration of patients' life quality that can necessitate surgical treatment modalities.

The prevalence of ID/OA in males and females is not well documented, but most of the patients seeking treatment are females [2–4]. Joint overloads, facial trauma, whiplash, clenching and bruxism may cause or aggravate TMJ pain and dysfunction [5, 6].

Traditional surgical treatments of ID include repositioning of the disc or discectomy. However, the introduction of minimally invasive TMJ arthroscopy in 1975

* Correspondence: cefeoglu@yahoo.com
[1]Oral Surgery Department, Ege University School of Dentistry, 35100 Izmir, Turkey
Full list of author information is available at the end of the article

was a turning point in the surgical management of ID. [7–9]. Remarkably successful results were achieved simply with arthroscopic lysis and lavage that allowed the removal of inflammatory cytokines and lysis of adhesions limiting joint mobility [9–12].

The success of arthroscopic TMJ lavage was followed by the introduction of arthrocentesis. This technique is also shown to be effective in the treatment of ID, particularly in cases of symptomatic closed lock [10–13].

This manuscript aims to retrospectively analyze the value of our stepped surgical treatment approach (arthrocentesis as the first line of treatment, followed by arthroscopic lysis and lavage in unresolving cases) in cases that are diagnosed to have symptomatic unilateral ID with or without OA of their TMJs. The null hypothesis tested is "the stepped approach is a successful treatment strategy in the management of symptomatic internal derangements of TMJ."

Methods

Study design and patient population

Case notes of patients referring to the Department of Oral Surgery in the School of Dentistry, Ege University for TMJ pain and dysfunction that were managed by the authors of this manuscript over a period of 3 years (2009–2012) were retrospectively reviewed. All the patients were managed with a standard protocol (Table 1). The local ethics committee approved this retrospective study and the treatments were carried out after obtaining verbal and written informed consents from the patients.

Inclusion criteria for the review process were unilateral ID with or without OA requiring surgical treatment and management according to the above given protocol. Patients who became asymptomatic by conservative measures and therefore did not require surgical intervention; patients with a history of orthognathic and/or TMJ operations, arthritis effecting other joints, bilateral TMJ problems, incomplete documentation of treatment details or inability to attend review appointments regularly, were excluded from this retrospective cohort study.

Diagnosis and data collection

All of the patients had a panoramic film at presentation and a magnetic resonance imaging (MRI) was requested from those who had ongoing symptoms refractory to conservative treatment (Table 1). MRI was taken to confirm internal derangement. According to our standard management protocol, an objective parameter and 4 different subjective parameters were recorded pre-operatively and on post-operative reviews. Pain-free inter-incisal opening (the difference between incisal edges of central incisors when the patient is asked to open their mouth as wide as possible without any discomfort or pain) is an objective parameter and it was recorded as an average of three

Table 1 Flow chart describing the standard treatment protocol of patients who have TMJ pain and dysfunction

1. A detailed history, evaluation of head and neck, panoramic films to demonstrate temporal bone and condylar morphology

⇓⇓

2. If indicated, consultations with ear, nose and throat surgery; neurology; physical medicine and rehabilitation; internal medicine; and restorative dentistry as appropriate

⇓⇓

3. Advices included soft diet, limiting their mouth opening and not to chew gum for 6 weeks

⇓⇓

4. Ibuprofen (200 mg tds for 6 weeks) was the drug of choice for TMJ pain, and if necessary muscle relaxants were added (maximum for a period of 10 days)

⇓⇓

5. Patients with a clenching habit were provided with mouth guards for use while sleeping

⇓⇓

6. Review appointment was within 6 to 8 weeks to monitor the patients' progress.

⇓⇓

7. MRIs were requested from symptomatic patients with a clinical diagnosis of internal derangement. Patients with ongoing symptoms refractory to conservative treatment and MRI confirmed internal derangement were listed for arthrocentesis of the effected joint under local anaesthesia

⇓⇓

8. Post-operatively patients were regularly reviewed and those with persisting symptoms beyond 6 months were listed for arthroscopic lysis and lavage

⇓⇓

9. Post-operative reviews

consecutive measurements done by the same clinician. Subjective parameters (spontaneous pain, pain on function, difficulty on chewing, perceived disability on jaw movements) were recorded pre-operatively and on post-operative reviews. For this purpose Modified VAS (visual anolgue scale) scales were printed on a scale of 4 on 4 separate sheets of paper with the subjective parameter in question as the running title and patients were asked to rate their discomfort or pain on these scales (none, mild, medium and severe). Staging (Wilkes) of internal derangement of TMJs were done according to clinical and MRI data pre-operatively and according to clinical data post-operatively [2–4]. AAOMS (American Association of Oral and Maxillofacial Surgeons) success criteria were used for post-op evaluation of outcomes and success rate.

Treatment

Technique of arthrocentesis: Auriculotemporal nerve block is achieved and 1.5 ml of Lidocaine HCL (20 mg/ml) is used for distension of the superior joint space. A technique described by Laskin [7] was utilized for access and irrigation (with saline) of the superior joint space. 150–500 ml of saline is used for lysis and lavage. During the procedure the patient is instructed by the surgeon to carry out exercises like protrusion of the lower jaw and stretch opening the mouth. At the end of the procedure 1 ml of Orthovisc® (Biomex GmbH, Germany) is injected intra-articularly. A non-steroidal anti-inflammatory drug is prescribed post-operatively. Mouth stretching exercise to maintain the achieved range of motion is instructed [7].

Technique of arthroscopic lysis and lavage: General anaesthesia and complete neuro-muscular relaxation is achieved. After surgical preparation a 21 G cannula is used for access and distension of the joint. Later two trocar sheaths are placed from superior posterolateral and superior anterolateral approaches. Under constant saline irrigation, a 30° forward oblique telescope (Hopkins® Karl Storz GmbH & Co Germany) and a blunt obturator is used interchangibly through both access holes for sweeping the upper joint space under telescopic vision to aid lysis of the adhesions [14]. A minimum amount of 500 ml saline is used for lysis and lavage. During the procedure the jaw is manipulated to aid in the lysis of adhesions. At the end of the procedure1ml of Orthovisc® is injected intra articularly. Prescription and exercises are identical to those preferred after arthrocentesis.

Statistical analysis

Pre-operative and post-operative (at the end of the follow up period) pain free maximum interincisal opening values were compared with paired t test. The subjective parameters and Clinical (Wilkes) staging of internal derangement pre-operatively and at discharge were evaluated with Chi-square analysis using SPSS 10.0. (SPSS Inc. Chicago, İllinois, USA) AAOMS success criteria ("parameters of care" 2017) are considered and surgical treatment outcome is calculated [15].

Results

The authors of this manuscript managed a total of 1414 patients with TMJ pain and dysfunction between January 2009 and January 2012 according to the standard protocol outlined in Table 1. A comprehensive review of the case notes revealed that only 43 patients were surgically treated over a period of 3 years. (Arthrocentesis +/− arthroscopic lysis and lavage) According to our inclusion and exclusion criteria, 33 patients (31 females, 2 males) were regarded to be eligible for inclusion and statistical analysis. Mean age was 33.8 (range 15–63). Symptoms of 24 patients were completely or partially resolved after arthrocentesis hence did not require further treatment, however 9 patients required further treatment with arthroscopic lysis and lavage.

The follow–up period is defined as the period starting from the final surgical intervention (arthrocentesis or arthroscopic lysis and lavage) to the date of discharge. Follow-up period ranged from 3 to 30 months (mean 15.5 and standard deviation 5.8).

Pain free maximum interincisal opening values measured pre-operatively and at the end of the follow-up period were found to be statistically significant (Paired t test; $p < 0.001$) (Table 2).

Subjective parameters; spontaneous pain, pain on function, difficulty on chewing, perceived disability of jaw movements values rated pre-operatively and at discharge were found to be statistically significant (Chi-square analysis; $p < 0.001$) (Table 3 and Table 4).

The number of patients with severe or medium rated subjective parameters pre-operatively was reduced at discharge. This reduction was from 57.6 to 6.1% for spontaneous pain; from 90.9 to 3% for pain on function; from 81.8 to 6.1% for difficulty on chewing; and from 78.8 to 21.2% for perceived disability of jaw movements.

Clinical (Wilkes) staging of internal derangement pre-operatively and at discharge is shown in Table 5. Accordingly clinical staging of;

Stage IV patients remained unchanged, although their subjective parameters improved significantly (Chi-square analysis; $p < 0.001$).

All stage III patients became either Stage II or Stage I with a significant improvement in their pain free maximum interincisal opening values and subjective parameters (Paired t test; $p < 0.001$ and Chi-square analysis; $p < 0.001$ respectively).

Five stage II patients remained unchanged while 4 patients became stage I or free of symptoms. Patients that were Stage I at the beginning were not included in the study and there were no stage V patients within the study population.

Pre-operative Wilkes staging according to MRI data showed that 9 patients were Stage II with early signs of disc deformity in a slightly forward position. Ten patients were Stage III with a reducing anterior disc displacement and thickening of their discs. Fourteen patients were Stage IV with a non-reducing anterior disc displacement, moderate deformity and thickening of their discs. The bony changes were detected in Stage III and IV patients ranging from beaking of the condyle to abnormal bone

Table 2 Mean values, standard deviation and standard error of mean for pain free maximum interincisal opening

	Mean	Standard deviation	Standard error of mean
Pre-op value (mm)	27.636	8.652	1.151
Value at discharge (mm)	33.363	6.827	1.189
Difference	5.727	7.989	1.380

Table 3 Distribution of patients' subjective parameter ratings pre-operatively. (Total $N = 33$)

Subjective parameters	None (n)	Mild (n)	Medium (n)	Severe (n)
Spontaneous pain	11	3	10	9
Pain on function	0	3	15	15
Difficulty on chewing	1	5	12	15
Perceived disability of jaw movements	1	6	12	14

Table 5 Distribution of patients' clinical staging (Wilkes) of internal derangement pre-operatively and at discharge (Total $N = 33$)

	Stage I	Stage II	Stage III	Stage IV	Stage V
Pre-op.	0	9	10	14	0
At discharge	9	10	0	14	0

contours around the articular eminence. Stage I and Stage V joints were not detected.

Arthroscopic examination revealed that 1 Wilkes Stage II patient had anterior disc displacement; 3 Wilkes Stage III patients had mild and localised thin fibrillations of the articular cartilage with antero-medial disc displacement; 5 Wilkes Stage IV patients had extensive, thick fibrillations of the articular cartilage with antero-medial disc displacement and creeping synovitis.

Findings of pre-operative clinical examination, pre-operative MRI and arthroscopic lysis and lavage were parallel; thus clinical, MRI and arthroscopic (under direct vision) Wilkes Staging of the 9 patients were identical.

When AAOMS success criteria [15] are considered, surgical treatment outcome in our group of patients is given in Table 6. The list of AAOMS criteria and the results applied to our study are below,

A. Masticatory function was improved in all, but 2 patients
B. Level of pain was of little or no concern for all, but 2 patients as measured by the modified visual analogue scale.
C. Mastication, deglutition, speech and oral hygiene hence mandibular function improved in all, but 7 of our patients had extended disability.
D. All of the patients had stable occlusion with no temporary or permanent premature contacts.
E. Recovery was uneventful and introduction of mouth stretching exercises immediately post-operatively limited period of disability.
F. No permanently disabling complications were encountered (further morbidity was limited).

G. Understanding and acceptance by patient (family) of favourable outcomes, known risks and complications is an imperative component of the informed consent process for surgical management of TMJ patients.
H. Symptoms and quality of life improved for most of the patients' through out the follow up period.

Discussion

The contemporary evidence based management of ID with or without OA include; no treatment, medical treatment, physical therapy, arthrocentesis and arthroscopic surgery [15–20]. Treatment costs are quite variable from none (no treatment) to several thousand British pounds (arthroscopic surgery under general anaesthesia). One might think that not treating patients would not involve any costs and all the patients would eventually become asymptomatic as shown by Schiffmann et al. [16]. "No treatment" can actually be more costly, because of the extended distress of the patients, resulting in loss of labour and prolonged use of analgesics. For this reason the authors of this manuscript believe that not offering treatment to symptomatic ID with or without OA cases is unethical because of the psychological burden this would place on the patients. However "no treatment" should definitely be an option to be discussed with the patient during the informed consent process.

Information gathered from clinical and radiological examinations might fail to point towards a best treatment approach; hence deciding on the most appropriate treatment option for ID is difficult. The reliability of panoramic radiography is known to be poor for detecting OA or other soft tissue pathologies of TMJ. However MRI is a reliable tool inorder to detect bone marrow oedema, disc displacement with or without reduction, increased fluid level in the joint and computerised tomography (CT) is reliable for radiological diagnosis of OA [21].

Table 4 Distribution of patients' subjective parameter ratings at discharge (Total $N = 33$)

Subjective parameters	None (n)	Mild (n)	Medium (n)	Severe (n)
Spontaneous pain	28	3	1	1
Pain on function	27	5	1	0
Difficulty on chewing	26	5	2	0
Perceived disability of jaw movements	22	4	7	0

Table 6 Treatment outcome according to the AAOMS (American Association of Oral and Maxillofacial Surgeons) criteria (2017)

Treatment outcome	Number of patients (n)
Excellent	14
Good	17
Poor	2
Success rate	94%

CT obviously yields valuable data regarding the osseous structures and Ahmad et al. [21] suggests that clinical or research studies of OA should use CT when possible, however we are focused on the symptoms of the patients and a CT scan would not have changed our treatment modality and therefore was not deemed to be necessary before arthrocentesis and/or arthroscopy routinely. Panaromic radiographs taken in the present study served as a screening tool for TMJ pathology. Presence of osteophytic lipping, subarticular radiolucent areas, and presence of remodelling of the condyle in panoramic films are findings leading to the diagnosis of OA, however because of the low sensitivity of panaromic films in detecting OA, one should consider CT or cone-beam computerised tomography (CBCT) for optimal diagnostic evaluation of bony changes of TMJ [21].

Treating patients arthroscopically while arthrocentesis or conservative treatment would be sufficient will result in a rise of treatment costs and exposure of the patients to unnecessary risks. Therefore we preferred a stepped approach to manage symptomatic ID patients that is also suggested by Schiffman et al. [17]. We acknowledge that assessment of patients with pain from both joints can be confusing and therefore we included only unilateral cases. The fact that this is a retrospective study and therefore a comparison group is missing is a limitation of this study. A prospective, randomised controlled clinical trial aiming to compare the outcomes of various conservative and surgical treatment modalities in patients with internal derangement would be invaluable.

The subjective parameters were rated on a scale of 4 by the patient in the presence of the attending surgeon. We avoided using the VAS scale owing to the literacy status of some of our patients. The 4-point scale that was printed on paper was handed and read to the patient. Later the patient was asked to choose the appropriate number that best quantifies the subjective parameter in question. Mistakes in scoring were thus eliminated.

It is well known that appropriate selection of patients requiring surgical intervention is essential for successful treatment results [7, 22]. Moses [22] reported that 10 out of 400 patients with TMJ pain and dysfunction need surgical treatment (2.5%). In our study 1414 patients with TMJ pain and dysfunction attended oral surgery clinic during the study period, and 1371 of these were managed conservatively according to our standard treatment protocol. The remaining 43 patients received arthrocentesis and/or arthroscopy. Therefore 3% of our patients required surgical treatment, which is in accordance with the literature.

The follow-up period for 33 patients showed a normal distribution with a mean of 15.5 months. The details of the case notes revealed that most of the patients failed to attend their review appointments once they were satisfied by the result. All of the patients had access to the secretaries' phones for booking a slot in the clinic if they thought it was necessary. Hence it could be argued that the duration of our follow-up period is adequate for a realistic and correct assessment of treatment outcomes. However we recognise that this is a limitation of the present study and studies with a prospective design can allow for longer follow-up periods.

The average increase in pain free inter incisal opening was 6 mm giving an average opening of 33 mm at discharge. Although this is lower then the normal values of inter incisal opening that is 35-45 mm and lower then the values achieved by Sorel et al. [23], the increase in our group is statistically significant. However clinical significance of the average increase in pain free inter incisal opening is debatable.

Ahmed et al. prospectively assessed the therapeutic benefits of arthroscopy and arthrocentesis in patients with internal derangement of their temporomandibular joints. They found that both treatment modalities improve mouth opening and reduce pain when conservative approaches have failed [24]. Emes et al. advocate that more invasive procedures should be considered for patients with TMJ pain who do not benefit from arthrocentesis [17]. Our findings are in accordance with these studies.

In their randomized controlled trial of 80 patients with arthralgia of the TMJ, Vos et al. showed that, arthrocentesis as initial treatment reduces pain and functional impairment more rapidly compared to conservative treatment. However, after 26 weeks, both treatment modalities achieved comparable outcomes [18].

Several studies report that arthroscopic TMJ lysis and lavage with or without anterolateral capsular release reduce arthralgia significantly. In accordance with these studies, our stepped treatment approach allowed a statistically significant improvement in our patients' suffering as evaluated by "the subjective parameters" [25–29].

Staging of internal derangement of TMJ does not seem to be related to the severity of subjective parameters and the amount of relief of these symptoms after arthrocentesis and/or arthroscopy in our setting. Regardless of their staging, all patients benefit from arthrocentesis and/or arthroscopy particularly in pain relief. However pain free inter incisal opening of Stage IV patients appear to improve less than Stage II and Stage III patients. Thus it can be possible to speculate that, Stage II and III patients are more likely to have an improved mouth opening than Stage IV patients after treatment. The null hypothesis tested here can not be rejected within the limitations of this study, as subjective parameters and mouth opening of the patients improved at discharge. However randomized, prospective and controlled clinical studies should be performed for more evidence.

AAOMS success criteria [22] ("parameters of care" 1995) offered limited amount of data for comparison across studies. Therefore, in this study a revised version of AAOMS "parameters of care" that listed the "General Favorable Therapeutic Outcomes For Temporomandibular Joint Surgery" including arthrocentesis and arthroscopy was preferred [15] (Table 6).

Ideally VAS rating and where possible quantitative measuring of the above mentioned "General Favorable Therapeutic Outcomes" would enable comparison across groups and/or different studies. Similarly the "subjective parameters" rated on a scale of 4 in our study, allow temporal monitorization of the outcomes listed in the AAOMS publication [15].

Ahmed et al. reported that 2 patients out of 244 TMJ patients that were treated with arthroscopy or arthrocentesis had temporary weakness of the temporal branch of the facial nerve [24]. In our group no permanently disabling complications were encountered. However one of our patients experienced an inferior alveolar nerve block during arthrocentesis that completely resolved in an hour. This inadvertent local anaesthesia was thought to be due to a needle puncture on the medial wall of the joint capsule, and the local anaesthetic administered in the joint, must have infiltrated to the infra-temporal fossa. It is well known that mandibular nerve lies close to the joint and it is possible that the local anaesthesia was achieved through this mechanism. We are not aware of any similar reported complications during arthrocentesis. On the other hand brutal manipulation of the thoracars during TMJ arthroscopy may lead to temporary weakness of the Vth and VIIth cranial nerves [30]. Accordingly one of our arthroscopy patients had temporary weakness of her eyelid with complete recovery at the end of 3 weeks. She was treated conservatively with eye lubricants during this period. Other reported complications of this procedure that were not seen in our group include perforation of the external auditory meatus and extradural haematoma [24].

Conclusion

The stepped approach for the management of symptomatic internal derangement with or without osteoarthritis is a predictable treatment strategy to reduce the suffering of our patients, hence improve the quality of their lives. However, it is imperative for the patients to understand the involved procedures and their outcomes, for developing realistic expectations and improving patient co-operation.

Acknowledgements

The authors of this manuscript would like to thank to Dr. Hayal Boyacıoğlu for statistical analyses and our scrub nurse Pervin Kaynar for her assistance in the theatre.

Funding

All treatment costs were covered by national health insurance that had no role in collection, analysis, and interpretation of data and in writing the manuscript.

Authors' contributions

Made substantial contributions to conception and design, or acquisition of data, or analysis and interpretation of data; (EC, SC). Been involved in drafting the manuscript or revising it critically for important intellectual content; (EC, SC, KH, YE). Given final approval of the version to be published. Each author should have participated sufficiently in the work to take public responsibility for appropriate portions of the content; and (EC, SC, KH, YE). Agreed to be accountable for all aspects of the work in ensuring that questions related to the accuracy or integrity of any part of the work are appropriately investigated and resolved (EC).

Competing interests

The authors declare that they have no competing interests.

Author details

[1]Oral Surgery Department, Ege University School of Dentistry, 35100 Izmir, Turkey. [2]Anesthesiology Department, Ege University School of Medicine, 35100 Izmir, Turkey.

References

1. Bont LD, Stegenga B. Pathology of temporomandibular joint internal derangement and osteoarthrosis. Int J Oral Maxillofac Surg. 1993;22:71–4.
2. Larheim TA, Westesson P-L, Sano T. Temporomandibular joint disk displacement: comparison in asymptomatic volunteers and patients. Radiology. 2001;218:428–32.
3. Wilkes CH. Surgical treatment of internal derangements of temporomandibular joint. A long term study. Arch Otolarngol Head Neck Surg. 1991;117:64–72.
4. Hall HD, Navarro EZ, Gibbs SJ. One-and three-year prospective outcome study of modified condylotomy for treatment of reducing disk displacement. J Oral Maxillofac Surg. 2000;58:7–17.
5. Werther JR, Hall HD, Gibbs SJ. Type of disc displacement and change in disc position after modified condylotomy in 80 symptomatic T-M joints. Oral Surg Oral Med Oral Pathol. 1995;79:668–79.
6. Presman B, Shellock F, Schames J. MR imaging of temporomandibular joint abnormalities associated with cervical hyperextension/hyperflexion (whiplash) injuries. J Magn Reson Imaging. 1992;2:569–74.
7. Laskin DM. Arthrocentesis for the treatment of internal derangements of the temporomandibular joint. Alpha Omegan. 2009;102:46–50.
8. Yıldız A, Esen E. Complications of the temporomandibular joint arthroscopy. Turkiye Klinikleri J Dental Sci. 2007;13:55–62.
9. Kisnisci RŞ, Tüz HH, Önder E. Clinical outcomes of temporomandibular joint disc surgery. Turkiye Klinikleri J Dental Sci. 2001;7:105–10.
10. Fridrich KL, Wise JM, Zeitler DL. Prospective comparison of atrhroscopy and arthrocentesis for temporomandibular joint disorders. J Oral Maxillofac Surg. 1996;54:816–20.
11. Goudot P, Jaquinet AR, Hugonnet S, Haefliger W, Richter M. Improvement of pain and function after arthroscopy and arthrocentesis of the temporomandibular joint: a comparative study. J Craniomaxillofac Surg. 2000;28:39–43.
12. Murakami K, Segami N, Okamoto M, Yamamura I, Takahashi K, Tsuboi Y. Outcome of arthroscopic surgery for internal derangements of the temporomandibular joint: long term results covering 10 years. J Craniomaxillofac Surg. 2000;28:264–71.
13. Nitzan DW, Dolwick MF, Heft MW. Arthroscopic lysis and lavage of the temporomandibular joint: a change in perspective. J Oral Maxillofac Surg. 1990;48:798–801.
14. Tarro AW. TMJ arthrocentesis and blunt sweeping of the superior joint space. Br J Oral Maxillofac Surg. 1997;35:446.
15. Bouloux G, Koslin MG, Ness G, Shafer D. Parameters of care: clinical practice guidelines for oral and maxillofacial surgery (AAOMS ParCare 2017). J Oral Maxillofac Surg. 2017;75:e195–223.
16. Schiffman EL, Look JO, Hodges JS, Swift JQ, Decker KL, Hataway KM, et al. Randomized effectiveness study of four therapeutic strategies for TMJ closed lock. J Dent Res. 2007;86:58–63.
17. Schiffman EL, Velly AM, Look JO, Hodges JS, Swift JQ, Decker KL, et al. Effects of four treatment strategies for temporomandibular joint closed lock. Int J Oral Maxillofac Surg. 2014;43:217–26.

18. Vos LM, Huddleston Slater JJR, Stegenga B. Arthrocentesis as initial treatment for temporomandibular joint arthropathy: a randomized controlled trial. J Craniomaxillofac Surg. 2014;42:e134–9.

19. Murakami K. Rationale of arthroscopic surgery of the temporomandibular joint. J Oral Biol Craniofac Res. 2013;3:126–34.

20. Machon V, Sedy K, Klima D, Hirjak D, Foltan R. Arthroscopic lysis and lavage in patients with temporomandibular anterior disc displacement without reduction. Int J Oral Maxillofac Surg. 2012;41:109–13.

21. Ahmad M, Hollender L, Anderson Q, Kartha K, Ohrbach RK, Truelove E, et al. Research diagnostic criteria for temporomandibular disorders (RDC/TMD): development of image analysis criteria and examiner reliability for image analysis. Oral Surg Oral Med Oral Pathol Oral Radiol Endod. 2009;107:844–60.

22. Moses J. TMJ arthroscopic surgery: rationale and technique. J Oral Maxillofac Surg. 2004;62:96–7.

23. Sorel B, Piecuch JF. Long term evaluation following temporomandibular joint arthroscopy with lysis and lavage. Int J Oral Maxillofac Surg. 2000;29:259–63.

24. Ahmed N, Sidebottom A, O'Connor M, Kerr HL. Prospective outcome assessment of the therapeutic benefits of arthroscpy and arthrocentesis of the temporomandibular joint. Br J Oral Maxillofac Surg. 2012;50:745–8.

25. Emes Y, Arpinar IŞ, Oncu B, Aybar B, Aktas I, Al Badri N, et al. The next step in the treatment of persistent temporomandibuar joint pain following arthrocentesis: a retrospective study of 18 cases. J Craniomaxillofac Surg. 2014;42:e65–9.

26. Kaneyama K, Segami N, Sato N, Murakami KI, Iizuka T. Outcomes of 152 temporomandibular joints following arthroscopic anterolateral capsular release by holmium:YAG laser or electrocautery. Oral Surg Oral Medicine Oral Pathol. 2004;97:546–51.

27. Indresano AT. Surgical arthroscopy as the preferred treatment for internal derangements of the temporomandibular joint. J Oral Maxillofac Surg. 2001;59:308–12.

28. Smolka W, Yanai C, Smolka K, Iizuka T. Efficiency of arthroscopic lysis and lavage for internal derangement of the temporomandibular joint correlated with Wilkes classification. Oral Surg Oral Med Oral Pathol Oral Radiol Endod. 2008;106:317–23.

29. Sidebottom AJ. Current thinking in temporomandibular joint management. Br J Oral Maxillofac Surg. 2009;47:91–4.

30. Koslin MG, Indresano AT, Mercuri LG. Temporomandibular joint surgery. J Oral Maxillofac Surg. 2012;70:e204–31.

33

Comparison of inhaled versus intravenous anesthesia for laryngoscopy and laryngeal electromyography in a rat model

M. Gazzaz[1*] (iD), J. Saini[2,3], S. Pagliardini[2,3,4], B. Tsui[5], C. Jeffery[1] and H. El-Hakim[1]

Abstract

Background: Propofol and remifentanil intravenous combination is one popular form of total intravenous anesthesia (TIVA) in mainstream clinical practice, but it has rarely been applied to a rat model for laryngoscopy and laryngeal electromyography (LEMG). Our objective was to establish a safe and reproducible general anesthetic protocol for laryngoscopy and endoscopic LEMG in a rat model. Our hypothesis is that TIVA allows a minimally morbid, and feasible laryngoscopy and LEMG.

Methods: Sprague Dawley rats were subjected to either inhalational anesthesia (IA) (isoflurane) or TIVA (propofol and remifentanil) and underwent laryngoscopy and LEMG. The primary outcome was a complete minimally interrupted rigid laryngoscopy and obtaining reproducible motor unit potentials from the posterior cricoarytenoid muscles. The secondary outcome was morbidity and mortality.

Results: Seventeen out of twenty-two rats underwent both TIVA and IA. Only two underwent IA only. All nineteen rats that underwent IA had a successful experiment. Seventeen rats underwent TIVA, however, only nine completed a successful experiment due to difficulty achieving a surgical plane, and respiratory events. Upon comparing the success of the two anaesthetic regimens, IA was superior to TIVA ($P = 0.0008$). There was no statistical difference between the amplitudes ($p = 0.1985$) or motor units burst duration ($p = 0.82605$) of both methods. Three mortalities were encountered, one of which was due to lidocaine toxicity and two were during anesthetic induction. Respiratory related morbidity was encountered in two rats, all seen with TIVA.

Conclusions: TIVA is not an ideal anesthetic regimen for laryngeal endoscopy and LEMG in rat models. Contrary to our hypothesis, IA did not affect the quality of the LEMG and allowed a seamless rigid endoscopy.

Keywords: Laryngeal mobility disorders, Laryngeal electromyography, Inhalational anesthesia, Total intravenous anesthesia

Background

The standards of general anesthesia for airway endoscopy in humans have evolved due to developing technological and pharmacological innovations. One of the most challenging diagnoses to establish in laryngology is mobility disorders, particularly in children where endoscopy under

general anesthesia, supplemented accordingly by laryngeal electromyography (LEMG) is the reference standard.

Traditionally, inhalational anesthesia (IA) was routinely employed for airway endoscopy in clinical practice. In the late 1990's, total intravenous anesthesia (TIVA) technique was introduced and gained popularity [1]. But to this day, proponents of both options argue their cases strongly. The claimed advantages of IA include speed, ease and comfortable induction using a mask in the absence of intravenous (IV) access, in addition to simple non-invasive evaluation of the blood tension of the inhaled agent [2]. On the other hand, TIVA is professed to lessen postoperative nausea and vomiting, act rapidly and independently from the alveolar ventilation, and is

* Correspondence: mgazzaz@ualberta.ca
This work was presented on the podium at the Poliquin Residents Research Competition (Canadian Society of Otolaryngology-Head and Neck Surgery Annual Meeting, June 2018, Quebec City, QC).
[1]Division of Otolaryngology-Head and Neck Surgery, Department of Surgery, University of Alberta, 2C3.57 Walter MacKenzie Centre, Edmonton, AB T6G 2R7, Canada
Full list of author information is available at the end of the article

administrable using peripheral locations away from airway instrumentation. It is also a non-pollutant for the operative room environment [2–4].

Some experts in airway endoscopy and electromyography studies support the notion that anesthetic agents may modify the findings. It is proposed that different concentration and duration of IA may modify LEMG findings and produce spurious abnormalities. Some rest this notion on evidence from literature pertaining to spine surgery [5–8]. However, many centers perform LEMG in humans under IA [9–12], especially that there are no head to head studies comparing the two techniques. In rats, LEMG has also been performed under IA [13], yet in most cases it has been used as an induction agent for sedation [14–17].

Propofol and remifentanil IV combination is one popular form of TIVA in mainstream clinical practice, but it has rarely been applied to a rat model for laryngoscopy and LEMG. We therefore set out to evaluate whether a TIVA protocol is applicable to the rat model for reproducible assessment of laryngeal function, with minimal morbidity. We specifically aimed to compare the mortality, morbidity, and reproducibility of two general anesthetic protocols for laryngoscopy and endoscopic LEMG in a rat model. Our hypothesis was that TIVA allows a minimally morbid, and feasible laryngoscopy and LEMG.

Methods

Study design

The experiment was conducted in accordance with the Canadian Council of Animal Care guidelines and policies, following approval from the University of Alberta Health Research Ethics Board (AUP00001311) and the Animal Care and Use Committee for health sciences at the University of Alberta.

This prospective comparative non-randomized, cross over experimental animal study was conducted at the Surgical Medical Research Institute and Katz Group - Rexall Centre for research at the University of Alberta, between April 2016 and February 2017.

After induction of general inhalation anesthesia using isofluorane (2% in air; IA) to set up vein cannulation, anesthesia was maintained under one of the two anesthetic options followed by the second one (i.e TIVA followed by IA or vice versa) allowing a washout period to occur in between, during which the animal shows a positive toe pinch reflex.

Study subjects

A total of 30 Sprague-Dawley rats were approved for this study. All rats were housed in pairs within the housing facility of Health Sciences Laboratory Animal Services at the University of Alberta. Eight rats were used initially as a pilot study.

Experimental procedure

Preparation and anesthesia

Pre-operatively, age, sex, and weight of the rats were documented and a unique identifying number was given. Rats were then placed in an induction chamber saturated with 2% isoflurane. Anesthesia was maintained using either inhaled isoflurane 1.5–5% or a combination of propofol (10 mg/ml and 40–50 mg/kg/h IV infusion) [18] and remifentanyl (5 mcg/ml and 0.4 mcg/kg/min IV infusion) [19] after establishing IV access (either via tail or femoral vein). Ampicillin (50 mg/kg SC), meloxicam (1-2 mg/kg SC) and ringer's lactate (1 ml/kg/hr. intraperitoneal) were administered preoperatively. The rat was then transferred to the surgical table and placed on a restraining board with an integrated circulating fluid heating pad with temperature set at 37 °C. A respiratory belt (Kent Scientific Co., USA), a rectal thermometer probe and a vital signs monitoring foot sensor (STARR Life Sciences® Mouse Ox® Plus) were attached. The depth of anesthesia was determined by eliciting a toe pinch reflex, observing the respiratory rate and pattern of breathing, and finally the tolerance and response to airway stimulation to endoscope insertion. If TIVA was used for maintenance, isoflurane concentration was reduced to 0.5%, and then turned off after a period of five minutes. The depth of the anesthesia was then assessed again and the rate of infusion was adjusted accordingly. Baseline and periodic readings of heart and respiratory rate, peripheral capillary oxygen saturation (SpO2), temperature and mucous membrane color were all recorded every five minutes.

Laryngoscopy and laryngeal EMG

Once the rat was adequately anesthetized under either IA or TIVA, room air (21% O2) was delivered through the nasal mask for 1–2 min to maintain SpO_2 above 90%. The rat was then positioned supine on the experimental workstation inside a Faraday cage. By retracting the tongue, the larynx was visualized and lidocaine 1% (1.67 mg/kg) was applied topically under telescopic guidance. A nebulizer was also connected to the nasal cone and lidocaine 1% was delivered for ~ 1 min. This step was aborted in future experiments after presumed lidocaine toxicity mortality was encountered.

Laryngoscopy

While the animal was spontaneously breathing, a zero degree 2.7 mm rod lens telescope (KARL-STORZ®, Germany) connected to an image capture unit, was used to visualize vocal cords' movements.

Laryngeal electromyography

Once the larynx was exposed, LEMG recordings from the posterior cricoarytenoid (PCA) muscle were obtained by inserting a monopolar needle electrode (29GA, 37 mm) (Rochester Electro-Medical, USA) transorally under direct rigid endoscopic visualization with each anesthetic regimen. Since the PCA muscle is responsible for vocal cord abduction during inspiration, in addition to the ease of electrode insertion in comparison to other adductor intrinsic laryngeal muscles in the tenuous rat airway, we elected to choose it as our muscle of choice to obtain LEMG recordings. A ground electrode (27G, 12 mm) (Ambu® Neuroline Subdermal, Malaysia) was secured into the chest. Electrodes were connected to amplifiers (AM Systems, Carlsborg, WA) and activity was filtered between 300 Hz and 1 kHz, amplified at x10k and sampled at 1 kHz (Powerlab 16/30; AD Instruments, Colorado Springs, CO). A piezoelectric chest belt was connected to the recording system in order to detect chest wall movements and correlate between LEMG signal and the respiratory cycle. A minimum of ten respiratory cycles was digitally recorded from the muscle for off-line analysis.

Recovery, postoperative care and euthanasia

Upon the conclusion of the experiment the rat was transferred to a new cage to allow recovery from anesthesia. Each rat was housed individually for 2 h post-operatively to be monitored and assessed clinically every fifteen minutes. This included activity, response to external stimuli, appearance and feeding. The animal was then euthanized by decapitation under isoflurane anesthesia.

Outcome measures
Primary outcomes: Proportion of complete rigid laryngoscopy and LEMG

A successful experiment was defined as completion of both laryngeal endoscopy and the ability to obtain a reliable LEMG recording. A complete laryngoscopy was defined as a minimally interrupted, well-tolerated rigid endoscopy of the respiratory action of the larynx while the subject goes through ten cycles of spontaneous breathing. For LEMG, ten consecutive respiratory related bursts of activity were required and the mean amplitudes and burst durations of the LEMG signal were analyzed and calculated using Lab ChartPro8.

Criteria used to abort the experiment included: signs of hemodynamic instability encountered during intraoperative monitoring (persistent maximal scores of respiratory distress, i.e. apnea/hypopnea, or sustained heart rate deviations) or a ninety minutes maximum duration as a cut-off point to achieve the appropriate depth of anesthesia.

Secondary outcomes: Mortality and morbidity

Mortalities encountered were documented. Morbidities experienced were defined as respiratory events during the procedure, which included laryngeal spasm, apnea and hypopnea requiring interruption of the procedure.

Statistical analysis

Demographics were summarized as means, standard deviation (SD), minimal and maximal values. Student t-test was used for comparing means, and 95% confidence intervals were provided. Fisher's exact test and chi square were used to compare proportions of mortality and morbidity between anesthetic regimens [20].

Based on a previous study from our laboratory using only propofol as TIVA [18], a 70% respiratory morbidity rate was demonstrated. A decision was made that a reduction to 15% would be statistically and clinically significant. Based on 16.67% mortality rate and accepting a p value of 0.05 and a power of 80%, the sample size would be ten per group. Allowing for unforeseen morbidity, five rats were added to each group for a total of 30 rats.

As part of the LEMG waveform evaluation, we included motor unit potential assessment in the form of amplitude and burst duration. The amplitude was calculated from the height, the burst duration from the period and 60 divided by the period to obtain the respiratory rate using peak analysis in Lab ChartPro8.

Results

A total of 30 rats were used. The mean age was 7.56 ± 5.79 months (3–18). Thirteen were males and seventeen were females. The mean weight was 509.02 ± 258.24 g (245–1200). The basic clinical parameters for the two groups are described in Table 1. All 8 rats from the pilot group underwent TIVA and two of them underwent a successful experiment.

Seventeen (77.3%) rats underwent both TIVA and IA, two (9.1%) underwent IA only. Three (13.6%) mortalities were encountered in total. Two of them occurred during anesthetic inhalational induction and one mortality was likely due to lidocaine toxicity while on IA. Eight rats (47.06%) were maintained with TIVA first followed by IA and twelve (52.94%) were maintained with IA first followed by TIVA. See Fig. 1.

All nineteen rats that underwent IA had a successful experiment requiring a maximum period of 15 min, i.e. tolerated endoscopy without major respiratory events and completed a reproducible LEMG. Out of the 17 rats that underwent TIVA, nine of them (52.94%) completed a successful experiment requiring a duration between 45 and 90 min. See Fig. 2. The eight unsuccessful experiments (47.06%) were mainly due to inability to achieve an appropriate anesthetic plane. Seven of these rats continued to be responsive and intolerant of endoscopy despite escalation of the TIVA dosage to as high as 3.5 times the weight and boluses, whereas one animal

Table 1 Parameters of the rats

Parameter	TIVA (n = 17)	IA (n = 19)
Age (months) Mean ± SD (range)	7.18 ± 6.1 (3–18)	6.74 ± 5.9 (3–18)
Males	9	9
Females	8	10
Weight (gm) Mean ± SD (range)	514.88 ± 219.28 (245–980)	488 ± 217.95 (245–980)

developed bradycardia down to 70 beats per minute and the SpO_2 dropped to 60%, and the procedure was aborted to ensure safety. In the nine successful experiments under TIVA, no mortalities were encountered. However, two rats (11.76%) developed apneic events for seconds during the procedure and recovered spontaneously.

While the rats were maintained on IA, no morbidities were encountered. Only one (5.26%) mortality took place (presumably due to lidocaine toxicity). Comparing both anesthetic regimens, no statistical significance was evident for morbidity ($p = 0.096$) or mortality ($p = 0.679$), however, IA proved to be superior to TIVA in performing successful experiments ($p = 0.0008$).

With regards to LEMG variables, it was noted that the mean amplitude of LEMG in TIVA is 66.9% that of IA. However, there was no significant difference between mean amplitudes – 1.79 ± 9.88 mV (95% CI -1.79-2.2, $p = 0.1985$) or mean burst duration 0.27 ± 0.75 s (95% CI -0.23-0.76, $p = 0.82605$). See in the Additional file 1: Table S1 for details.

Two rats had the electrode maintained in the same position without manipulations while the anesthetic regimens were switched. No statistical difference in mean amplitude or mean burst duration was evident individually ($p > 0.05$) despite the amplitude being lower on TIVA. The PCA contraction displays a pre-inspiratory pattern of activity in both IA and TIVA consistently. See Fig. 3.

Of note, the time required to perform a full experiment using IA was 10–15 min compared to 45–90 min when using TIVA.

When comparing clinical parameters during the recovery period, no morbidities or mortalities occurred during recovery.

Discussion

This study compared the use of TIVA and IA during laryngoscopy and LEMG recording in rat models. Our endpoints were the ability to perform a complete endoscopy and neurophysiological recordings with the least morbidity and mortality. Our results show that TIVA is unlikely to be the anesthetic of choice for endoscopy and LEMG recordings in a rat model.

Balancing adequate depth of anesthesia and stability of spontaneous respiration during pediatric endoscopic surgery may be difficult to maintain using TIVA [21, 22]. Additionally, drug dosing appears more demanding with TIVA and higher infusion rates are sometimes necessary to provide the desired plasma concentrations [2]. Malik and Sen [23] reported 5.3% respiratory related morbidity manifested as brief episodes of desaturation due to malposition of the airway and laryngospasm with intermittent TIVA for pediatric endoscopic procedures. On the other hand, evidence suggests that TIVA reduces airway reactivity; decreases bronchospasm and laryngospasm in children [4, 24].

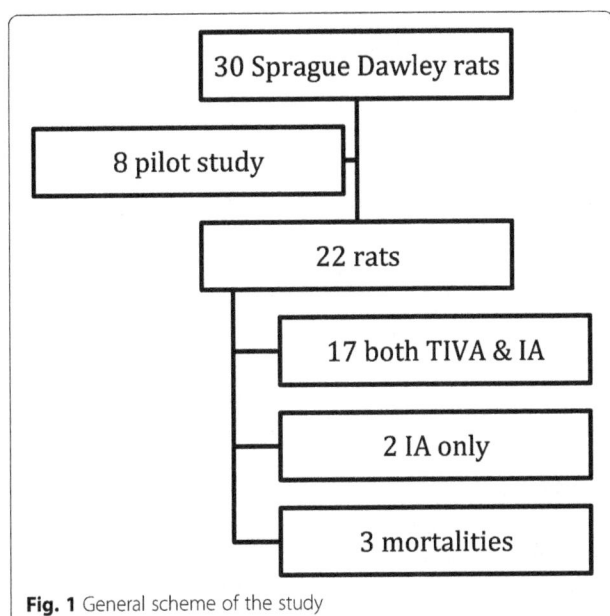

Fig. 1 General scheme of the study

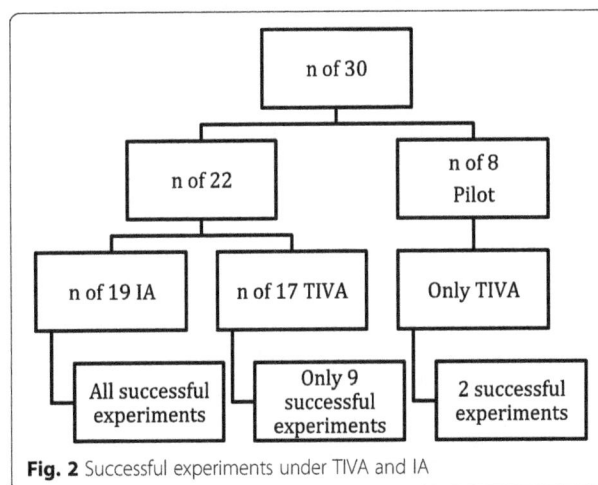

Fig. 2 Successful experiments under TIVA and IA

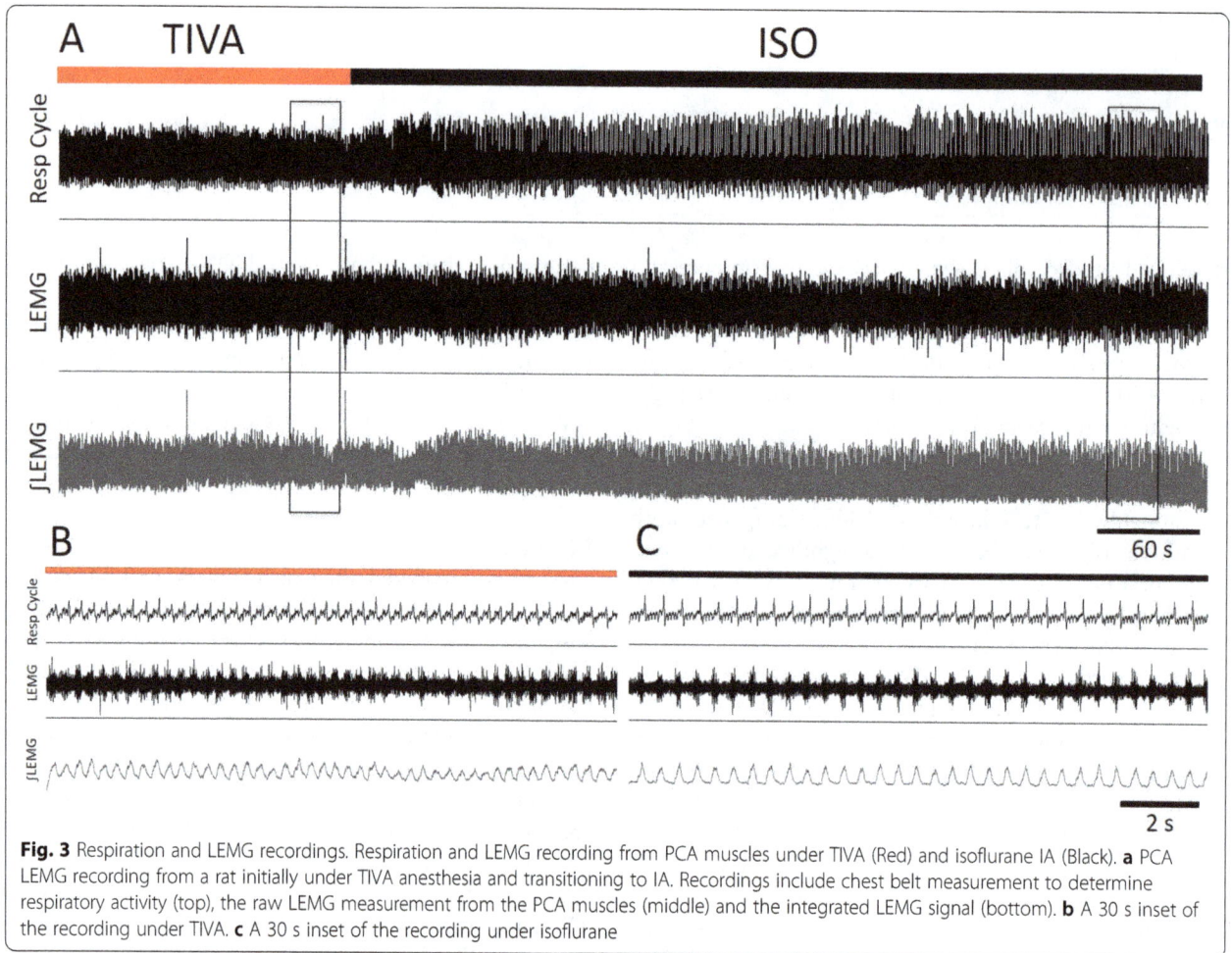

Fig. 3 Respiration and LEMG recordings. Respiration and LEMG recording from PCA muscles under TIVA (Red) and isoflurane IA (Black). **a** PCA LEMG recording from a rat initially under TIVA anesthesia and transitioning to IA. Recordings include chest belt measurement to determine respiratory activity (top), the raw LEMG measurement from the PCA muscles (middle) and the integrated LEMG signal (bottom). **b** A 30 s inset of the recording under TIVA. **c** A 30 s inset of the recording under isoflurane

In the current study, the morbidity rate was reduced from 70% based on previous experiments performed by the senior author HE [18] to 11.7% which is considered clinically significant in the current experiment. This may be due to the effect of adding remifentanyl.

Several studies have compared different types of anesthetics regimes in pediatric otolaryngology surgeries. A direct comparison between TIVA (propofol plus remifentanil) and volatile anesthetics indicated that TIVA is superior for induction, maintenance and recovery from anesthesia in children undergoing flexible fiberoptic bronchoscopy, adenoidectomy and/or tonsillectomy [25, 26].

Evidence in pediatric IA suggests that it may cause apnea following induction, especially if great concentrations were delivered [2]. This may explain the unexpected mortalities encountered during induction under IA in our current study.

Several anesthetics in experimental animal models have been used to perform safe, interpretable and reliable endoscopy and/or LEMG, but direct comparisons and proof of reproducibility are limited [13–17, 27–32]. These included intraabdominal barbitone sodium [27], mixture of intramuscular ketamine hydrochloride and xylazine hydrochloride [14, 15, 30] intramuscular ketamine only [28], combination of inhaled isoflurane and intraperitoneal ketamine and xylazine [16, 17, 29, 31], intraperitoneal/intravenous pentobarbital sodium [32], and isoflurane only [13]. With the exception of ketamine and isoflurane, none of these drugs are used in clinical practice. Interestingly, only scant reports on mortality and morbidity have been previously described given the fragility of the animal and its delicate airway, with prior experience indicating up to 20% mortality [13, 18, 33, 34].

Our results indicate that LEMG can be reliably performed under IA in a rat model. Despite previous studies in human spinal surgery [5–8] and animal studies [35] suggesting that the duration and concentration of IA affect evoked electromyogram parameters, specifically amplitude and latency, our results showed no difference in spontaneous LEMG variables between anesthetics. Several LEMG clinical studies [36–39] have used TIVA instead of IA when studying laryngeal disorders. The exact reasons are unclear, perhaps due to the increased use of TIVA among pediatric anesthetists or the potential effect of IA on LEMG.

One important observation in our study is the reduction in the duration of a complete experiment using IA (10–15 min) compared to TIVA (45–90 min). The advantages of using IA compared to TIVA in terms of reduction in induction time, maintenance of stable breathing, lack of laryngeal bronchospasm and emergence from anesthesia has been also reported previously in pediatric studies [21, 40]. In our study, the longer duration required while on TIVA was mainly due to inability to achieve an appropriate anesthetic plane to perform the experiment. This may well be due to IV agents displaying excessive inter-individual variability to TIVA maintenance that cannot be easily estimated [2] or perhaps associated with the large body weight of some rats used for this study and the accumulation of fat mass that may alter the dose necessary to establish the optimal surgical plane.

Tsai and colleagues [41] compared the recovery from laryngoscopy procedures under propofol TIVA and conventional isoflurane in a canine model. The TIVA group was significantly better than the isoflurane group in terms of smoothness of recovery from surgery, defined as absence of struggling, vocalization, or excitement and requiring little or no physical restraint to prevent self-injury. However, the isoflurane group recovered faster from anesthetic. No significant difference was observed between the two groups in terms of adverse effects, which was comparable to our findings.

LEMG is considered a valuable clinical and research tool to assess different pathologies in laryngeal motor function. Its' use has been described in the literature for humans and in experimental models as an outcome measure following a specific laryngeal intervention. As part of the reporting practice, the type of anesthetic used throughout the procedure should be documented [42]. Proponents of LEMG argue its prognostic and diagnostic values that may guide treatment decisions in patients with vocal fold mobility disorders [37, 43].

Multiple intrinsic laryngeal muscles were described in the literature as a point for recording LEMG activity in both animals and humans. This includes thyroarytenoid [9–12, 15–18, 33, 36–39, 44–49], cricothyroid [44, 46, 48, 50], PCA [11–13, 15, 16, 18, 27, 32, 33, 37, 38, 44, 45, 49, 51, 52] and lateral cricoarytenoid [15] either individually or in combination. The authors have selected the PCA muscle, as it's the single laryngeal muscle responsible for vocal fold abduction. PCA contraction has been pre-inspiratory on a consistent basis noted by the piezoelectric chest belt in our study.

One of the study limitations is the wide range of weight (245 g–980 g) and the large weight potentially contributing in the rat's morbidity and/or mortality while under general anesthesia. Despite the known typical weight of laboratory rats ranging between 300 g and 500 g, mortalities encountered were amongst smaller animals weighing equal to or less than 400 g and morbidities were seen within the mean of weight.

We acknowledge that the monopolar needle electrode was inserted in different locations within the PCA muscle with each anesthetic regimen, which may have affected the LEMG recordings. We are aware that recordings depend on the size of muscle fibers, the proximity of the electrode to large muscles, and the depth of electrode insertion. However, maintaining the electrode in the same position is practically difficult to achieve. A proper washout period between the two anesthetic methods cannot be feasible. Still, we were able to keep the electrode in the same location without manipulation in 2 rats and found no statistical difference in mean amplitude or burst duration.

An additional limitation is the fact that the rats were not blindly randomized for the anesthetic regimens, nor were the results concealed due to the nature of the experiment. However, we used a cross over trial instead. In such case, randomization or which anesthetic was started first does not matter, as the rat will undergo both anesthetic regimens regardless. Also, TIVA and IA are known to have rapid onset/offset action, the effect of anesthetic is reversible, the period of administration is short; the condition is relatively stable as the rats were completely healthy, and the carry-over is not an issue [53]. This permitted convenience and efficiency of the project [54]. This design also allowed amplification of the sample size used.

In the future, we aim to replicate the same experiment in pediatric patients and compare anesthetic regimens and their effect on laryngoscopy and LEMG, as IA is a useful translational model for laryngoscopy and LEMG experiments.

Conclusion

Contrary to our hypothesis, IA did not affect the quality of LEMG and allowed a seamless rigid endoscopy in rat models superior to TIVA. It proved to be quick, easy and safe to administer. We conclude that this is a reliable translational model for laryngoscopy and LEMG experiments.

Abbreviations
IA: Inhalational anesthesia; IV: Intravenous; kg/min: Kilogram/minute; L/min: Liters/minute; LEMG: Laryngeal electromyography; mcg/kg/min: Microgram/kilogram/minute; mcg/ml: Microgram/milliliter; mg/kg: Milligram/kilogram; mg/ml: Milligram/milliliter; min: Minutes; ml: Milliliter; ml/kg/hr: Milliliter/kilogram/hour; mm: Millimeter; O_2: Oxygen; PCA: Posterior cricoarytenoid; SC: Subcutaneous; SD: Standard deviation; SpO_2: Oxygen saturation; TIVA: Total intravenous anesthesia

Funding

This study has been funded by the Edmonton Civic Employees Grant. Malak Jamal Gazzaz acknowledges her residency scholarship through Umm Al-Qura University, Makkah, Saudi Arabia. SP laboratory is funded by NSERC, CIHR, Canadian Lung Association and Women and Children Health Research Institute.

Authors' contributions

MJG contributed to the experimental procedures, data analysis and interpretation, and manuscript preparation. She has approved the final manuscript in its current form. JS contributed to the experimental procedures, data analysis and interpretation. She has approved the final manuscript in its current form. SP contributed to the experimental procedures, oversaw the technical aspects of the research and contributed to manuscript preparation. She has approved the final manuscript in its current form. BT contributed to the experiment conception and design and contributed to the pilot study. He has approved the final manuscript in its current form. CJ contributed to the conception and design of the study, and provided input to the manuscript. She has approved the final manuscript in its current form. HE was responsible for the conception, design, and overall execution of the study. He contributed to the manuscript preparation and has approved the final manuscript in its current form.

Competing interests

The authors declare that they have no competing interests.

Author details

[1]Division of Otolaryngology-Head and Neck Surgery, Department of Surgery, University of Alberta, 2C3.57 Walter MacKenzie Centre, Edmonton, AB T6G 2R7, Canada. [2]Neuroscience and Mental Health Institute, University of Alberta, Edmonton, AB, Canada. [3]Women and Children Research Institute, University of Alberta, Edmonton, AB, Canada. [4]Department of Physiology, University of Alberta, Edmonton, AB, Canada. [5]Stanford University Pediatric Regional Anesthesia, Stanford University, Stanford, California, USA.

References

1. Malherbe S, Whyte S, Singh P, Amari E, King A, Mark Ansermino J. Total intravenous anesthesia and spontaneous respiration for airway endoscopy in children - a prospective evaluation. Paediatr Anaesth. 2010;20:434–8.
2. Lerman J, JÖhr M. Inhalational anesthesia vs total intravenous anesthesia (TIVA) for pediatric anesthesia. Paediatr Anaesth. 2009;19:521–34.
3. McCormack JG. Total intravenous anaesthesia in children. Curr Anaesth Crit Care. 2008;19:309–14. https://doi.org/10.1016/j.cacc.2008.09.005.
4. Gaynor J, Ansermino JM. Paediatric total intravenous anaesthesia. BJA Educ. 2016;16:369–73.
5. Chen X, Xu L, Wang Y, Xu F, Du Y, Li J. Sevoflurane affects evoked electromyography monitoring in cerebral palsy. Open Med. 2016;11:138–42. https://doi.org/10.1515/med-2016-0027.
6. Banoub M, Tetzlaff JE, Schubert A. Pharmacologic and Physiologic Influences Affecting Sensory Evoked Potentials: implications for perioperative monitoring. Anesthesiology. 2003;(3):716–37.
7. Chong CT, Manninen P, Sivanaser V, Subramanyam R, Lu N, Venkatraghavan L. Direct comparison of the effect of desflurane and sevoflurane on intraoperative motor-evoked potentials monitoring. J Neurosurg Anesthesiol. 2014;26:306–12.
8. Chen Z. The effects of isoflurane and propofol on intraoperative neurophysiological monitoring during spinal surgery. J Clin Monit Comput. 2004;18:303–8.
9. Gartlan MG, Peterson KL, Hoffman HT, Luschei ES, Smith RJH. Bipolar hooked-wire electromyographic technique in the evaluation of pediatric vocal cord paralysis. Ann Otol Rhinol Laryngol. 1993;102:695–700.
10. Wohl DL, Leshner RT, Kilpatrick JK, Shaia WT. Intraoperative pediatric laryngeal electromyography: experience and caveats with monopolar electrodes. Ann Otol Rhinol Laryngol. 2001;110:524–31.
11. Berkowitz RG. Laryngeal electromyography findings in idiopathic congenital bilateral vocal cord paralysis. Ann Otol Rhinol Laryngol. 1996;105:207–12.
12. Berkowitz RG, Ryan MM, Pilowsky PM. Respiration-related laryngeal electromyography in children with bilateral vocal fold paralysis. Ann Otol Rhinol Laryngol. 2009;118:791–5.
13. McRae BR, Kincaid JC, Illing EA, Hiatt KK, Hawkins JF, Halum SL. Local neurotoxins for prevention of laryngeal Synkinesis after recurrent laryngeal nerve injury. Ann Otol Rhinol Laryngol. 2009;118:887–93. https://doi.org/10.1177/000348940911801210.
14. Tessema B, Roark RM, Pitman MJ, Weissbrod P, Sharma S, Schaefer SD. Observations of recurrent laryngeal nerve injury and recovery using a rat model. Laryngoscope. 2009;119:1644–51.
15. Pitman MJ, Weissbrod P, Roark R, Sharma S, Schaefer SD. Electromyographic and histologic evolution of the recurrent laryngeal nerve from transection and anastomosis to mature reinnervation. Laryngoscope. 2011;121:325–31.
16. Tessema B, Pitman MJ, Roark RM, Berzofsky C, Sharma S, Schaefer SD. Evaluation of functional recovery of recurrent larymgeal nerve using transoral laryngeal bibopar electromyography: a rat model. New York. 2008; 117:604–8.
17. Kupfer RA, Old MO, Oh SS, Feldman EL, Hogikyan ND. Spontaneous laryngeal reinnervation following chronic recurrent laryngeal nerve injury. Laryngoscope. 2013;123:2216–27. https://doi.org/10.1002/lary.24049.
18. Jomah MA, Jomah MA. Does botulinum toxin type a alter the consequences of recurrent laryngeal nerve transection in the rat model ? By master of science in experimental Surgery University of Alberta. 2014.
19. Ismaiel NM, Chankalal R, Zhou J, Henzler D. Using remifentanil in mechanically ventilated rats to provide continuous analgosedation. J Am Assoc Lab Anim Sci. 2012;51:58–62.
20. SISA. Simple Interactive Statistical Analysis. http://www.quantitativeskills.com/sisa/index.htm. Accessed 10 Feb 2018.
21. Xu J, Yao Z, Li S, Chen L. A non-tracheal intubation (tubeless) anesthetic technique with spontaneous respiration for upper airway surgery. Clin Investig Med. 2013;36:151–7.
22. Dilos BM. Anesthesia for pediatric airway endoscopy and upper gastrointestinal endoscopy. Int Anesthesiol Clin. 2009;47:55–62.
23. Malik M, Sen S. Propofol anesthesia is an effective and safe strategy for pediatric endoscopy [4]. Paediatr Anaesth. 2006;16:220–1.
24. Lauder GR. Total intravenous anaesthesia will supercede inhalational anesthesia in pediatric anesthetic practice. Paediatr Anaesth. 2015;25:52–64.
25. Chen L, Yu L, Fan Y, Manyande A. A comparison between total intravenous anaesthesia using propofol plus remifentanil and volatile induction/maintenance of anaesthesia using sevoflurane in children undergoing flexible fibreoptic bronchoscopy. Anaesth Intensive Care. 2013;41:742–9.
26. Grundmann U, Uth M, Eichner A, Wilhelm W, Larsen R. Total intravenous anaesthesia with propofol and remifentanil in paediatric patients: a comparison with a desflurane-nitrous oxide inhalation anaesthesia. Acta Anaesthesiol Scand. 1998;42:845–50. https://doi.org/10.1111/j.1399-6576.1998.tb05332.x.
27. Liu HJ, Dong MM, Chi FL. Functional remobilization evaluation of the paralyzed vocal cord by end-to-side neurorrhaphy in rats. Laryngoscope. 2005;115:1418–20.
28. Motoyoshi K, Hyodo M, Yamagata T, Gyo K. Restoring vocal fold movement after transection and immediate suturing of the recurrent laryngeal nerve with local application of basic fibroblast growth factor: an experimental study in the rat. Laryngoscope. 2004;114:1247–52.
29. Rubin AD, Hogikyan ND, Oh A, Feldman EL. Potential for promoting recurrent laryngeal nerve regeneration by remote delivery of viral gene therapy. Laryngoscope. 2012;122:349–55.
30. Shiotani A, Nakagawa H, Flint PW. Modulation of myosin heavy chains in rat laryngeal muscle. Laryngoscope. 2001;111:472–7. https://doi.org/10.1097/00005537-200103000-00017.
31. Old MO, Oh SS, Feldman E, Hogikyan ND. Novel model to assess laryngeal function, innervation, and reinnervation. Ann Otol Rhinol Laryngol. 2011;120:331–8.
32. Berkowitz RG, Chalmers J, Sun QIJ, Pilowsky PM. Respiratory activity of the rat posterior cricoarytenoid muscle. Ann Otol Rhinol Laryngol. 1997;106:897–901.
33. Xu W, Han D, Hu I, Fan E. Characteristics of experimental recurrent laryngeal nerve surgical injury in dogs. Ann Otol Rhinol Laryngol. 2009;118:575–80.

34. Sakowski SA, Heavener SB, Lunn JS, Fung K, Oh SS, Spratt SK, et al. Neuroprotection using gene therapy to induce vascular endothelial growth factor-a expression. Gene Ther. 2009;16:1292–9.

35. Haghighi SS, Madsen R, Green KD, Oro JJ, Kracke GR. Suppression of motor evoked potentials by inhalation anesthetics. J Neurosurg Anesthesiol. 1990;2:73–8.

36. Scott A, Chong P, Randolph G, Hartnick C. Intraoperative laryngeal electromyography in children with vocal fold immobility: a simplified technique. Int J Pediatr Otorhinolaryngol. 2008;72:31–40.

37. AlQudehy Z, Norton J, El-Hakim H. Electromyography in children's laryngeal mobility disorders: a proposed grading system. Arch Otolaryngol - Head Neck Surg. 2012;138:936–41.

38. Jacobs IN, Finkel RS. Laryngeal electromyography in the management of vocal cord mobility problems in children. Laryngoscope. 2002;112:1243–8.

39. SC M, Braun N, DJ B, Chong P, JE K, CJ H. Intraoperative laryngeal electromyography in children with vocal fold immobility: results of a multicenter longitudinal study. Arch Otolaryngol Neck Surg. 2011;137:1251–7. https://doi.org/10.1001/archoto.2011.184.

40. Liao R, Li JY, Liu GY. Comparison of sevoflurane volatile induction/maintenance anaesthesia and propofol-remifentanil total intravenous anaesthesia for rigid bronchoscopy under spontaneous breathing for tracheal/bronchial foreign body removal in children. Eur J Anaesthesiol. 2010;27:930–4.

41. Tsai Y-C, Wang L-Y, Yeh L-S. Clinical comparison of recovery from total intravenous anesthesia with propofol and inhalation anesthesia with isoflurane in dogs. J Vet Med Sci. 2007;69:1179–82.

42. Blitzer A, Crumley RL, Dailey SH, Ford CN, Floeter MK, Hillel AD, et al. Recommendations of the Neurolaryngology study group on laryngeal electromyography. Otolaryngol - Head Neck Surg. 2009;140:782–793.e6. https://doi.org/10.1016/j.otohns.2009.01.026.

43. Munin MC, Heman-Ackah YD, Rosen CA, Sulica L, Maronian N, Mandel S, et al. Consensus statement: using laryngeal electromyography for the diagnosis and treatment of vocal cord paralysis. Muscle Nerve. 2016;53:850–5.

44. García-López I, Santiago-Pérez S, Peñarrocha-Teres J, del Palacio AJ, Gavilan J. Laryngeal Electromyography in Diagnosis and Treatment of Voice Disorders. Acta Otorrinolaringol. 2012;63:458–64. https://doi.org/10.1016/j.otoeng.2012.11.008.

45. Mu L, Yang S. An experimental study on the laryngeal electromyography and visual observations in varying types of surgical injuries to the unilateral recurrent laryngeal nerve in the neck. Laryngoscope. 1991;101(7 Pt 1):699–708.

46. Park HS, Jung SY, Yoo JH, Park HJ, Lee CH, Kim HS, et al. Clinical usefulness of ultrasonography-guided laryngeal electromyography. J Voice. 2016;30:100–3. https://doi.org/10.1016/j.jvoice.2015.03.009.

47. Paniello RC, West SE, Lee P. Laryngeal Reinnervation with the hypoglossal nerve. Ann Otol Rhinol Laryngol. 2001;110:532–42.

48. Kianicka I, Diaz V, Renolleau S, Canet E, Praud JP. Laryngeal and abdominal muscle electrical activity during periodic breathing in nonsedated lambs. J Appl Physiol. 1998;84:669–75.

49. Watts TL, Wozniak JA, Davenport PW, Hutchison AA. Laryngeal and diaphragmatic activities with a single expiratory load in newborn lambs. Respir Physiol. 1997;107:27–35.

50. Rex MA. Laryngeal activity during the induction of anaesthesia in the cat. Aust Vet J. 1973;49:365–8.

51. Carlo WA, Kosch PC, Bruce EN, Strohl KP, Martin RJ. Control of laryngeal muscle activity in preterm infants. Pediatr Res. 1987;22:87–91.

52. Bliss MR, Wark H, McDonnall D, Smith ME. Functional electrical stimulation of the feline larynx with a flexible ribbon electrode array. Ann Otol Rhinol Laryngol. 2016;125:130–6.

53. Senn S, Ezzet F. Clinical cross-over trials in phase I. Stat Methods Med Res. 1999;8:263–78.

54. Lui K-J. Notes on crossover design. Enliven Biostat Metr. 2015;1:1–2.

34

Resection versus preservation of the middle turbinate in surgery for chronic rhinosinusitis with nasal polyposis

Marc-Antoine Hudon[1], Erin D. Wright[2], Etienne Fortin-Pellerin[3] and Marie Bussieres[1*] (iD)

Abstract

Background: Chronic rhinosinusitis (CRS) affects up to 16% of the population. When medical treatment fails, endoscopic sinus surgery (ESS) is considered. The value of resecting the middle turbinate to optimize surgical outcomes has been hypothesized but remains controversial and unproven. Whether the middle turbinate should be left in place or resected is controversial. Our objective is to determine if middle turbinectomy improves objective surgical outcomes after ESS.

Methods: Sixteen patients (15 men, 15 primary surgery) undergoing bilateral complete ESS for CRS with nasal polyposis were recruited. Nasal cavities were randomized so that middle turbinectomy was performed on one side while the middle turbinate was preserved on the other. Each participant acted as their own control. Nasal cavities were compared using Perioperative Sinus Endoscopy (POSE) and Lund-Kennedy (LKES) scores pre-operatively, and at 1, 3 and 6 months after ESS. Results were analyzed using Wilcoxon signed-rank test.

Results: Pre-operatively, the POSE (12.4 ± 2.9 vs 12.8 ± 2.6, $p = 0.33$, for the preserved side and the resected side, respectively) and LKES (5.0 ± 1.0 vs 4.8 ± 1.2, p = 0.33) scores were similar between sides. During follow up, resection was associated with more crusting at 1 month following ESS (1.0 ± 0.7 vs 0.4 ± 0.6, $p = 0.02$). There was a small, but statistically significant, difference between the nasal cavities at 3 months, where the resected side showed better endoscopic appearance (2.0 ± 2.2 vs 3.4 ± 2.8, $p = 0.01$). No difference was found at 6 months. Frontal sinus scores were similar between sides at 6 months (0.7 ± 0.5 vs 0.7 ± 0.5, $p = 1.00$).

Conclusion: Our results show no sustained objective endoscopic benefit of routine middle turbinectomy, at least within the first six postoperative months, in patients undergoing primary ESS for CRS with polyposis.

Keywords: Chronic rhinosinusitis, Nasal polyposis, Endoscopic sinus surgery, Middle turbinate

Background

Chronic rhinosinusitis (CRS) is a common disease affecting up to 16% of the population [1]. Medical expenses related to CRS reach more than 60 billion dollars per year in the United States alone [2], with an additional 13 billion dollars per year [3] in loss of productivity.

Medical treatments, consisting of nasal saline irrigations, topical and systemic corticosteroids, are first offered to the patients. If symptoms persist, endoscopic sinus surgery (ESS) can be recommended [4]. The surgery has multiple goals such as removal of gross disease, marsupialization of sinus cavities, clearance of inspissated secretions and improved access of post-operative topical medical therapies [5]. The role of middle turbinectomy in ESS remains controversial. Traditionally, this structure has been preserved in order to maintain the integrity of the nasal cavity as much as possible. Removal of

* Correspondence: marie.bussieres@usherbrooke.ca
[1]Université de Sherbrooke, 580 Rue Bowen S, Sherbrooke, QC J1G 2E8, Canada
Full list of author information is available at the end of the article

the middle turbinate was deemed to be hazardous, with some authors advocating it could lead to increased risk of iatrogenic frontal sinusitis [6, 7]. This, however, has been refuted by Saidi et al. [8]. Removal of the middle turbinate might also increase the difficulty of revision surgeries, since it is an important anatomic landmark [6]. On the other hand, some authors have suggested resection could allow for more efficient nasal irrigations and topical corticosteroids owing to improved access, potentially leading to reduced polyp recurrence in the long term [5]. Retrospective studies have demonstrated longer time lapse before revision surgery [9], better endoscopic scores [10] and less synechiae with resection of the middle turbinate [11]. Unfortunately, there is very limited prospective data specifically looking at this issue [12]. More importantly, available studies were not randomised, leaving the decision as to whether to resect or preserve the turbinate at the surgeon's discretion, thus introducing a significant bias [10].

Our goal was to prospectively evaluate the role of middle turbinectomy on endoscopic outcomes of patients undergoing ESS for CRS with polyposis. Our hypothesis was that resection of the middle turbinate would improve sinonasal cavities appearance, as assessed by the POSE and the LKES scores.

Methods

A randomized controlled trial was conducted on patients undergoing bilateral complete ESS for CRS with nasal polyposis in a rhinology tertiary care center (Centre Hospitalier de l'Université de Sherbrooke, Sherbrooke, Canada). Ethics approval was obtained from the institutional ethics board (Comité d'éthique de la recherche en santé chez l'humain du CIUSSS de l'Estrie – CHUS). The protocol was registered prior to patient enrollment (clinicaltrials.gov - NCT02855931).

Sample size calculation was based on a study using a similar design [13]. Thirty-two nasal cavities were required to detect a difference of 3.5 points in POSE score (alpha 0.05, 80% power). A difference of 3.5 points in the POSE score is considered clinically significant [14].

Patients were recruited if they were above 18 years of age with a diagnosis of CRS with nasal polyposis. Patients undergoing both primary and revision surgeries were included. Patients were excluded if they had a diagnosis of allergic fungal rhinosinusitis, if the middle turbinate had been resected during a previous surgery, or if they were pregnant. General data on age, sex, asthma, smoking, airborne allergies and postoperative epistaxis were collected. Prior to the surgery, the Lund-Mackay radiologic scoring system [15] was used to assess the degree of opacification of the sinus cavities, a higher score correlating with more severe disease (six regions evaluated on each side, scored 0–2, total maximum score of 12).

Informed consent was obtained prior to surgery, which consisted of bilateral polypectomy, maxillary antrostomy, sphenoethmoidectomy and frontal sinusotomy (Draf 2a surgery). Each participant had the middle turbinate resected completely on one side and preserved on the other and were consented accordingly. Participants acted as their own control. Treatment allocation for choice of nasal cavity was done using computer-based block randomization, irrespective of the appearance of the middle turbinate (ex. polypoid, destabilized or with paradoxical curvature). At the end of surgery, Nasopore (Stryker Canada, Hamilton, Canada) impregnated with triamcinolone (40 mg/mL) was inserted in each ethmoid cavity. Patients were given a 7-day course of antibiotics and gentle saline irrigations. As per our routine postoperative protocol, they were seen 1 week after surgery for debridement of their sinonasal cavities and then were instructed in using budesonide nasal irrigations twice daily on a long-term basis (2 ml of 0.5 mg/ml budesonide in 240 ml of saline water). The study was single-blinded as participants were unaware of which side was resected. The investigators could not be blinded during follow-up due to the nature of the intervention.

Patients were evaluated at 1, 3 and 6 months postoperatively by the main investigator. Two clinically validated endoscopic scores were used to assess the nasal cavities. The Lund-Kennedy Endoscopic Scoring system (LKES) was used to evaluate the presence of polyps, edema, secretions, synechia and crusting in the sinonasal cavities (5 items scored 0–2 for a total maximal score of 10 on each side) [16]. The Peri-Operative Sinus Endoscopy (POSE) score adds information on the appearance of different parts of the sinonasal cavities. The middle turbinated is examined for synechia, lateralization or narrowing of the middle meatus. The maxillary, frontal and sphenoid sinuses are scored separately with regards to their healthiness or the presence and severity of mucosal edema and secretions (thin or mucoid vs purulent or mucinous). The ethmoid cavity is further inspected for signs of crusting, polypoid changes or frank polyposis. There are 10 items scored 0–2 for a maximal score of 20 on each side [17]. Higher values indicate worse disease in both scores.

Statistical analysis was performed with SPSS 19 (IBM, Chicago, IL, USA). A non-parametric statistical approach (Wilcoxon signed-rank test) was chosen due to the relatively small number of patients. However, data distribution was qualitatively fairly normal and thus the authors have decided to present the results as average ± standard deviation (SD) for ease of understanding.

Results

Sixteen patients (47.5 ± 13.6 years old) were recruited between April 2016 and July 2017. Our cohort mostly consisted of middle-aged men who had primary surgery (Table 1). None presented post-operative epistaxis.

At baseline, POSE and LKES scores were very similar between the 2 nasal cavities (12.4 ± 2.9 vs 12.8 ± 2.6, $p = 0.33$ and 5.0 ± 1.0 vs 4.8 ± 1.2, $p = 0.33$, for the side allocated to resection and the side allocated to preservation, respectively $n = 16$). Compared to pre-operative score, there was a significant improvement in the POSE score postoperatively on both sides which persisted throughout the 6-month follow-up period ($p < 0.001$) (Fig. 1a). The differences between the 2 sides at each time point, however, were minimal. Three months after ESS, there was a statistically significant but clinically limited difference favoring the resected side (2.0 ± 2.2 vs 3.4 ± 2.8, $p = 0.01$, $n = 12$) that was not present at 1 month (3.5 ± 2.0 vs 2.7 ± 2.4, $p = 0.06$, $n = 13$) and did not persist at 6 months (3.5 ± 3.3 vs 3.9 ± 4.0, $p = 0.76$, $n = 15$). The LKES scores globally followed the same trend as the POSE scores, showing better endoscopic appearance for both sinus cavities after surgery as compared to pre-operatively ($p < 0.001$). LKES values were higher (worse) at one month on the resected side (2.4 ± 1.3 vs 1.5 ± 1.2, $p = 0.03$, $n = 13$) but lower (better) at 3 months (1.2 ± 1.5 vs 1.8 ± 1.3, $p = 0.05$, $n = 12$). Scores were the same in both groups at 6 months (1.7 ± 1.5 vs 1.7 ± 1.6, $p = 0.83$, n = 15) (Fig. 1b).

Analysis of individual POSE scores' criteria showed significantly more crusting on the resected side at one month (1.0 ± 0.7 versus 0.4 ± 0.6, $p = 0.003$), but not afterwards. Synechia were seen in 3 patients on the

Table 1 Patient characteristics

	Number of participants n (%)	p-value
Age (mean ± SD)	48.5 ± 13.6 years	
Sex		
Male	15 (94)	
Female	1 (6)	
Surgery type		
Primary	15 (94)	
Revision	1 (6)	
Asthma	4 (25)	
Aspirin-exacerbated respiratory disorder	1 (6)	
Environmental allergies	4 (25)	
Smoking status		
Yes	1 (6)	
No	15 (94)	
Baseline radiologic Lund-MacKay score		
Resected side (mean ± SD)	8.8 ± 2.1	p = 0.24
Preserved side (mean ± SD)	8.8 ± 2.5	

preserved side at 6 months after surgery compared to none on the resected side. The frontal recess and sinus scores were better at every follow up visit after ESS compared to the baseline data on both sides ($p = 0.001$) (Fig. 2). Still in the frontal recess and sinus region, resected and preserved sides were similar at 1 (0.6 ± 0.5 vs 0.5 ± 0.5, $p = 0.32$, preserved and resected side, respectively), 3 (0.6 ± 0.5 vs 0.8 ± 0.6, $p = 0.18$) and 6 (0.7 ± 0.5 vs 0.7 ± 0.5, $p = 1.00$) months after surgery.

Discussion

The role of middle turbinectomy during ESS is a matter of debate for the treatment of CRS. Some authors have found advantages to resection, as discussed earlier. Unfortunately, most of the available evidence comes from retrospective studies and were not randomized, thus introducing a significant bias [9, 18, 19]. To our knowledge, this is the first prospective randomized controlled trial to evaluate the potential of middle turbinectomy in improving outcomes after ESS for CRS with polyposis. Although there were transient differences between the 2 approaches, we found no objective persistent advantage of middle turbinectomy in the surgical treatment of CRS patients.

We found a statistically significant difference in POSE scores in favour of middle turbinate resection 3 months after surgery. The amplitude of this difference, however, was small enough to be arguably of limited clinical relevance. Moreover, it did not persist at 6 months. This was an unexpected finding. Since there is evidence of better access of topical medication in a completely marsupialized sinus cavity [20], we were expecting a sustained improvement on the side of middle turbinate resection after ESS. More specifically, we thought the improved access of postoperative medication would make a difference in the region of the frontal recess where early recurrence of polyposis is usually seen. Even though we found no significant added benefit of resection, it is noteworthy that there was no adverse effect of resection, showing the middle turbinate can be removed safely if deemed clinically indicated. Despite our negative findings at 6 months, we believe there could still be a role for middle turbinectomy in selected, more severe cases. Revision surgeries and/or patients with 'floppy' or polypoid turbinates could still be candidates for a future prospective study looking specifically at this topic.

Analysis of individual criteria of both scores showed an increase in crusting in the first month after surgery with resection. Crusts were predominantly seen at the anterior attachment site of the resected middle turbinate, which can be explained by the increased surface of exposed bone during healing. However, this was a transient effect that disappeared once healing was completed and was not associated with adverse outcomes.

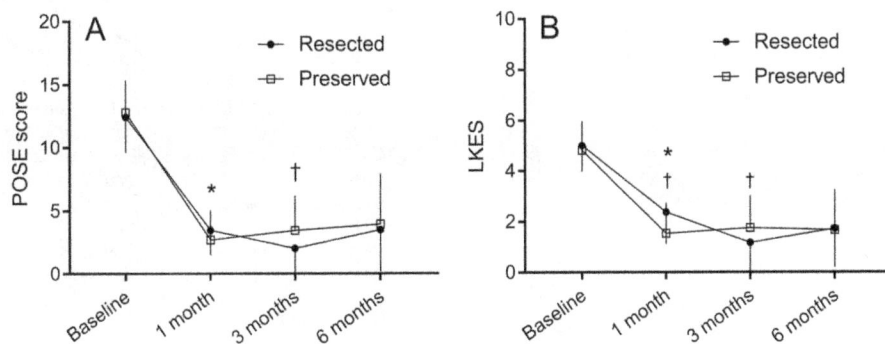

Fig. 1 Sinonasal endoscopic outcomes after surgery. Trends for POSE (**a**) and LKES (**b**) scores over time. * First timepoint where scores within the same groups are statistically different from baseline. † Significant difference between groups at the indicated timepoint. POSE: Peri-Operative Sinus Endoscopy, LKES: Lund-Kennedy Endoscopic Score

This pattern is different from the diffuse ethmoid crusting that can be seen in a pathologic sinus cavity plagued with bacterial proliferation, which has a worse prognostic implication. Finally, the proportion of postoperative synechia was unsurprisingly higher on the preserved side.

Our study has some limitations. Because of its design, surgeons could not be blinded to the treatment, the presence or absence of the middle turbinate being obvious at endoscopic evaluation. Symptomatic evaluation of the participants was not possible because of the absence of available tools evaluating nasal symptoms from each nasal cavity independently. This could have been overcome by randomizing patients instead of nasal cavities, but would have taken at least twice the number of participants. The majority of patients underwent primary surgeries, thus results could have been different if revision-only cases were studied, as suggested by Scangas

et al. [21]. Finally, a six-month follow-up period may be short considering the chronic course of CRS. Wu et al. showed a longer time interval between sinus surgeries in patients who had undergone middle turbinectomy than in those who had not, but this was shown to happen 4 to 5 years after the first surgery [9]. Our cohort will be followed to assess revision rates.

Conclusion

Despite previous evidence of increased delivery of nasal topical medication to the sinus cavities after ESS, our results show no objective endoscopic benefits of routine middle turbinectomy in the context of primary surgeries, at least within the first six postoperative months. Limiting the indications for middle turbinectomy to revision surgeries or cases with already problematic turbinates would be a legitimate research question for future prospective studies.

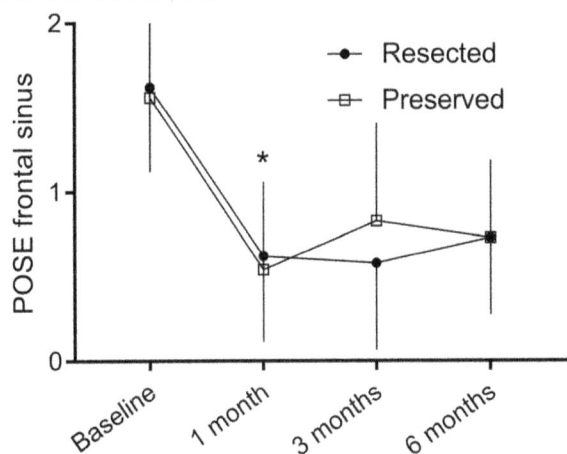

Fig. 2 Endoscopic outcomes of the frontal sinus/recess. Trends for frontal sinus/recess subcategory of the POSE score over time. * First timepoint where scores within the same groups are statistically different from baseline. POSE: Peri-Operative Sinus Endoscopy

Abbreviations
CRS: Chronic rhinosinusitis; ESS: Endoscopic sinus surgery; LKES: Lund-Kennedy endoscopic score; POSE: Peri-operative sinus endoscopy; SD: Standard deviation

Acknowledgements
No acknowledgements.

Funding
No funding was necessary for this study.

Authors' contributions
MB and EDW both worked on conception and design of the current study. MB and MAH collected the data. MB, MAH and EFP analyzed and interpreted the data. All authors were major contributors in writing the manuscript. They all read and approved the final version of the manuscript.

Competing interests

The authors declare that they have no competing interests.

Author details

[1]Université de Sherbrooke, 580 Rue Bowen S, Sherbrooke, QC J1G 2E8, Canada. [2]University of Alberta, Room 1E4, W.C.M. Health Sciences Centre, 8440-112 Street, Edmonton, AB T6G 2B7, Canada. [3]Université de Sherbrooke, 3001, 12e avenue Nord, Sherbrooke, QC J1H 5N4, Canada.

References

1. Halawi AM, Smith SS, Chandra RK. Chronic rhinosinusitis: epidemiology and cost. Allergy Asthma Proc. 2013;34:328–34.
2. Caulley L, Thavorn K, Rudmik L, Cameron C, Kilty SJ. Direct costs of adult chronic rhinosinusitis by using 4 methods of estimation: results of the US medical expenditure panel survey. J Allergy Clin Immunol. 2015;136:1517–22.
3. Rudmik L, Soler ZM, Smith TL, Mace JC, Schlosser RJ, DeConde AS. Effect of continued medical therapy on productivity costs for refractory chronic rhinosinusitis. JAMA Otolaryngol Head Neck Surg. 2015;141:969–73.
4. Dautremont JF, Rudmik L. When are we operating for chronic rhinosinusitis? A systematic review of maximal medical therapy protocols prior to endoscopic sinus surgery. Int Forum Allergy Rhinol. 2015;5:1095–103.
5. Jang DW, Lachanas VA, Segel J, Kountakis SE. Budesonide nasal irrigations in the postoperative management of chronic rhinosinusitis. Int Forum Allergy Rhinol. 2013;3:708–11.
6. Kennedy DW. Middle turbinate resection: evaluating the issues--should we resect normal middle turbinates? Arch Otolaryngol Head Neck Surg. 1998; 124:107.
7. Fortune DS, Duncavage JA. Incidence of frontal sinusitis following partial middle turbinectomy. Ann Otol Rhinol Laryngol. 1998;107:447–53.
8. Saidi IS, Biedlingmaier JF, Rothman MI. Pre- and postoperative imaging analysis for frontal sinus disease following conservative partial middle turbinate resection. Ear Nose Throat J. 1998;77:326–8 330, 332 passim.
9. Wu AW, Ting JY, Platt MP, Tierney HT, Metson R. Factors affecting time to revision sinus surgery for nasal polyps: a 25-year experience. Laryngoscope. 2014;124:29–33.
10. Marchioni D, Alicandri-Ciufelli M, Mattioli F, Marchetti A, Jovic G, Massone F, Presutti L. Middle turbinate preservation versus middle turbinate resection in endoscopic surgical treatment of nasal polyposis. Acta Otolaryngol. 2008; 128:1019–26.
11. Havas TE, Lowinger DS. Comparison of functional endonasal sinus surgery with and without partial middle turbinate resection. Ann Otol Rhinol Laryngol. 2000;109:634–40.
12. Clement WA, White PS. Trends in turbinate surgery literature: a 35-year review. Clin Otolaryngol Allied Sci. 2001;26:124–8.
13. Cote DW, Wright ED. Triamcinolone-impregnated nasal dressing following endoscopic sinus surgery: a randomized, double-blind, placebo-controlled study. Laryngoscope. 2010;120:1269–73.
14. Soler ZM, Smith TL. Quality of life outcomes after functional endoscopic sinus surgery. Otolaryngol Clin N Am. 2010;43:605–12 x.
15. Hopkins C, Browne JP, Slack R, Lund V, Brown P. The Lund-Mackay staging system for chronic rhinosinusitis: how is it used and what does it predict? Otolaryngol Head Neck Surg. 2007;137:555–61.
16. Lund VJ, Kennedy DW. Quantification for staging sinusitis. The staging and therapy group. Ann Otol Rhinol Laryngol Suppl. 1995;167:17–21.
17. Wright ED, Agrawal S. Impact of perioperative systemic steroids on surgical outcomes in patients with chronic rhinosinusitis with polyposis: evaluation with the novel perioperative sinus endoscopy (POSE) scoring system. Laryngoscope. 2007;117:1–28.
18. Byun JY, Lee JY. Middle turbinate resection versus preservation in patients with chronic rhinosinusitis accompanying nasal polyposis: baseline disease burden and surgical outcomes between the groups. J Otolaryngol Head Neck Surg. 2012;41:259–64.
19. Soler ZM, Hwang PH, Mace J, Smith TL. Outcomes after middle turbinate resection: revisiting a controversial topic. Laryngoscope. 2010;120:832–7.
20. Kidwai SM, Parasher AK, Khan MN, Eloy JA, Del Signore A, Iloreta AM, Govindaraj S. Improved delivery of sinus irrigations after middle turbinate resection during endoscopic sinus surgery. Int Forum Allergy Rhinol. 2017;7: 338–42.
21. Scangas GA, Remenschneider AK, Bleier BS, Holbrook EH, Gray ST, Metson RB. Does the timing of middle turbinate resection influence quality-of-life outcomes for patients with chronic rhinosinusitis? Otolaryngol Head Neck Surg. 2017;157:874–9.

Permissions

All chapters in this book were first published in JO-H&NS, by BioMed Central; hereby published with permission under the Creative Commons Attribution License or equivalent. Every chapter published in this book has been scrutinized by our experts. Their significance has been extensively debated. The topics covered herein carry significant findings which will fuel the growth of the discipline. They may even be implemented as practical applications or may be referred to as a beginning point for another development.

The contributors of this book come from diverse backgrounds, making this book a truly international effort. This book will bring forth new frontiers with its revolutionizing research information and detailed analysis of the nascent developments around the world.

We would like to thank all the contributing authors for lending their expertise to make the book truly unique. They have played a crucial role in the development of this book. Without their invaluable contributions this book wouldn't have been possible. They have made vital efforts to compile up to date information on the varied aspects of this subject to make this book a valuable addition to the collection of many professionals and students.

This book was conceptualized with the vision of imparting up-to-date information and advanced data in this field. To ensure the same, a matchless editorial board was set up. Every individual on the board went through rigorous rounds of assessment to prove their worth. After which they invested a large part of their time researching and compiling the most relevant data for our readers.

The editorial board has been involved in producing this book since its inception. They have spent rigorous hours researching and exploring the diverse topics which have resulted in the successful publishing of this book. They have passed on their knowledge of decades through this book. To expedite this challenging task, the publisher supported the team at every step. A small team of assistant editors was also appointed to further simplify the editing procedure and attain best results for the readers.

Apart from the editorial board, the designing team has also invested a significant amount of their time in understanding the subject and creating the most relevant covers. They scrutinized every image to scout for the most suitable representation of the subject and create an appropriate cover for the book.

The publishing team has been an ardent support to the editorial, designing and production team. Their endless efforts to recruit the best for this project, has resulted in the accomplishment of this book. They are a veteran in the field of academics and their pool of knowledge is as vast as their experience in printing. Their expertise and guidance has proved useful at every step. Their uncompromising quality standards have made this book an exceptional effort. Their encouragement from time to time has been an inspiration for everyone.

The publisher and the editorial board hope that this book will prove to be a valuable piece of knowledge for researchers, students, practitioners and scholars across the globe.

List of Contributors

M. F. Griffin
Division of Surgery and Interventional Science, University College London (UCL), London, UK
Anatomy Department, St Georges University, London, UK
Plastic and Reconstructive Surgery Department, Royal Free Hospital, London, UK

B. C. Leung and P. E. Butler
Division of Surgery and Interventional Science, University College London (UCL), London, UK
Plastic and Reconstructive Surgery Department, Royal Free Hospital, London, UK

Y.Premakumar and M.Szarko
Anatomy Department, St Georges University, London, UK

Monika Wojtera
Schulich School of Medicine and Dentistry, Western University, 1151 Richmond St, London N6A 5C1, ON, Canada

Josee Paradis, Murad Husein, Anthony C. Nichols, John W. Barrett and Julie E. Strychowsky
Schulich School of Medicine and Dentistry, Western University, 1151 Richmond St, London N6A 5C1, ON, Canada
Department of Otolaryngology-Head and Neck Surgery, Victoria Hospital B3-400, 800 Commissioners Rd E, London N6A 5W9, ON, Canada

Marina I. Salvadori
Schulich School of Medicine and Dentistry, Western University, 1151 Richmond St, London N6A 5C1, ON, Canada
Department of Paediatrics, Children's Hospital at London Health Sciences Centre, 800 Commissioners Rd E, London, ON N6A 5W9, Canada

Yaeesh Sardiwalla
Faculty of Medicine, Dalhousie University, Halifax, NS, Canada

David P. Morris
Faculty of Medicine, Dalhousie University, Halifax, NS, Canada
Division of Otolaryngology – Head and Neck Surgery, Dalhousie University, Halifax, NS, Canada
QEII Health Science Center - VG Site Otolaryngology, 5820 University Ave - Rm 3037, Halifax, NS B3H 2Y9, Canada

Nicholas Jufas
Division of Otolaryngology – Head and Neck Surgery, Dalhousie University, Halifax, NS, Canada
Discipline of Surgery, Sydney Medical School, University of Sydney, Sydney, Australia

Manohar Bance
Division of Otolaryngology – Head and Neck Surgery, Dalhousie University, 3rd Floor Dickson Building, VG Site, QE II Health Sciences Centre, 5820 University Ave, Halifax, NS B3H 2Y9, Canada

Nicholas Jufas
Division of Otolaryngology – Head and Neck Surgery, Dalhousie University, 3rd Floor Dickson Building, VG Site, QE II Health Sciences Centre, 5820 University Ave, Halifax, NS B3H 2Y9, Canada
Kolling Deafness Research Centre, University of Sydney and Macquarie University, Sydney, Australia
Sydney Endoscopic Ear Surgery (SEES) Research Group, Sydney, Australia

Brittany Barber, Hadi Seikaly, Shannon Rychlik, Vincent Biron, Jeffrey Harris and Daniel O'Connell
Division of Otolaryngology-Head and Neck Surgery, University of Alberta, Edmonton, Canada

K. Ming Chan
Department of Physical Rehabilitation Medicine, University of Alberta, Edmonton, Canada

Rhys Beaudry
Department of Physical Therapy, University of Texas, Arlington, Texas, USA

Jaret Olson and Matthew Curran
Division of Plastic Surgery, University of Alberta, Edmonton, Canada

Peter Dziegielewski
Department of Otolaryngology, University of Florida, Gainesville, FL, USA

Margaret McNeely
Faculty of Rehabilitation Medicine, University of Alberta, Edmonton, Canada

Grace Margaret Scott
Laurentian University, 935 Ramsey Lake Rd, Sudbury, ON P3E 2C6, Canada

Corliss Ann Elizabeth Best and Damian Christopher Micomonaco
Northern Ontario School of Medicine, 935 Ramsey Lake Rd, Sudbury, ON P3E 2C6, Canada

Hiroshi Hosoi
Department of Otolaryngology-Head and Neck Surgery, Nara Medical University, Kashihara, Japan

Takahiro Kimura
Department of Otolaryngology-Head and Neck Surgery, Nara Medical University, Kashihara, Japan Department of Head and Neck Surgery, Aichi Cancer Center Hospital, 1-1 Kanokoden, Chikusaku, Nagoya 464-8681, Japan

Taijiro Ozawa
Department of Oto-Rhino-Laryngology, Toyohashi Municipal Hospi-tal, Toyohashi, Japan

Nobuhiro Hanai, Hidenori Suzuki and Yasuhisa Hasegawa
Department of Head and Neck Surgery, Aichi Cancer Center Hospital, 1-1 Kanokoden, Chikusaku, Nagoya 464-8681, Japan

Hitoshi Hirakawa
Department of Otorhinolaryngology, Head and Neck Surgery, University of the Ryukyus, Nakazu, Japan

Nicole L. Lebo, Lisa Caulley, Hussain Alsaffar and Stephanie Johnson-Obaseki
Department of Otolaryngology - Head and Neck Surgery, University of Ottawa, S3, 501 Smyth Road, Ottawa, ON K1H 8L6, Canada

Martin J. Corsten
Department of Otolaryngology, Aurora Health Care, Aurora St. Luke's Hospital, Milwaukee, WI, USA

Krupal B. Patel, Anthony C. Nichols, Kevin Fung, John Yoo and S.Danielle MacNeil
Department of Otolaryngology – Head and Neck Surgery, Schulich Medicine and Dentistry, London Health Sciences Centre, Western University, Victoria Hospital, London, ON, Canada

Milan Kostal Milan Bláha and Miriam Lánská
4th Department of Internal Medicine, University Hospital Hradec Kralove Charles University, Faculty of Medicine in Hradec Kralove, Hradec Králové, Czech Republic

Jakub Drsata and Viktor Chrobok
Department of Otorhinolaryngology and Head and Neck Surgery, University Hospital Hradec Kralove Charles University, Faculty of Medicine in Hradec Kralove, Hradec Králové, Czech Republic

Nina Ariani
Department of Prosthodontics, Faculty of Dentistry, Universitas Indonesia, Jakarta, Indonesia

Division of Preventive Dentistry, Niigata University Graduate School of Medical and Dental Sciences, Niigata, Japan

Harry Reintsema
Department of Oral and Maxillofacial Surgery, University of Groningen, University Medical Center Groningen, Groningen, The Netherlands

Kathleen Ward
Creighton University School of Dentistry, Omaha, NE, USA

Cortino Sukotjo
Department of Restorative Dentistry, University of Illinois at Chicago, College of Dentistry, Chicago, IL, USA

Alvin G. Wee
Department of Prosthodontics, Creighton University School of Dentistry, Omaha, NE, USA
Department of Surgery, Dental Service, Veterans Affairs Nebraska-Western Iowa Healthcare System, 4101 Woolworth Ave, Omaha, NE 68105, USA

Shubhi Singh and Brian Blakley
Division of Otolaryngology-Head and Neck Surgery, University of Manitoba, Health Sciences Centre GB421, 820 Sherbrook Street University of Manitoba, Winnipeg, MB R3T 2N2, Canada

Robert E. Brown, Mary F. McGuire and Jamie Buryanek
Department of Pathology and Laboratory Medicine, at UT Health McGovern Medical School, Houston, TX, USA

Syed Naqvi and Ron J.Karni
Department of Otorhinolaryngology, Head and Neck Surgery at UT Health McGovern Medical School, Houston, TX, USA

Ingo Todt, Julica Utca, Dania Karimi, Arne Ernst and Philipp Mittmann
Department of Otolaryngology, Head and Neck Surgery, Unfallkrankenhaus Berlin, Warenerstr.7, 12683 Berlin, Germany

Fabio Medas, Ernico Erdas, Gian Luigi Canu, Alessandro Longheu, Giuseppe Pisano and Pietro Giorgio Calò
Department of Surgical Sciences, University of Cagliari, Cittadella Universitaria, SS554, Bivio Sestu, 09042 Monserrato (CA), Italy

Massimiliano Tuveri
Istituto Pancreas, Policlinico Borgo Roma, AOUI Verona, Piazzale L.A. Scuro, 10, 37134 Verona, Italy

Nathan Yang and Sarah Hosseini
Faculty of Medicine, McGill University, Montreal, QC,
Canada

Marco A. Mascarella
Department of Otolaryngology – Head and Neck
Surgery, McGill University, Montreal, QC, Canada

Lily H. P. Nguyen
Department of Otolaryngology – Head and Neck
Surgery, McGill University, Montreal, QC, Canada
Center for Medical Education, McGill University,
Montreal, QC, Canada

Meredith Young
Center for Medical Education, McGill University,
Montreal, QC, Canada
Department of Medicine, McGill University, Montreal,
QC, Canada

Nancy Posel
McGill Molson Medical Informatics, McGill University,
Montreal, QC, Canada

Kevin Fung
Department of Otolaryngology – Head and Neck
Surgery, Western University, London, ON, Canada

Yael Bensoussan
Department of Otolaryngology Head and Neck
Surgery, University of Toronto, Toronto, ON, Canada

Jennifer Anderson
Department of Otolaryngology-Head and Neck
Surgery, University of Toronto, St-Michael's Hospital,
30 Bond Street, Toronto, ON M5B 1W8, Canada

Changxing Liu, Uttam K.Sinha and Niels C. Kokot
USC Tina and Rick Caruso Department of
Otolaryngology-Head and Neck Surgery, Keck
Medicine of USC, University of Southern California,
Los Angeles, CA 90033, USA

Daljit Mann
Keck School of Medicine, University of Southern
California, Los Angeles, CA 90033, USA

N. Alsufyani
Department of Dentistry, Faculty of Medicine and
Dentistry, University of Alberta, Edmonton, Canada
Department of Oral Medicine and Diagnostic Sciences,
College of Dentistry, King Saud University Division of
Otolaryngology-Head and Neck Surgery Department
of Surgery, Riyadh, Saudi Arabia
University of Alberta, Edmonton, AB, Canada

Anderson, A. Isaac, M. Gazzaz and H. El-Hakim
University of Alberta, Edmonton, AB, Canada

Division of Pediatric Surgery, Department of Surgery,
Stollery Children's Hospital, Edmonton, AB, Canada
Division of Otolaryngology-Head and Neck Surgery,
Department of Surgery, University of Alberta, 2C3.57
Walter MacKenzie Centre, 8440 112 St NW, Edmonton,
AB T6G 2R7, Canada

James P. Bonaparte
Department of Otolaryngology – Head and Neck
Surgery Senior Clinical Investigator, The Ottawa
Hospital Research Institute, University of Ottawa,
1919 Riverside Drive, Suite 308, Ottawa, Ontario K1H
7W9, Canada

Ross Campbell
Department of Otolaryngology – Head and Neck
Surgery, The University of Ottawa, Ottawa, Canada

David W. Cote
Division of Otolaryngology-Head and Neck Surgery,
University of Alberta, 8440-112 st, 1E4 Walter
Mackenzie Centre, Edmonton, AB T6G 2B7, Canada

Jeffrey Harris, Hadi Seikaly and Daniel A.O'Connell
Division of Otolaryngology-Head and Neck Surgery,
University of Alberta, 8440-112 st, 1E4 Walter
Mackenzie Centre, Edmonton, AB T6G 2B7, Canada
Alberta Head and Neck Centre for Oncology and
Reconstruction, Walter MacKenzie Health Sciences
Centre, Edmonton, AB, Canada

Vincent L. Biron
Division of Otolaryngology-Head and Neck Surgery,
University of Alberta, 8440-112 st, 1E4 Walter
Mackenzie Centre, Edmonton, AB T6G 2B7, Canada
Alberta Head and Neck Centre for Oncology and
Reconstruction, Walter MacKenzie Health Sciences
Centre, Edmonton, AB, Canada
Otolaryngology-Head and Neck Surgery Research
Laboratory of Alberta, University of Alberta,
Edmonton, AB, Canada

Ashlee Matkin
Alberta Head and Neck Centre for Oncology and
Reconstruction, Walter MacKenzie Health Sciences
Centre, Edmonton, AB, Canada
Faculty of Medicine and Dentistry, Undergraduate
Medical Education, University of Alberta, Edmonton,
AB, Canada

Morris Kostiuk
Alberta Head and Neck Centre for Oncology and
Reconstruction, Walter MacKenzie Health Sciences
Centre, Edmonton, AB, Canada
Otolaryngology-Head and Neck Surgery Research
Laboratory of Alberta, University of Alberta,
Edmonton, AB, Canada

Jordana Williams
Otolaryngology-Head and Neck Surgery Research Laboratory of Alberta, University of Alberta, Edmonton, AB, Canada

Sherif Idris, Khalid Ansari, Jeffrey R. Harris, Nabil Rizk, David Cote, Daniel A. O'Connell, Heather Allen and Hadi Seikaly
Division of Otolaryngology — Head and Neck Surgery, University of Alberta, 1E4 Walter Mackenzie Center, 8440 112 Street, Edmonton, AB T6G 2B7, Canada

Alex M. Mlynarek
Department of Otolaryngology — Head and Neck Surgery, McGill University, Montréal, Quebec, Canada

Peter Dziegielewski
Department of Otolaryngology — Head and Neck Surgery, University of Florida, Gainesville, Florida, USA

Vinay Fernandes and Vincent Lin
Division of Otolaryngology – Head and Neck Surgery, Faculty of Medicine, University of Toronto, Toronto, Canada

Yiqiao Wang
Faculty of Medicine, University of Ottawa, Ottawa, Canada

Robert Yeung and Sean Symons
Division of Radiology, Faculty of Medicine, University of Toronto, Toronto, Canada

D. S. Chan, M. G. Roskies, V. I. Forest, M. P. Hier and R. J. Payne
Department of Otolaryngology Head and Neck Surgery, Jewish General Hospital, McGill University, 3755 Côte-Ste-Catherine Road, Montreal H3T 1E2, Canada

K. Gong
Faculty of Medicine, McGill University, Montreal, Canada

Rachelle A.LeBlanc, Andre Isaac, Vincent L. Biron, David W. J. Côté, Matthew Hearn, Daniel A. O'Connell, Hadi Seikaly and Jeffrey R. Harris
Division of Otolaryngology — Head and Neck Surgery, University of Alberta, 1E4 Walter Mackenzie Center, 8440 112 Street, Edmonton, AB T6G 2B7, Canada

Jonathan Abele
Department of Radiology and Diagnostic Imaging, Royal Alexandra Hospital, 1046 Royal Alexandra Hospital – Diagnostic Treatment Center, 2J2.00 WC Mackenzie Health Sciences Centre, 8440 112 Street, Edmonton, AB T6G 2R7, Canada

Lisa Caulley, Scott Kohlert and Matthew Bromwich
Faculty of Medicine, University of Ottawa, Ottawa, ON, Canada
Department of Otolaryngology-Head and Neck Surgery, The Ottawa Hospital, Ottawa, ON, Canada
Division of Otolaryngology – Head and Neck Surgery, Children's Hospital of Eastern Ontario, 400 Smyth Road, Ottawa, ON K1H 8L1, Canada

Hazen Gandy
Faculty of Medicine, University of Ottawa, Ottawa, ON, Canada
Department of Psychiatry, Children's Hospital of Eastern Ontario, University of Ottawa, Ottawa, ON, Canada

Janet Olds
Faculty of Medicine, University of Ottawa, Ottawa, ON, Canada
Department of Psychology, Children's Hospital of Eastern Ontario, University of Ottawa, Ottawa, ON, Canada

Vincent Wu
School of Medicine, Faculty of Health Sciences, Queen's University, Kingston, Ontario, Canada

Jennifer Siu and Jonathan Yip
Division of Rhinology, Department of Otolaryngology – Head and Neck Surgery, St. Michael's Hospital, University of Toronto, Toronto, Ontario, Canada

John M. Lee
Division of Rhinology, Department of Otolaryngology – Head and Neck Surgery, St. Michael's Hospital, University of Toronto, Toronto, Ontario, Canada
Li Ka Shing Knowledge Institute, St. Michael's Hospital, Toronto, Ontario, Canada

Pichit Sittitrai, Donyarat Reunmarkkaew and Saisaward Chaiyasate
Department of Otolaryngology, Chiang Mai University, Chiang Mai 50200, Thailand

Justin M.Pyne and Tarek Ibrahim Lawen
Faculty of Medicine, Dalhousie University, Halifax, NS, Canada
Department of Surgery, Division of Otolaryngology – Head and Neck Surgery, Dalhousie University, Faculty of Medicine, Halifax, NS, Canada

Manohar Bance
Faculty of Medicine, Dalhousie University, Halifax, NS, Canada
Department of Surgery, Division of Otolaryngology – Head and Neck Surgery, Dalhousie University, Faculty of Medicine, Halifax, NS, Canada

Department of Clinical Neurosciences, University of Cambridge, Cambridge, UK

Duncan D. Floyd
Department of Surgery, Division of Otolaryngology – Head and Neck Surgery, Dalhousie University, Faculty of Medicine, Halifax, NS, Canada

Lisa M. Evangelista, Maggie A. Kuhn and Peter C. Belafsky
Center for Voice and Swallowing, Department of Otolaryngology – Head and Neck Surgery, University of California Davis, Sacramento, CA, USA

Derrick R. Randall
Center for Voice and Swallowing, Department of Otolaryngology – Head and Neck Surgery, University of California Davis, Sacramento, CA, USA
Section of Otolaryngology – Head and Neck Surgery, Department of Surgery, University of Calgary, Calgary, AB T2W 3K2, Canada

Chang-Hee Kim and Jung Eun Shin
Department of Otorhinolaryngology-Head and Neck Surgery, Konkuk University School of Medicine, Konkuk University Medical Center, 120-1 Neungdong-ro (Hwayang-dong), Gwangjin-gu, Seoul 143-729, Republic of Korea

Candan Efeoglu, Aylin Sipahi Calis and Huseyin Koca
Oral Surgery Department, Ege University School of Dentistry, 35100 Izmir, Turkey

Esra Yuksel
Anesthesiology Department, Ege University School of Medicine, 35100 Izmir, Turkey

M. Gazzaz, C. Jeffery and H. El-Hakim
Division of Otolaryngology-Head and Neck Surgery, Department of Surgery, University of Alberta, 2C3.57 Walter MacKenzie Centre, Edmonton, AB T6G 2R7, Canada

J. Saini
Neuroscience and Mental Health Institute, University of Alberta, Edmonton, AB, Canada
Women and Children Research Institute, University of Alberta, Edmonton, AB, Canada

S. Pagliardini
Neuroscience and Mental Health Institute, University of Alberta, Edmonton, AB, Canada
Women and Children Research Institute, University of Alberta, Edmonton, AB, Canada
Department of Physiology, University of Alberta, Edmonton, AB, Canada

B. Tsui
Stanford University Pediatric Regional Anesthesia, Stanford University, Stanford, California, USA

Marc-Antoine Hudon and Marie Bussieres
Université de Sherbrooke, 580 Rue Bowen S, Sherbrooke, QC J1G 2E8, Canada

Erin D. Wright
University of Alberta, Room 1E4, W.C.M. Health Sciences Centre, 8440-112 Street, Edmonton, AB T6G 2B7, Canada

Etienne Fortin-Pellerin
Université de Sherbrooke, 3001, 12e avenue Nord, Sherbrooke, QC J1H 5N4, Canada

Index